Global Health

The health of human populations around the world is constantly changing and the health profiles of most nations in the early twenty-first century global health landscape are unrecognizable compared with those of just a century ago.

This book examines and explains these health changes and considers likely future patterns and changes. While the overall picture charted is one of progress and improvement, certain unfortunate regressions and stubbornly persistent health inequalities are shown to be part of the evolving patterns of global health. The chapters of the book are organized in three major parts:

- The first part introduces readers to the principal concepts of global health, and to the idea of populations having distinctive health profiles. In particular, it explores how those profiles can be measured, and how they change, using the umbrella concepts and theories of epidemiological and health transition.
- Building on the first section, the second part focuses on the evolution of health states, as well as paying particular attention to the reasons for the many subnational inequalities in global health. It also examines health challenges, such as the continuing infectious disease burden and current emerging 'epidemics'.
- The final part transports readers from the current health scene to future possible and probable health scenarios, acknowledging the challenges presented by global environmental change, as well as issues centred on geopolitics and human security.

Using clear and original explanations of complex issues, this text makes extensive use of case studies and international examples, with thought-provoking discussion questions posed for readers at the end of each chapter. *Global Health* is essential reading for students of global health, public health and development studies.

Kevin McCracken is an Honorary Fellow at Macquarie University, Australia and an Honorary Professor at Lingnan University, Hong Kong.

David R. Phillips is a Chair Professor at Lingnan University, Hong Kong and an Adjunct Professor at Macquarie University, Australia.

Global Health

An introduction to current and future trends

Kevin McCracken and David R. Phillips

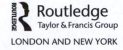

LONDON AND NEW YORK

First published 2012
by Routledge
2 Park Square, Milton Park, Abingdon, Oxon, OX14 4RN

Simultaneously published in the USA and Canada
by Routledge
711 Third Avenue, New York, NY 10017

Routledge is an imprint of the Taylor & Francis Group, an informa business

British Library Cataloguing in Publication Data
A catalogue record for this book is available from the British Library

Library of Congress Cataloging-in-Publication Data
McCracken, Kevin, 1946-
   Global health : an introduction to current and future trends /
   Kevin McCracken and David R. Phillips.
      p. ; cm.
   I. Phillips, David R. II. Title.
   [DNLM: 1. World Health—trends. WA 530.1]
   362.1—dc23   2012000459

ISBN13: 978-0-415-55756-6 (hbk)
ISBN13: 978-0-415-55757-3 (pbk)
ISBN13: 978-0-203-10944-1 (ebk)

Typeset in Goudy by Keystroke, Station Road, Codsall, Wolverhampton

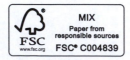
MIX
Paper from
responsible sources
FSC   FSC® C004839
www.fsc.org

Printed and bound in Great Britain by
TJ International Ltd, Padstow, Cornwall

Contents

   What determines population health?   42
   A multi-level model   43
   Feedback effects: health as the driver   49
   Positioning the determinants of health   49
   Discussion topics   52

**Part II Global health and health transition – past and present –
places and groups**   **53**

   4 Global health: where we are and how we got there   55

      Introduction   55
      Health transitions: past and present   57
      Life expectancy reversals   75
      Health and economic development   76
      Health and income inequality   77
      Global health . . . widening the explanatory net   79
      The global health divide: convergence or divergence?   81
      Epidemiological profiles   81
      Adding morbidity to epidemiological profiles   86
      Alternative epidemiological profiles: the 'real causes' of death and ill-health 86
      Concluding notes – continuing and emerging challenges to global health 89
      Discussion topics   89

   5 Global health: sub-national inequalities   90

      Introduction   90
      Dimensions of health inequality within countries   92
      Discussion topics   118

   6 Age and lifecourse transitions in health   119

      Introduction: health and related changes over the lifecourse   119
      Lifecourse and lifespan perspectives   119
      Age and life changes in health   122
      Health changes and transitions over life: some examples   124
      Discussion topics   146

   7 Major contemporary challenges in global health   147

      Risk factors and contemporary disease control priorities   147
      Grand challenges in health today: Millennium Development Goals   148
      Infectious challenges: not yet 'on the retreat'?   152
      Non-communicable diseases and global health   158
      Disabilities: the global picture   160
      Emerging 'lifestyle' challenges to health   162
      Discussion topics   187

Figures

Tables

Boxes

About the authors

Kevin McCracken did his Bachelor's and Master's degrees at the University of Otago, New Zealand, and his Ph.D. at the University of Alberta, Canada. He was a faculty member at Macquarie University, Sydney, Australia from 1973 to 2008, teaching and researching population and health studies. He retired from Macquarie as Dean of Environmental and Life Sciences at the end of 2008 and is now an Honorary Fellow at Macquarie and an Honorary Professor at Lingnan University, Hong Kong.

David R. Phillips did his Bachelor's degree and Ph.D. at the University of Wales, Swansea. He was Reader in Health Studies at the University of Exeter to 1994 and also Director of the Institute of Population Studies and of its WHO Collaborating Centre in Human Reproduction. He was then Professor of Human Geography at the University of Nottingham, to 1997, and Director of its WHO Collaborating Centre in Spatial Health Modelling. Since then, he has been Chair Professor of Social Policy at Lingnan University, Hong Kong, where he was Founder Director of the Asia–Pacific Institute of Ageing Studies. He is an Adjunct Professor at Macquarie University, Sydney, Australia.

Preface

Global health, as a broad shorthand, covers topics and developments of importance to everyone, everywhere. It not only concerns people's health but often affects global and local wealth and well-being. Issues related to the health and well-being of individuals, groups, regions, nations and humanity as a whole perhaps form the largest-growing body of academic publications and popular media attention in the current world. This book is one of a growing number with the term 'global health' in the title, but one which we believe offers a fresh and distinctive view of the subject. In short, our aim has been to provide a concise but detailed and thought-provoking introduction to current and future trends. While the book thoroughly examines the 'here and now' of global health it is also very much concerned with how global health issues may develop over the coming decades of the twenty-first century.

The genesis of this book arose from our years of experience as researchers and university teachers of health- and population-related topics. Increasingly, also, we have both been focusing on the interwoven influences of society, demography, politics, economics and the environment on health, features often collectively termed the 'social determinants' of health. Likewise, we have increasingly come to appreciate the reverse: that is, the role health plays in influencing local, national and international demographic, economic, political and other sectoral outcomes. Working and publishing together over some years, we have found we have particularly complementary interests: Kevin has strong interests in health geography and social demography and has frequently published on these topics in the press as well as academic outlets. David has longstanding teaching, research, training and policy involvement in various areas of general health, social epidemiology, reproductive health and demographic ageing internationally, especially in Asia and parts of Africa. We both have strong interests in inequalities in health status and healthcare opportunities, in environmental issues and health, and in health policies and their impacts. In this book we have therefore done our best to present to readers wide international coverage of key global health issues, with an up-to-date, strong futures orientation. In several chapters, and in the organizational conceptual model shown in Figure 3.1, we especially recognize the importance for global health of health disparities *within* nations as well as between them.

We have structured the book in three main sections, following a hopefully logical sequence. Part I introduces the principal concepts of global health as we see them, plus issues related to data, measurement and health determinants.

The second part builds on these and has a particular interest in the evolution of health status, sometimes called epidemiological or health transition. In this, we trace where we are now in global health, and how we got there. We then acknowledge and analyse the many sub-national inequalities in health around the world. As it is increasingly recognized that demographic ageing and age structure changes (not age per se, but the cumulative effects) are major influences on health status and health needs, we also analyse lifecourse transitions in health. Last in this section, we identify a number of the major contemporary challenges in global health, and discuss some such as malaria, measles, HIV/AIDS and other infections that currently provide huge burdens of global disease, and others, such as non-communicable diseases and especially dementias, that are likely to become the major challenges of the future.

In Part III, we examine possible global health futures, with the future starting tomorrow and looking forward longer term over the rest of this century. Here, we consider how health systems have evolved and how they might – and should – develop, especially in finance, planning and management terms. The huge topic of current and forthcoming global environmental change and its intersections with health is outlined. We then focus on issues mainly, though not exclusively, impacting on 'developing areas' (if this is a meaningful label), in the interrelations among geopolitics, human security and health. Here we cover such topics as population movements, armed conflict, gender inequality and food security and their complex relations with physical and psychological health. Finally, we end with a contemplation of 'global health futures', some aspects of which are fairly certain bets, others more speculative, including how far, effectively and equitably technology will assist global health developments in the next few decades.

Who might read this book? Our aim has been to deliver often detailed, sometimes complex material in a way that will appeal to readers across a wide range of disciplines and interests. We hope that students, researchers, policy-makers and general readers will find it informative, interesting and useful. In terms of specific courses, a number of disciplines may be attracted to the book as a main text or for additional readings. These include under-graduate and postgraduate global health programmes, courses in public health, epidemiology, international studies, geography, and personnel in a number of international agencies. For students and instructors, we have posed discussion topics at the end of each chapter.

Throughout, we have attempted to make the book as up-to-date and comprehensive as possible, while trying to avoid superficiality. The book naturally draws and builds on much existing population health research, but we also provide substantial original analyses of our own: for example, on epidemiological variability, health disparities within countries, health and income inequality, and population ageing and health. We hope this adds to the originality and interest of the volume for readers. We have also included a wide and com-prehensive bibliography for readers who wish to pursue any topics further. Moreover, we have provided a list of websites relevant to global health, and have provided the web addresses (URLs) of a substantial number of items in the References. Some of these URLs, however, will inevitably become inactive during the lifespan of the book.

A volume of this nature would have been very difficult to complete without cooperation from many organizations and individuals as global health has a wide publication footprint. In this context, we would like to note the generosity of many international organizations, especially the World Health Organization (WHO), for permission to reproduce material from various publications. Similarly, Alzheimer's Disease International and the Alzheimer's Association have kindly given permission to use their material, as have Elsevier (*The Lancet*) and others. All sources are acknowledged as appropriate in the text, figures, tables and text boxes.

Several individuals in our respective universities have provided us with great support and assistance at various stages over the past two years or so. In particular, we would like to acknowledge Judy Davis and Frank Siciliano at Macquarie University for assistance in cartographic and graphical work, and Ivy Tsang at Lingnan University for excellent help in extracting tables and illustrations from many sources. On the 'home front', our respective spouses Lyn and Frances have endured many days of 'writing widowhood' and we wish to thank them for their enduring patience.

To the global health community, and those studying and researching these topics, we dedicate this text.

Kevin McCracken, Macquarie University, Sydney, Australia
David R Phillips, Lingnan University, Hong Kong
March 2012

Abbreviations

ACT	Artemisinin-based combination therapies
AD	Alzheimer's disease
ADI	Alzheimer's Disease International
ADL	Activities of daily living
AMI	Acute myocardial infarction
AMR	Adult mortality rate
ASDR	Age-specific death rate
BBC	British Broadcasting Corporation
BMI	Body Mass Index
CDC	Centers for Disease Control and Prevention
CDR	Crude death rate
CFCs	Chlorofluorocarbons
CIOMS	Council for International Organizations of Medical Sciences (WHO)
CMR	Child mortality rate
COPD	Chronic obstructive pulmonary disease
CSDH	Commission on Social Determinants of Health
CT	Computerized tomography
DALY	Disability-adjusted life year
DFLE	Disability-free life expectancy
DHS	Demographic and Health Surveys
DM	Diabetes mellitus
DMM	Dispersion Measure of Mortality
Dollars ($)	US dollars, unless otherwise specified
DOT	Directly observed therapy/treatment (in TB)
DRC	Democratic Republic of Congo
DSP	Disease surveillance points
DSS	Demographic surveillance sites
EDPLN	Emerging and Dangerous Pathogens Laboratory Network (WHO)
EID	Emerging infectious disease
ELB	Expectation of life at birth (usually called life expectancy at birth)
EMRSA	A strain of MRSA
ENCR	European Network of Cancer Registries
EPI	Expanded Programme on Immunization
ESBLs	Extended-spectrum beta-lactamases
ESKAPE	*Enterococcus faecium, Staphylococcus aureus, Klebsiella pneumoniae, Acinetobacter baumannii, Pseudomonas aeruginosa, Enterobacter* species
ET	Epidemiological transition
FAO	Food and Agricultural Organization (United Nations)
FDA	Food and Drug Administration (United States)

GAR	Global Alert and Response (WHO)
GARP	Global Antibiotic Resistance Partnership
GAVI	Global Alliance for Vaccines and Immunization (GAVI Alliance)
GBD	Global burden of disease
GBV	Gender-based violence
GDP	Gross Domestic Product (pc = per capita)
GEGA	Global Equity Gauge Alliance
GFRP	Global Food Crisis Response Program (World Bank)
GH	Global Health
GNP	Gross National Product (pc = per capita)
GOARN	Global Outbreak Alert and Response Network (WHO)
GPHIN	Global Public Health Intelligence Network
GVF	Global Viral Forecasting
H1N1	A subtype of Influenza A virus ("swine flu")
H5N1	A subtype of Influenza A virus ("bird flu")
HAB	Harmful algal bloom
HAART	Highly active antiretroviral therapy (for HIV/AIDS)
HALE	Health-adjusted life expectancy (healthy life expectancy)
Hib	*Haemophilus influenzae* type b
HIV/AIDS	Human Immunodeficiency Virus/Acquired Immune Deficiency Syndrome
HLY	Healthy life year (European Union)
HPV	Human papillomavirus
IACR	International Association of Cancer Registries
IADL	Instrumental activities of daily living
IAEA	International Atomic Energy Agency
ICD	International Statistical Classification of Diseases and Related Health Problems
ICF	International Classification of Functioning, Disability and Health
ICRC	International Committee of the Red Cross
IDF	International Diabetes Federation
IFRC	International Federation of Red Cross and Red Crescent Societies
IHD	Ischaemic heart disease
IGT	Impaired glucose tolerance
ILO	International Labour Office
IMF	International Monetary Fund
IMR	Infant mortality rate
IOM	Institute of Medicine (Washington, DC)
IPCC	Intergovernmental Panel on Climate Change
IPPF	International Planned Parenthood Federation
LAMIC	Low- and middle-income countries
LGBT	Lesbian, gay, bisexual and transgender
MDGs	Millennium Development Goals
MDR-TB	Multidrug-resistant tuberculosis
MHP	Maternal health promoter
MMR	Maternal mortality ratio
MRI	Magnetic resonance imaging
MRSA	Methicillin/oxacillin-resistant *Staphylococcus aureus*
MSF	Médecins sans Frontières (Doctors without Borders)
NCD	Non-communicable disease
NCHS	National Center for Health Statistics
NIA	National Institute on Aging (Washington, DC)

NIAID	National Institute of Allergy and Infectious Diseases
NMR	Neonatal mortality rate
NTD	Neglected Tropical Diseases (WHO)
ODA	Official development assistance
ODS	Ozone-depleting substances
OECD	Organization for Economic Cooperation and Development
ORT	Oral rehydration therapy
PAHO	Pan-American Health Organization (WHO)
PET	Positron emission tomography
PHEIC	Public Health Emergencies of International Concern
PM	Particulate matter (air pollution)
POP	Persistent organic pollutant
PPP	Purchasing power parity
PRSP	Penicillin-resistant *Streptococcus pneumoniae*
PYLL	Potential years of life lost
RDT	Rapid diagnostic tests (malaria)
SARS	Severe acute respiratory syndrome
SMPH	Summary measures of population health
SRS	Sample Registration System (India)
STD	Sexually transmitted disease
SUN	Scaling Up Nutrition
TB	Tuberculosis
TBA	Traditional birth attendant
TCAM	Traditional, complementary or alternative medicine/medical practice
TEPHINET	Training in Epidemiology and Public Health Intervention Network
TFR	Total fertility rate
TM	Traditional medicine
U5MR	Under-five mortality rate
UK	United Kingdom
UN	United Nations
UNAIDS	Joint United Nations Programme on HIV/AIDS
UNCCD	United Nations Convention to Combat Desertification
UNDESA	United Nations Department of Economic and Social Affairs
UNDESA-PD	United Nations Department of Economic and Social Affairs, Population Division
UNDP	United Nations Development Programme
UNESCAP	United Nations Economic and Social Commission for Asia and the Pacific
UNFPA	United Nations Population Fund
UNICEF	United Nations Children's Fund
US	United States
USAID	United States Agency for International Development
USCB	United States Census Bureau
USSR	Union of Soviet Socialist Republics
VA	Verbal autopsy
VRE	Vancomycin-resistant *Enterococci*
WHO	World Health Organization
WHS	World Health Survey (WHO)
XDR-TB	Extensively drug-resistant tuberculosis
YLD	Years of healthy life lost due to poor health or a disability

Part I

Concepts, data, measurement, explanations

1 Global health

An introduction

The genesis of global health (GH)

Terminologies change, enter and exit fashion. The concepts underlying the changing health needs, status and situations of groups and nations are becoming ever better understood, and terms to describe them are changing. In this context, *global health* (GH) is gaining popularity and momentum. The term has emerged from many perspectives and disciplines and may well yet be varyingly interpreted in the coming years in different countries. To some scholars and policy-makers, GH refers generally to emerging global shifts in health status and apparent convergences of health experience across the world. Others apply GH more technically, in relation to particular diseases or conditions: for example, the attainment of specific health-related objectives, the reduction, prevention or elimination of specific, often infectious, diseases (such as HIV, malaria, schistosomiasis) or groups of chronic conditions (heart disease, cancers, or wider non-communicable diseases), or in the reduction in incidence and extent of specific health problems, such as maternal or infant mortality. Others see GH as implying some sort of generality in evolution and variation in human behaviour, such as drug and alcohol misuse, under- or over-nutrition, obesity or behaviour leading to the spread of sexually transmitted diseases. Yet others see GH in the context of policies for widespread targeting of particular groups or geographical areas: for example, the young, women, refugees, migrants, victims of disasters, or older people. 'Although universities, government agencies, and private philanthropies are all using the term in highly visible ways, the origin and meaning of the term "global health" are still unclear' (Brown *et al.*, 2006, p. 62). But it has a huge and critical reality, as former Director of the WHO G.H. Brundtland (2003) noted almost a decade ago.

Where, then, can the researcher or student start? Today, many, including the *Journal of Public Health Policy*, refer to Wikipedia definitions, which in this case has a useful array of measures of global health but surprisingly few concrete references and definitions. Web searches likewise reveal a range of interesting but not always globally relevant issues. What of the international, academic and policy literature? There is a rapidly growing number of academic papers with the term in the title, although as yet relatively few books specifically using it.

Among current books, Kathryn Jacobsen (2008), for example, in her *Introduction to Global Health*, adopts a structured approach to specific issues. She raises a number of epidemiological questions, such as: 'What are the key diseases and health conditions that cause death and disability in different parts of the world? What are the theories and methods that allow us to study population health? What can be done to create a healthier global population?' Her text is a useful starting point as it looks at possible ways forward in global health as well as focusing on problems. Skolnik (2008; 2012) provides a helpful discussion on health-development links and the health needs of developing countries and poor and disadvantaged groups. Crisp (2010) is more visionary, seeing the search for 'global health' as something requiring radical policies, as health systems everywhere appear practically and financially inadequate and unable to deliver adequate care. New ways of thinking are required, with much greater co-development and learning. His book emphasizes interdependence, rich countries learning from poor as well as the usual vice versa, introducing some novel potential socio-economic and geopolitical approaches. Birn *et al.* (2009) use the two terms 'global health' and 'international health' in the title of their book and provide a useful discussion of the distinctions.

The emergence of global health as a term

In recent years, many academic and policy writers have noted that a common definition of global health will be useful. If not, used shorthand, the term might overlook important differences in philosophies, strategies and priorities among the various parties (including policy-makers, practitioners, funders, researchers, the media and the public). Koplan *et al.* (2009, p. 1993), working to such a common definition, contend that GH has at least three facets:

- as a notion (the state of global health);
- as an objective (aiming for a condition of global health, a world of healthy people); and
- as a mix of scholarship, research, and practice (with multidisciplinary issues, questions and participants).

Definitions will need to set GH apart from earlier related approaches. Koplan and others note that GH has evolved from, and alongside, a century-old tradition of *public health*, which was then and is now a broad and largely comprehensible concept, through to the more recent conceptualization of *international health*. 'International health' (IH) also has a long history and tended to focus mainly on the control of epidemics in developing countries, especially across the boundaries between nations (Brown *et al.*, 2006; Birn *et al.*, 2009). Birn *et al.* (2009) provide a third-edition update of Basch's classic *Textbook of International Health*, published in 1990. IH as a term is retained by many teachers, researchers and practitioners and today probably focuses, validly, as much on differences as similarities between health policies, practices and systems in different countries. Merson *et al.* (2006), in a text combining the terms – *International Public Health* – stress the practical and very interdisciplinary origins of public health and the application of its principles, particularly in low- and middle-income countries. However, over the past decade or more, the term 'global health' – to be defined – has been overtaking international health, especially given a greater understanding of global interrelatedness, interdependence and an awareness that the health and well-being of people and groups in all nations and regions are increasingly interdependent, probably through a popular conception of globalization. The US Global Health Council was an interesting multi-sectoral policy and research initiative that, until it ceased operation in 2012, focused on US and international health issues, including communicable diseases, NCDs, maternal and child health and HIV/AIDS. It published the magazine *Global Health*.

'Global health', to Brown *et al.* (2006, p. 62), in general 'implies consideration of the health needs of the people of the whole planet above the concerns of particular nations'. They view 'global' as 'associated with the growing importance of actors beyond governmental or intergovernmental organizations and agencies, including, for example, the media, internationally influential foundations, non-governmental organizations and transnational corporations'.

Koplan *et al.* (2009) compare and contrast the characteristics of global health, international health and public health (Table 1.1). All are population based, though the first

Table 1.1 Comparison of global, international and public health

	Global health	International health	Public health
Geographical reach	Focuses on issues that directly or indirectly affect health but that can transcend national boundaries	Focuses on health issues of countries other than one's own, especially those of low income and middle income	Focuses on issues that affect the health of the population of a particular community or country
Level of cooperation	Development and implementation of solutions often requires global cooperation	Development and implementation of solutions usually requires binational cooperation	Development and implementation of solutions does not usually require global cooperation
Individuals or populations	Embraces both prevention in populations and clinical care of individuals	Embraces both prevention in populations and clinical care of individuals	Mainly focused on prevention programmes for populations
Access to health	Health equity among nations and for all people is a major objective	Seeks to help people of other nations	Health equity within a nation or community is a major objective
Range of disciplines	Highly interdisciplinary and multidisciplinary within and beyond health sciences	Embraces a few disciplines but has not emphasized multidisciplinarity	Encourages multidisciplinary approaches, particularly within health sciences and with social sciences

Source: Koplan *et al.*, 2009, p. 1994

two can include clinical care for individuals; they have a preventive focus, and tend to concentrate on poorer, vulnerable and underserved populations. They are generally multidisciplinary, and global health is particularly interdisciplinary. All place health as a public good involving the participation of many stakeholders. Global health focuses on issues that directly or indirectly affect health but can transcend national boundaries. Public health tends to focus more on the health of particular communities or a country. International health tends to concentrate on countries other than one's own, and especially the health issues of low- and middle-income countries. Koplan *et al.*'s paper (pp. 1994–5)identifies several key issues to be resolved in reaching a definition of global health, which we consider below:

- What is global?
- Does a health crisis have to cross national borders to be defined as a global health issue (geographical reach)?
- Is global health aimed principally at infectious diseases and maternal and child issues, or does it also address chronic diseases, injuries, psychological health and the environment?
- Does GH relate to globalization and, if so, how?
- Must GH operate only within a framework or goal of socio-economic equity (access)?
- What is the range of disciplines involved in global health?

Based on their review of the evolution of the various subjects, and in light of these questions, Koplan *et al.* (2009, p. 1995; our emphases) offer the following formulation:

> *global health* is an area for study, research, and practice that places a priority on improving health and achieving *equity in health for all people worldwide*. Global health emphasizes *transnational* health issues, determinants, and solutions; involves *many disciplines* within and beyond the health sciences and promotes interdisciplinary collaboration; and is a *synthesis* of population-based prevention with individual-level clinical care.

A concise version based on this definition is offered by Beaglehole and Bonita (2010, p. 1), in which GH is 'collaborative trans-national research and action for promoting health for all'; and a similar perspective is echoed by Skolnik (2008, 2012). This perspective stresses the need for collaboration and action, and refrains from calling itself global public health to avoid an implication that global health focuses only on 'classical, and nationally-based, public health actions' (Beaglehole and Bonita, 2010, p. 1). This is a useful practical distinction. '*Global health* implies a global perspective on public health problems' which suggest many issues people almost everywhere face, to a greater or lesser extent, 'such as the impact of a growing and aging worldwide population on health or the potential risks of climate change to health' (Skolnik, 2012, p. 7). A similar sentiment is seen in the statement on the de facto global reach and demands of public health by former Director-General of the WHO G.H. Brundtland (Box 1.1). This is very much the approach we adopt in this book, as we try to explain patterns of global health change, seeking commonalities and looking forward to how future common health issues will emerge, although probably with varied expressions and solutions in different places and groups.

One of the most interesting cross-disciplinary perspectives is in the UK government's 2008 policy document *Health is Global*, which reviews the major areas involved in and influencing GH, with a focus on the cross-national and international. Here, GH refers to 'health issues where determinants circumvent, undermine or are oblivious to the territorial boundaries of states, and are thus beyond the capacity of individual countries to address through domestic institutions' (HM Government, 2008, p. 5). *Health is Global* notes that the UK was the first nation to publish a cross-government strategy in global health, and an updated version of the document, *Health is Global: An Outcomes Framework for Global Health 2011–2015* (HM Government, 2011), points out that there were substantial international developments in the short period between 2008 and 2011. Global conditions had changed, especially in terms of deepening global economic crisis and with economic power and opportunity shifting towards many countries in the East and South. This later document mentions especially the increasing importance of Brazil, India, China, Indonesia, other parts of Asia, and Turkey.

The UK government's 2011 vision of global health is particularly useful for this book. It starts by mentioning examples of the range of health issues influenced by factors that can extend beyond, or 'transcend', state borders, such as preparedness for pandemic influenza and emerging infections, climate change, international development and a hugely valuable

---

BOX 1.1 Global challenges need global solutions

'The reality is that public health is, as never before, a priority on the global agenda, for the simple reason that so many of the challenges we face now have a global impact, requiring global solutions and a global response.'

(Source: Brundtland, 2003, p. 8)

worldwide healthcare industry worth more than US$3 trillion annually. Most crucially, it considers that global health 'interacts with all the core functions of foreign policy: achieving national and global security, creating economic wealth, supporting development in low-income countries and promoting human dignity through the protection of human rights and the delivery of humanitarian assistance' (HM Government, 2011, p. 3). We touch on almost all of these issues in this book.

The 2008 statement recognizes the concerns of global health focus on people across the whole planet rather than in particular nations, though clearly local context must be crucial too. In geopolitical terms, the UK strategy explicitly acknowledges that global health security is crucial for economic and political stability and that health is vulnerable to a wide range of complex, 'often daunting' issues. To improve global health security, the strategy advocates a focus on key practical issues, many of which we follow in subsequent chapters (HM Government, 2008, p. 9):

- global poverty and health inequalities;
- climate change and environmental factors;
- the effects of conflict on health and healthcare;
- reducing the threat from infectious disease; and
- human trafficking and the health of migrants.

These were conflated to three action areas in 2011, with a particular focus on outcomes:

- global health and security;
- international development; and
- trade for better health.

Similar to the Millennium Development Goals (MDGs) that will be discussed in subsequent chapters, twelve outcomes are aimed for under these three areas. These are cited in some detail in Box 1.2, because they highlight many issues we discuss in subsequent chapters. It is interesting to note that trade, health and development are identified as closely interrelated,

---

BOX 1.2 UK Government: twelve global health outcomes wished for by 2015

Area for Action I: Global health and security

1 MDGs – food and water security: a greater proportion of the world's people will enjoy improved food and water security; increase agricultural productivity in developing countries; raise food security; improve nutrition for most vulnerable.
2 Climate change: support low- and middle-income countries to assess/address health vulnerability in relation to climate change.
3 Health and conflict: reduced humanitarian and health impact of conflict.
4 Emergency preparedness: the UK and the rest of the world should be better able to predict, avoid and respond to emerging global health threats, including epidemic and pandemic infections, natural disasters and bioterrorism.
5 Research: achieve deeper scientific understanding of the effects on health of changes in climate, water and food resources; use this to inform options for action.

---

continued

Area for Action II: International development

6 MDGs – health systems and delivery: combat HIV/AIDS, tuberculosis (TB), malaria and improve reproductive, maternal, newborn and child health, resources will be used to support health systems strengthening to ensure greater coverage and access to quality essential health services that are safe, effective and efficient; moving to reduce the global gap in healthcare workers.

7 Non-communicable diseases: stronger integrated strategies and actions, and effective support from international agencies, for tackling and preventing some non-communicable diseases and their drivers (obesity and diet, substance abuse, alcohol and smoking, pollution, etc.) as well as violence and injury in low- and middle-income countries.

8 Learning from other countries: improving the UK's population health outcomes through learning from international experience.

9 Research: better coordination of UK and European Union (EU) global health research; enhanced, low-cost access to research knowledge for researchers and policy-makers in developing countries, strengthening evidence–policy linkages in developing countries; research more available to end users, e.g. through electronic media.

Area for Action III: Trade for better health

10 MDGs – access to medicines: increased access to safe, high-quality, affordable treatments and medicines, including for HIV/AIDS, malaria and TB, especially for the world's poorest (strengthening access to markets and safeguarding transparent provision).

11 Trade and investment: UK life sciences and healthcare sectors make the most of global trade opportunities, particularly in key emerging markets and support the growth of foreign direct investment in UK life sciences and healthcare sectors.

12 Research: partnerships to address challenges in scaling up innovation and evidence-based interventions to achieve universal coverage, especially for the poor and in hard-to-reach areas.

(Source: Based on HM Government, 2011, pp. 7, 8, 9)

and the imbalances engendered in the global economy in relation to trade are implicit. However, though considerable advances have been achieved this century, funding problems in particular threaten programmes and a 'golden window' for global health developments may be closing (see Box 1.3).

Similar strategic, and certainly cross-national, issues and causes were identified in the 1990s by the Board on International Health of the US Institute of Medicine (1997), although with a more restricted perspective. There, GH was seen as involving rather defined issues and causes, most of which remain valid and will also be considered later in this book:

- economic globalization and the transfer of risks;
- demographic change and the epidemiologic transition;
- poverty and health;
- rising costs of healthcare and the need for health system reform; and
- changes in international health agencies.

What is global?

The term 'global' has been much used, and probably abused, in recent literature, sometimes employed accurately, sometimes perhaps to give an air of importance or emphasis. Dictionary definitions specify global as being 'worldwide', referring to comprehensive events affecting or taking into consideration the whole world. In the health field, the use of the term is by no means novel, although its meaning was not necessarily the dictionary one. Brown *et al.* (2006) note that 'global' has been used over decades with respect to specific conditions or health programmes, such as the WHO's Global Malaria Eradication Programme, launched in the mid-1950s. This would, of course, have referred to eradication plans for malaria *where it occurred* and the prevention of its spread beyond such zones. So, while malaria posed a slight risk for those outside such places, and huge numbers within, it would hardly be *global* in the sense of directly affecting people everywhere. One can, of course, argue its economic consequences and impacts were even at the time, in a sense, global. More comprehensive in meaning, perhaps, was the WHO's Global Battle against Disease in 1958, although its focus was again mainly on the types of diseases prevalent mainly in developing countries, so, arguably, it was not truly global. Yet nearer to the dictionary meaning may have been a 1971 report for the US House of Representatives, *The Politics of Global Health*, and so too were many studies of the 'global population problem' in the 1970s and 1980s (Brown *et al.* 2006), as the consequences of population growth in some countries were seen as a phenomenon challenging rich and poor nations alike due to increasing interdependence and potential for instability. However, while population stagnation and decline are today recognized as very important in many countries, the earlier population policies had a focus on specific groups of high-fertility developing nations. Banta (2001) and Brown *et al.* (2006), among others, consider that, at this stage, the term 'global' tended to be restricted and generally occurred in official statements and documents. Since the 1990s, however, there has been an increasing frequency of popular as well as quasi-official policy and academic references to *global* health.

Earlier the question was posed: does a condition have to be transnational to be considered global? According to the UK government's definition, it does, although its global health

---

BOX 1.3 A golden window closing for global health?

A cross-cutting approach is needed to meet the challenges of the global financial crisis . . . The past decade has been a 'golden window' for global health. New disease specific health initiatives and major new funding programmes have contributed to impressive gains. In 2008, for example, 10,000 fewer children were dying each day than in 1990. But there are disturbing signs that the window may be closing.

(Feachem *et al.*, 2010, p. 1)

Donor agencies have warned that financial help cannot be assured and many face serious funding shortfalls. 'How will the global health community respond? One risk is that the various sub-communities . . . will advocate and compete for their own stake in the shrinking pot of donor money' (p. 2). Loss of sustained, guaranteed funding to strengthen fragile health infrastructures in many developing countries may mean MDGs will not be reached. The community needs to unite, avoid competition and agree on a cross-cutting agenda for global health and maximize the returns for all funds allocated.

(Source: After Feachem *et al.*, 2010)

strategy is interesting in that it emphasizes interlinkages between areas with rather different health profiles and problems. However, even when we start to discuss specific health issues today, many, such as cancers, obesity and diabetes, are now becoming so commonplace and ubiquitous that they can be called global. The nature of their local expression, causes, evolution, trends and transition in different places or among different population groups may be what are important, rather than there being a simultaneous carbon-copy occurrence or worldwide blueprint. As we discuss below, people may exist in a global world but the vast majority live and act locally, so local conditions, environments and services are often the key to understanding the impact of the much wider influences.

Globalization

We all see the term 'globalization' used with increasing frequency and, commonly, as a shorthand for change (positive and negative) on a broad range of fronts (Cockerham and Cockerham, 2010). Today, the term is often used as summary for the nebulous but evident and continuing, probably accelerating, processes through which regional economies, societies, and cultures have become integrated via rapid communication and exchange networks that are (almost) totally global. Many people appear to take the term as meaning *economic* globalization, but with concomitant cultural spread associated with the diffusion of 'Westernization' of lifestyle and consumption patterns an important subsidiary feature. This is a type of de facto acknowledgement of increasing interdependence, possibly integration, but also the basis for competition among national economies or interests within the international economic framework. Competition almost inevitably occurs through the different loci of production and consumption. These are facilitated by networks of communication, transport, trade, foreign exchange, foreign direct investment, capital and labour flows and, crucially, twenty-four-hour, technology-driven financial markets. Increasingly, however, globalization is acknowledged as involving much more than just the economic, as the linkages involve technological, socio-cultural, political, environmental and bio-medical factors (see Box 1.4).

Globalization in popular terms, to most people, is therefore as much a socio-cultural as an economic phenomenon, involving the evolution of common understanding of ideas, languages, foods and popular culture. To this extent, the influence of the internet today and, to date, the influence of Western (especially American) media, television, films and corporations have been positively or negatively defined as driving forces. The most common evidence cited tends to be the spread of fast-food outlets and consumption, usually personalized as McDonald's. In this respect, globalization has its supporters and detractors. Many protagonists see globalization as a principally beneficial or benign phenomenon, bringing additional developmental, socio-cultural, political and public health improvements. By contrast, critics of globalization indict the process of undermining local economies and

---

BOX 1.4 Globalization, seen as . . .

'The widening, deepening and speeding up of worldwide interconnectedness in all aspects of contemporary social life. These global processes are changing the nature of human interaction across a wide range of social spheres including the economic, political, cultural and environmental.'

(Source: HM Government, 2008, p. 5)

cultures, replacing them with bland variants on the United States and blended elements of European cultures, a type of neocolonialism by stealth. Such critiques are found in both Western and non-Western countries. The Taliban form just one extreme wing that identifies Western expression and the trend as abhorrent. At the other end of a spectrum (if such can be said to exist) are multinational companies, some evangelical religions and many academics, who applaud the globalization of culture, development, consumption and (to corporations) profit.

In subsequent chapters, we note that the effectively global networks of the internet, worldwide web and, increasingly, mobile phone communication have been a driving force in globalization that have already had wide-ranging health impacts. The internet feeds much international health knowledge and is becoming ever more influential in dissemination of health news and information (even if sometimes dubious). It has effectively become essential to academic and commercial research and development in health, in cross-checking treatment options and, to an extent, in health promotion. These issues are explored later, especially in Chapters 8–11. The drive to extend internet addresses into non-Western scripts is an example of cultures wishing to communicate in their own languages, maybe even therefore side-stepping certain elements of the global scene.

It is indisputable that technology has, over just a couple of decades, enabled huge and increasing interconnectivities, both virtual via email, internet and telecommunications and subsequently often real connections. The 'global village' is in many ways a technological reality several decades after the term was first coined. Nevertheless, the digital divide between nations and socio-economically within countries remains considerable, although mobile phone networks and messaging are increasingly leapfrogging former infrastructural and cost barriers. But other barriers remain, with the governments of some countries, such as China, monitoring or censoring access to various parts of the web and mobile phone networks, and others, such as Burma and North Korea, severely restricting internet access for most of their populations.

In addition, on top of enormous increases in virtual communications, there are ever-increasing 'real' contacts, via international business, travel, tourism and longer- or shorter-term migration. These real contacts may often be beneficial but, of course, a side-effect of any international travel is the huge potential for affecting human health. This can be immediate, via the spread of infectious diseases but also longer term through the spread of more common lifestyles to many parts of the world. The socio-cultural aspects of globalization have been held variously responsible for drifts towards Western styles of life, consumption and morals. Many alleged by-products of such globalized lifestyles include attitudinal and behavioural change, environmental damage, global warming/climate change, and some direct health-status outcomes, such as widespread obesity, diabetes and heart disease. Less tangible changes involve those within societies more generally, such as altered family relations and social contexts for life and morality, as well as health and welfare.

Globalization and health

Stemming from this, if globalization refers to some form of fairly evident but nebulous spread of socio-economic and cross-cultural connectivity, how does it intersect with health? How extensive must be the reach of a health problem or crisis to be considered as an issue of global health? Koplan *et al.* (2009) pose a geographical question, partly answered as above by HM Government (2008, 2011), whether a health crisis must cross national borders to be deemed a global health issue. Here, the defining feature need not be a *literal global reach*; rather, in this context, *global* can refer to any health issue that concerns many countries or is affected by transnational determinants. These could include climate change or urbanization, or solutions requiring more than immediately local interventions, such as the eradication of polio (Koplan *et al.*, 2009) – an example of effective and extensive cross-national research and intervention. Clearly, this 'global reach' potential is an important characteristic, which we endorse for this book, along with Beaglehole and Bonita's variants, discussed above.

The world's population reached seven billion in 2011, so, does a health condition need to affect millions or even billions before it is considered global? Here, again, the extent of impact, the numbers affected (the prevalence), could be a factor, but so too could the incidence (the number of new cases) and the impact potential. A relatively low-incidence condition or disease could have global reach and hold the potential for much higher incidence and subsequent prevalence. An interesting example is the series of SARS outbreaks in 2003–04. Despite initial fears and some officially stoked panic, the condition ultimately affected only tens of thousands people worldwide and caused relatively few attributable deaths. Nevertheless, the corona virus possessed – and still possesses – the *potential* to be much more widespread and dangerous. Likewise, many epidemic infectious diseases, such as various strains of influenza (and sub-types of influenza A, such as H1N1 'swine flu' and H5N1 'avian influenza'), have global spread and some possess the potential to mutate, perhaps become stronger and severely threaten humans. HIV infection is also clearly global in both prevalence and geographical spread although its consequences and treatment options differ somewhat between richer and poorer countries and groups. Similarly, many types of non-communicable conditions, such as many common cancers, can have locally different distributional patterns and prevalence, yet affect enormous numbers of people in total in countries at different stages of development. Ruit *et al.* (2006) provide a specific example of how a slow-emerging, chronic condition, such as unoperated cataracts, affects the vision of millions of people in poor populations throughout both the developed and developing world. Its reach is global by any definition.

Clearly, global health as an approach must therefore address the interlinked socio-cultural, behavioural, socio-political and environmental factors related to health change. Many have been thought of as the social determinants of health (see Chapter 3). They include what are often (though not always accurately) termed 'lifestyle factors', such as alcohol, tobacco and other drug consumption and control; micronutrient deficiencies, overweight and obesity; injury prevention, health of migrants, the migration of health workers and the health of people affected by political and natural disasters. So, 'the global in global health refers to the scope of problems, not their location' (Koplan *et al.*, 2009, p. 1994). To this we add the *potential* scope and the *changing patterns* that are discussed in later chapters under epidemiological and health transition.

Think global but live local?

Similar health trends, problems and challenges are to be clearly seen in many, perhaps most, countries of the world. Their exact timing and prevalence ('amount') may differ but common trends are often visible. However, even if one thinks 'globally', most people effectively live locally. They are therefore primarily influenced by their local environment – natural and social, urban, suburban or rural – but numerous factors with origins well beyond any local residential area very substantially affect people's well-being. These can be regarded as the framing features of the local, regional and national situation. This was officially recognized in 2010, when the first report of Britain's Equality and Human Rights Commission articulated many regional, local and individual variations in social conditions, health and well-being opportunities, but explicitly acknowledged that many were obviously influenced by factors well beyond the scope even of British national control (let alone that of any local neighbourhood). But, as people tend to live, and even work, within specific localities, the key is often to identify how, within this wider nexus, the *local* natural environment is changing and may affect health, and how socio-economic conditions are changing, such as local public services, healthcare provision and access to many basic services. Both these major environmental nets will be affected by local, national, regional and international social-economic conditions and the real physical climate.

Take the example of clean water, a long-recognized human right but, as we see in Chapter 9, one to which almost a billion of the world's inhabitants still have no reliable access. So, however healthily they may try to live, their locality still denies them safe potable water to drink. Furthermore, the local environment offers different people very different faces: even within relatively restricted local areas, someone's opportunities for health are still heavily influenced by their income, education and employment, all of which are nowadays increasingly influenced by global forces. In Chapter 3, we develop a determinants-of-health model that encapsulates the various forces, ranging from global to sub-national or local, that can affect health which illustrates the strong interlinkages at all levels.

How did global health emerge?

Much research and many publications looking internationally in the 1980s and 1990s considered either specific types of health conditions, or health and healthcare in the developing world, or examined the relationships between health and development. Today, these are increasingly seen as artificial separations as everyone in almost every location is subject to varying degrees to infectious, non-infectious and mental health conditions and everywhere healthcare systems are under varying degrees of strain (albeit at very different levels of resourcing). Two or three decades ago, while evidence was starting to emerge, it was hard to envisage, say, cancers, heart diseases and psychiatric/psychological conditions becoming as high a burden – or a higher burden – in the poorer countries as they already were in richer countries. Likewise, it was only in some emergency plans that rich countries were deemed at risk of widespread infectious diseases, especially something as common as a new influenza strain. Over these few decades, it has been ever more recognized that many people and places are essentially 'in the same boat', and that global similarities in health are arguably becoming more common than differences. Looking at Yack and Bettcher's papers on the globalization of public health, Brown *et al.* (2006, p. 63) note they saw the origins of globalization going back a century or more and, as it gathered momentum, implicitly assuming increasingly importance for health. In particular:

> In 1998, Derek Yach and Douglas Bettcher came closer to capturing both the essence and the origin of the new global health in a two-part article on 'The Globalization of Public Health' in the *American Journal of Public Health*. They defined the 'new paradigm' of globalization as 'the process of increasing economic, political, and social interdependence and integration as capital, goods, persons, concepts, images, ideas and values cross state boundaries.

Using the fairly approximate measure of citations including the terms 'international health' and 'global health', Brown *et al.* (2006) detected a huge increase between the decade of the 1950s and 2000–05. Earlier, over 1,000 papers cited terms including 'international health' and only 54 cited 'global health' whereas, by 2000–mid-2005, 52,000 used 'IH' and almost 40,000 used 'GH'. Apart from this exponential increase in analysed articles, the balance between papers using the two terms evolved to being much nearer equal.

Grand challenges in global health

Global health now looks at a range of themes and topics, many large, others relatively small. The major areas are increasingly seen as those affecting the most people globally, and sometimes with the best possibility of being effectively addressed. These are sometimes termed *grand challenges*, envisioned as distinct from a simple statement of the many 'big problems' in global health, such as HIV/AIDS, malnutrition, the lack of access to medical care, or the lack of adequate resources. In 2003, Bill Gates announced a series of fourteen grand challenges in global health, based on a 100-year-old mathematical grand challenge formulation (Varmus *et al.*, 2003; Grand Challenges in Global Health, 2012). A grand challenge is one that will hopefully 'direct investigators to a specific scientific or technical breakthrough that would be expected to overcome one or more bottlenecks in an imagined path towards a solution to one, or preferably several, significant health problems' (Varmus *et al.*, 2003, p. 398). The Bill and Melinda Gates Foundation now sponsors scientific and technological research in these areas with a number of other organizations, under the Grand Challenges in Global Health initiative, looking specifically at the developing world, although some of these topics clearly have global interest (Box 1.5). These were established by polling many interdisciplinary and international researchers and practitioners, looking at a number of goals. It's clear that the goals and the eventually selected original fourteen challenges strongly emphasize the control of infectious diseases, though it is welcome to see that some chronic conditions are also targeted, as is the need for affordable health data in developing countries. Infectious diseases were principal challenges as they remain major causes of health problems in developing countries and account for many developed–developing world disparities in health. Moreover, their causes are often well recognized yet their defeat often needs technical as well as social breakthroughs (Varmus *et al.*, 2003). Many need research and investment that might be uneconomic without the encouragement of such initiatives. It was always intended that the list of challenges would grow as scientists identified new topics within the scope of the initiative. By 2012, two extra challenges had been added: No. 15: Discover biomarkers of disease; and No. 16: Discover new ways to achieve healthy birth, growth and development (Grand Challenges in Global Health, 2012). Both of these reflect the importance of research and identification of problems in foetal and child development so they underscore how common challenges can be met as science and technology advance. We follow up some of these issues in Chapters 7 and 11, as well as other major contemporary and emerging challenges that have yet to be addressed.

BOX 1.5 Grand challenges in global health (showing original goals)

- To improve childhood vaccines

    1 Create effective single-dose vaccines that can be used soon after birth
    2 Prepare vaccines that do not require refrigeration
    3 Develop needle-free delivery systems

- To create new vaccines

    4 Devise reliable tests in model systems to evaluate live attenuated vaccines

5 Solve how to design antigens for effective, protective immunity
6 Learn which immunological responses provide protective immunity

- To control insect vectors of disease

    7 Develop a biological strategy to deplete or incapacitate a disease-transmitting insect population
    8 Develop a chemical strategy to deplete or incapacitate a disease-transmitting insect population

- To improve nutrition to promote health

    9 Create a full range of optimal, bioavailable nutrients in a single staple plant species

- To improve drug treatments (infectious diseases)

    10 Discover drugs and delivery systems that minimize the likelihood of drug-resistant micro-organisms

- To cure latent and chronic conditions

    11 Create therapies that can cure latent infection
    12 Create immunological methods that can cure chronic infections

- To measure disease and health status accurately and economically in poor countries

    13 Develop technologies that permit quantitative assessment of population health status
    14 Develop technologies that allow assessment of multiple conditions, pathogens at point-of-care
        (Source: Varmus *et al.*, 2003; Grand Challenges in Global Health, 2011)

Millennium Development Goals (MDGs)

The Millennium Development Goals were identified and agreed in 2000 by the United Nations and many member states. They were effectively new, quantifiable – and ambitious – international development targets, most to be achieved by 2015. They included fundamental goals with targets, such as reducing extreme poverty, child and other mortality levels, and fighting many forms of epidemic disease, including HIV/AIDS, and improving maternal health (see Box 7.2). A number of goals are wide ranging and reflect development ideology up to the time, as well as being ambitious: for example, Goal 7, ensuring environmental sustainability, and, Goal 8, to build a global partnership for development. Some MDGs reflect the specific grand challenges noted above but they are generally broader. We discuss the MDGs, with risk factors, in Chapters 6 and 7. It should be noted here, however, that it was fairly widely acknowledged that, from the outset, many of the MDGs were unattainable in totality within the timescale to 2015. Nevertheless, they have been significant in introducing a degree of focus in the specification of twenty-one targets, and a series of measurable indicators for each, several of which have been attainable in some places. The details are on the UN's *Millennium Development Goals Indicators* website.

The MDGs and how they were derived have not escaped criticism, although most critiques turn to how to improve the derivation of principles for future goal-setting after 2015. An important achievement of the MDG 'concept' has been, as Waage *et al.* (2010) note, to foster an unprecedented global consensus about measures to reduce poverty. The existence of MDGs has also helped encourage greater global political consensus within international assistance, with a focus on advocacy, improving targeting of aid, and the monitoring of development projects, though of course these still have some way to go. The MDGs themselves have nevertheless had problems and are recognizable as an assembly of sector-specific and often quite narrowly focused targets, the origins of some harking back to development concepts and campaigns of the 1980s and 1990s. Waage *et al.* (2010) also note they were not derived from an inclusive analysis and prioritization of development needs.

Clearly, the goals all have greater or lesser implications for global health. Many which focus on environmental safety, access to safe water, education, especially of young girls, and the like are fundamental to equity, equality and human development. The goals are thus very interlinked and to a considerable degree interdependent. Three goals focus very explicitly on health (Goals 4, 5 and 6, with specific targets within the reduction of child mortality, improvement of maternal health and combating specific diseases, such as HIV/AIDS and malaria). But all MDGs would contribute in an integral manner towards the improvement or otherwise of health and well-being.

As we discuss in Chapter 7, progress towards reaching the principal MDG goals and many of the specific targets has been uneven. Some regions and countries have achieved many of the goals while others are unlikely to realize many within the time frame or even in the foreseeable future. Some major countries, such as China, have been achieving goals in poverty and hunger reduction, if not poverty eradication. But many countries where there is the greatest need for reduction, including several in sub-Saharan Africa, have yet to make any substantial changes or progress towards most targets. Considerable geographical unevenness remains evident in well-being, gender differences, governance, corruption, insecurity, widespread poverty and a lack of basic services that would contribute to achieving the goals. The challenges of gender equity in the social determinants of health within the international health context continue in many places and form an important intersectoral development agenda (Sen *et al.*, 2002).

Global health: epidemiology and medicine

At this stage it is useful to mention the different ways in which medical practitioners and epidemiologists look at health issues but to note that these are converging, to an extent. The specialisms of clinical medicine in general have to focus on the health and illness of individuals, and sometimes families and groups within local communities. Public health, epidemiology and many other areas of policy and research tend to focus more broadly on the health of wider groups and places and to examine trends in and detection of new and existing conditions. They have a particular interest in the identification and reduction or elimination of risk factors. In Chapters 2 and 3, we examine these issues, measuring health and the wide-ranging factors influencing or determining human health. Increasingly, however, the distinctions between clinical practice and social medicine, public and global health are becoming blurred, as interests overlap. Most practising doctors, especially family physicians and those working in the community, want and need to understand the social and family contexts within which their patients live, to deliver their healthcare as effectively as possible. In some places, social factors strongly influence the operation of healthcare as a business. Practitioners and planners need to know patterns of work, behaviour, travel, residence, consumption, vacationing, sexual predilections, and therefore increasingly they move into the spheres of behaviour and variables beyond those of the individual patient. So, almost everyone must have a knowledge of social epidemiology and its global reach.

The epidemiological triad

For many – perhaps most – infectious diseases, the classical 'epidemiological triad' is a useful model or framework for thinking about how the disease develops, spreads and, crucially, can be controlled (i.e. at what point can intervention 'break' the triad?). In particular, the interaction of hosts who acquire or incubate diseases, agents that cause diseases, and the environments (physical and social) in which these interact combine within the concept of the epidemiological triad. This very useful way of looking at a wide variety of health conditions, especially but not exclusively infectious diseases, is discussed in Chapter 3 (see Box 3.1).

Epidemiological (health) transition

One of the most noticeable global trends over many decades has been shifting patterns of health and especially the causes of morbidity (illness) and mortality (death). In Chapter 4 (Box 4.1) we summarize the general trend, to date, away from infectious diseases and famine as the major causes of illness and death towards longer-term, more chronic conditions, all of which are influenced, at least in part, by human behaviour. The term 'epidemiologic(al) transition' (ET) has been widely used as a shorthand for this shift, after the term was coined by Abdel Omran in a 1971 paper that, because of the research it has subsequently generated, has come to be regarded as a public health classic.

The basic concepts of ET are widely recognized and some prefer to term them 'health transition', as this implies a greater attention to the social, economic and healthcare contexts of the changes. Omran certainly deserved credit for the formulation of the transition, but its basic ideas of transitions in health (or, more accurately as far as ET is concerned, in types of diseases) can be seen in earlier work, such as that of the United Nations (UN, 1962) and Frederiksen (1969), who developed a typology outlining 'predominant patterns of disease, mortality, and fertility' in association with 'state of society'. Omran's initial concept and framework have been substantially extended and widened. Today, epidemiological transition is recognized as part of a wider 'health transition', and one strand of a group of interconnected other transitions in fertility, age structure, nutrition, urbanization, technology, and social and economic development.

As a concept (some call it a model), ET may be too deterministic in its linear stages and therefore rather diverse variants are discussed further in Chapter 4 and elsewhere. However, its ramifications are very significant to the concept of global health. First, while ET certainly operates differently in different areas and times, transition is clearly a global trend. Second, if one overlooks its emphasis on changing patterns of causes of *death* and broadens ET to encompass *health status* (to include morbidity and lifecourse changes in health), then it takes on a much more practical significance. Third, ET can help us understand health (as well as disease) changes in different social, ethnic and demographic groups, as well as considerable related spatial variation within and between countries and regions, and, say, within urban areas (Chapters 4 and 5). So, it can help us identify transitions in sub-groups and even counter-transitions if health trends deteriorate. Finally, these variants provide insights into potential health consequences of many forms of social development and the diffusion of combinations of medical, social and economic changes globally.

ET has even greater importance when viewed in conjunction with demographic, ageing and nutrition transitions, and changes (usually, but not always, increases) in life expectancy, especially at a global scale. The early model implied some sort of final end point would be reached for epidemiological transition but today's experience, and especially looking forward, indicates that health and illness patterns are evolving in many ways far beyond any envisaged end point. For example, the evolution in developed and some developing countries has seen a (very large) decline in cardiovascular disease mortality, with a pronounced delaying of deaths from the leading degenerative diseases (heart disease, cancer, stroke) to later ages (the 'rectangularization of the survival curve'), the rise of 'social pathology' deaths, and the dual emergence of new infectious diseases (such as HIV/AIDS and hepatitis C) and, perhaps unexpectedly, a resurgence of some old foes (such as tuberculosis) in drug and multidrug resistant forms. There are not universally agreed terms for these later stage(s) but they generally involve delayed degenerative diseases and emerging infections and socially induced conditions. ET also has complex parallels with other transitions, notably demographic and in ageing and nutrition (see Figure 4.2; McCracken and Phillips, 2009).

Demographic ageing

It is now becoming commonplace to see statements that the world is greying, 'growing older', and that soon older people will form the major group in many countries. The whole future of global health will undoubtedly be influenced by the *ageing transition*. As we will see at many points in the book, the demographic ageing of populations is occurring in almost every nation of the world, with a steady, almost universal, ageing of most countries' populations (National Institute on Aging, 2007; McCracken and Phillips, 2009). Last century, demographic ageing was mainly a phenomenon of the richer world but, ultimately, the bulk of older populations will be located in today's developing nations. This has enormous implications for health, welfare and support services as well as labour supplies in these places. The ageing transition, the underlying causes of demographic ageing, and the associations among older age and health status and health expenditures are arguably the most important global health issues that will confront almost all countries over the coming decades. These will be discussed in more detail in several subsequent chapters.

Healthier or less healthy futures?

Perhaps the foremost single question looking to the future is, as populations generally live longer and fertility in many countries declines, will people be more or less healthy as they age? Some decades ago, L.M. Verbrugge (1984) and others questioned, given lifestyle and technological changes, whether health statistics would show increasing morbidity for non-killer conditions. Potentially,

1   future cohorts of middle-aged and older people might experience healthier lifestyles, and safer work/home environments, with fewer hazards for chronic disease development;
2   medical diagnosis and treatment for potentially fatal conditions could slow or even arrest many diseases;
3   public attitudes and financial support could make it easier for people to adopt the 'sick role', take early retirement and obtain home long-term care, although these conditions are by no means universal.

Compression of morbidity issues

Therefore, the subsidiary question becomes: will people have longer lives but worse health, or will there be a compression of morbidity into a short period of late life (Verbrugge, 1984; Fries, 1980, 2003)? This has huge implications not only for the well-being of ageing populations worldwide, but also for the social support requirements, the ability for people to live alone and need for long-term care, and the associated huge financial costs. As a result, whether older populations will cost more medically and in welfare terms is a question vexing many disciplines, professions and politicians. Many are of the rather pessimistic view that older populations will be a considerable social and economic burden, as older people live longer in declining physical – and especially mental – health. Others suggest there will be declines in disability, on average, in old age (Wolf *et al.*, 2005) and yet others estimate that the alleged high medical costs of old age and dying are a myth (Pan *et al.*, 2007). We discuss the implications of issues of population ageing at many points in the book, and return to them in Chapter 11.

Globalization and health issues in transition

Throughout the book, we look at the many related issues within the global–local health web. These include the many trends in global health that are sometimes called 'social epidemics' or even 'pandemics', such as of non-communicable diseases, particularly heart disease, cancers, obesity, diabetes and dementias. We also consider the *potential*, perhaps more readily recognizable, pandemics, of infectious or communicable diseases, such as various types of influenza and the resurgence of conditions such as tuberculosis, especially drug-resistant types, and of diseases of poverty, such as leprosy, once thought almost eliminated in many countries. We also do our best to counsel readers to be alert to the potential for moral panic – unrealistic alarm or fear raised, often in the media, for instance with regard to alleged lifestyle conditions, such as obesity, population ageing, epidemic infectious conditions, drug resistance and the like. While these are undoubtedly major causes for concern, it is nevertheless important to keep a critical eye on some reports and alleged research-based findings.

We also introduce the concept of *risk factors* for many conditions. We consider the growing potential for global linkages, especially modern travel, to spread both diseases and lifestyle awareness through various forms of business, tourist and migration interactions. As we suggest in Chapter 3, many determinants operate at many levels, from the global to sub-national and personal (Figure 3.1).

In concluding this section, we should note that, globally and locally, many health risks are in transition, and so is health status. Conditions are constantly changing – take the example of new environmental challenges facing many people in developing countries where agricultural extension is occurring. Population structures are also changing, bringing different lifecourse and age-related patterns of health as well as considerable changes in support networks. In most countries, populations are ageing due to a combination of longer life but especially falling birth rates, a very socially based matter and one that has changed over relatively short time spans. Yet there are still many countries with predominantly youthful demographic profiles, where older people still make up only a small percentage of growing populations. So, such nations often face broad-ranging health and social care challenges from both the younger and older age cohorts. In terms of infectious diseases, successes against certain microbes have been balanced by failures against others, some of which have appeared newly, reappeared or even evolved to become almost untreatable by medicines. Social and consumption patterns are also changing in terms of physical activity;

food, alcohol and tobacco consumption; lifestyle and recreational activities. Many low- and middle-income countries are already increasingly facing a *double burden* of increasing incidence and prevalence of chronic, non-communicable conditions, as well as the many communicable diseases that traditionally affect poorer countries and groups. So, in terms of global–local health, understanding the role and likely *evolution* of the many risk factors is probably the key for developing effective strategies for improving health. We will return to these in subsequent chapters.

International assistance and policy in global health

Changes in global health patterns affect everyone and have fostered a huge amount of academic, official and popular engagement. The range of academic, policy and practice interest varies from the local to the international. There is concomitantly a huge number and variety of organizations researching biomedical features, healthcare, epidemiology, policies and social services. We will consider the role of some of these lead agencies and governments at a number of points in the book, especially when we consider health sector organization, management and financing in Chapter 8 and future developments in Chapter 11. These 'global players', as they are sometimes called, include some governments, international agencies in the public sector, NGOs, private corporations (especially in the pharmaceutical field) and private and charitable foundations. They include local, regional and national governments and supra-national groupings such as the EU. Of course, every national government has its various departments and ministries involved in areas of health and welfare at the national level and at sub-national levels. Some are tasked to plan and monitor healthcare services, but others often also deliver healthcare (one of the best-known examples of publicly provided healthcare being the National Health Service in the United Kingdom).

Policy and international assistance organizations in the health and related sectors are numerous. Some are official, others supported by charitable and other sources. Some have official funding and standing and work internationally, a prominent example being the US government's Centers for Disease Control and Prevention, established in 1942. Some governmental health bodies of course focus primarily on their own citizens and within their own borders but, increasingly and inevitably, many have to monitor population movements, especially of people in risk categories, and remain on the alert for infectious diseases. Other organizations are more independently funded, raising money from a range of sources, and some deliver health services in the field, often in difficult circumstances. A well-respected example is the international medical and humanitarian not-for-profit organization Médecins sans Frontières (Doctors without Borders), established in 1971. Sadly, they are not always well received by host nations; for example, in October 2011, MSF reluctantly decided to cease operations in Thailand after thirty-five years of providing healthcare to refugees and needy people. This was because they were unable to gain permission from the government to continue delivery of services to an estimated 1.5–2 million undocumented migrants and people in border areas they believed were in most need of assistance.

Of the official multilateral international organizations, the United Nations' World Health Organization (WHO), established 1948, is resurging as a global voice. Many sister UN organizations also have prominent roles in health, including, among others, UNAIDS, UNFPA and UNICEF, and the UN's regional social and economic commissions, such as UNESCAP. Other agencies essentially have international status representation at government level, such as the World Bank, which has been involved in health from time to time and especially in the past two decades. Many international NGOs, charities and service providers-cum-research bodies focus on particular aspects of health, or groups requiring services. Examples include the International Planned Parenthood Federation (IPPF), Save the Children, Orbis, and others directly or indirectly involved in health (Oxfam, World Vision, ActionAid, and numerous other large and small organizations).

As we shall see from many examples and data sources cited throughout the book, the role of the WHO has been gaining prominence in recent years. Brown *et al.* (2006, p. 62) suggest that the WHO is effectively 'an intergovernmental agency that exercises international functions with the goal of improving global health'. The WHO's opinion in research, advice and policy development is becoming increasingly important, given international media coverage. This is especially important with regard to the increasing issues of global reach, such as potential pandemics, global ageing and NCDs, and it has a Global Alert and Response (GAR) system for epidemics and other public health emergencies. The WHO's regional offices and spokespeople can provide advice and perspectives, especially on the possibilities of rapid spread of some established conditions (pandemic seasonal influenza, tuberculosis, etc.) and new emerging and potential threats, such as avian influenza (H5N1), more severe forms of seasonal flu and 'swine' flu (H1N1) and, previously, SARS. This is somewhat of a contrast to the situation around the turn of the century. In an analysis of the transition from international to global public health, Brown *et al.* (2006, p. 62) observe:

> Between 1948 and 1998, WHO moved from being the unquestioned leader of international health to being an organization in crisis, facing budget shortfalls and diminished status, especially given the growing influence of new and powerful players. We argue that WHO began to refashion itself as the coordinator, strategic planner, and leader of global health initiatives as a strategy of survival in response to this transformed international political context.

From this perspective, the global role of certain key international and UN agencies, especially the WHO, is growing as part of the wider socio-political twenty-first-century evolution of world relations, as well as changes in global health threats. Some commentators, such as Laurie Garrett (2000, 2007), see current global public health (and especially that in the USA) as in a crisis. Public health concerns are seen as paramount and even able to override certain individual liberties for the greater good. Of course, this is viewed as a controversial opinion by those who feel governments and international organizations already wield too much influence.

Last, but by no means least, the importance of academic and policy-related research in health is enormous. Added to the nexus of international agencies and national-level assistance or aid organizations (sometimes, sadly, competing and conflicting with each other), there is an enormous and growing raft of university-based research centres and institutes. An increasing number make reference to global health in their titles. In addition, the medical schools in almost every country are inevitably involved in research, training and collaboration on global health issues: the WHO listed over 1,640 worldwide in 2000, teaching Western or allopathic styles of medicine. There are many more university schools teaching various traditional or alternative forms of healthcare, sometimes (as in China) in combination with allopathic medicine. Almost every medical school will have its version of public or community medicine and interests in clinical and social epidemiology. In addition, there are many varieties of biomedical and social science research and teaching units in almost every nation that cover topics in global health at undergraduate and postgraduate levels. Their local, national, regional and international research foci and findings feed into our expanding knowledge of global–local health.

Our own view of global health naturally reflects the formal views above, 'health problems, issues and concerns that transcend national boundaries', to which concerted actions of public and clinical health, and education, can be addressed. In Chapter 3 (especially Figure 3.1, our conception of the determinants of health), we consider the issue of scale. Expressions of, and the genesis of, many global health issues can be seen locally, and common knowledge and experience can help in facing them, drawing on the collective experience of other places. The influence of local–regional social and physical environments is of the utmost importance, setting the scene as they often do for the development of many health conditions, as well as human and natural disasters. In particular, we acknowledge the transitions in health and demography that have occurred over the past century or more, and which will occur in the future, have commonalities that are truly global.

Discussion topics

1 Why should people care about health in other countries around the world?
2 'Globalization of health is as much to do with the spread of common lifestyles and diets as it is with the spread of infectious diseases.' To what extent do you agree?
3 'Much talk but little action.' Is this a fair assessment of how most Western governments approach the issue of global health in their political and economic agendas?

2 Measuring population health and disease

The initial reaction of most readers to the above chapter title is probably not one of great excitement. We accept that, specialists aside, data and the statistical measures derived from them have a low 'interest quotient' for most people. However, we argue this subject is in fact one of the most important discussed in the book and we hope we can convey that importance to you in the course of the volume. Put bluntly, the current global population health data situation can only be described as seriously incomplete and highly variable in quality, and without major improvements in data collection, processing, access, analysis and application, desired improvements in global health will inevitably be retarded.

Some will no doubt ask: why, though, do we need good global population health data and measures? Our answer is simply that without adequate health information databases (i.e. comprehensive, reliable, comparable, timely, relevant), population health actors, whether local, national or international, are forced to 'fly partially (sometimes almost totally) blind' in their health enhancement efforts.

All aspects of population health decision-making – policy development, programme planning, monitoring and evaluation – should ideally be guided by accurate, pertinent and up-to-date empirical data. For example, without knowing the magnitude and distribution of different health problems, determining priorities in health policies and planning (at whatever level) is blinkered and runs the risk of resources being poorly directed. Which countries have the greatest burden of disease from particular causes of ill-health and need for external aid? How have health patterns changed in different countries over the past decade? Which countries have the largest spatial inequalities in health status? Which provinces/districts in those countries most deserve special resourcing? Which countries have the steepest social gradients to health, and how might these be effectively addressed? If an extra one billion dollars of health funding suddenly became available to the World Health Organization, allocating that money to which health problem(s) would achieve the greatest global health gains? How do the respective health problems and associated resource needs of young children, adolescents, adults and the elderly compare across the countries of Asia? What progress has been made in sub-Saharan Africa towards meeting the health-related Millennium Development Goals? How effective has health-system intervention 'X' been? These are all important health questions, and answering them requires high-quality data. Unfortunately, such data are frequently unavailable and decision-making often has to proceed from a very weak evidence base. In some cases important questions simply cannot be answered.

Health status

As outlined in Chapter 1, population health is a multidimensional concept. Both what people in a population die of (*mortality*) and the health conditions (*morbidity*) they live with are important components and ideally should be incorporated in any assessment and comparisons of health status. The degree to which this is possible, however, varies greatly between (and within) countries, depending on the availability and quality of data sources.

Data sources

A scan of population health articles in such journals as *The Lancet*, the *British Medical Journal* and the *Bulletin of the World Health Organization* will quickly show the wide range of data sources used in charting the health status of populations. These include civil registration records of births and deaths and medically certified causes of death, sample registration systems, demographic surveillance sites, demographic and health surveys, disease surveillance systems, disease registers, healthcare utilization data and population censuses.

The best starting point for readers seeking convenient access to comprehensive collated global health data is the 'Data and statistics' page of the WHO website (http://www.who.int/research/en). In using the various data files available there the comments that follow on mortality and morbidity data sources should be kept in mind.

Mortality

In what may strike some readers as an irony, the most widely used comparative marker of population health is in fact the ultimate loss of health – namely, death. Statistics on the number of people who die, the age and sex of those people, and the causes of their deaths are key to understanding and trying to improve the health of all populations.

Civil vital registration systems

Ideally, every country in the world would have a national system for efficiently registering all deaths (and births) in its population, with accompanying accurate certification and internationally standard coding of the causes of the deaths. Those collated records would then be used informatively to guide health decision-making. Unfortunately, however, this desired situation is nowhere near being achieved globally.

Rich, developed countries generally come reasonably close to satisfying the above ideal, having civil vital registration systems in place that routinely capture details of all, or very nearly all, deaths in the population. Deaths are usually required to be medically certified on standard death certificate forms, with details recorded of the time, date and place of death, the age, sex and place of usual residence of the decedent, and the cause of death.

Beyond these countries, though, the completeness, detail and reliability of national civil registration systems-derived vital statistics drop away. In a few middle-income nations improvements have been made in recent years, but overall most still have a long way to go. Meanwhile, in low-income countries, civil registration systems, if in place at all, are in the main seriously incomplete and the vital statistics produced from them highly unreliable. In aggregate, millions of births and deaths occur around the world every year which are never officially recorded; a 'scandal of invisibility' in the words of a recent *Lancet* writing team (Box 2.1).

Sample registration systems

Due to the problems of achieving complete nationwide civil registration, a number of developing countries have introduced sample birth and death registration schemes. India's Sample Registration System (SRS) (http://www.censusindia.gov.in/Vital_ Statistics/SRS/Sample_

BOX 2.1 A scandal of invisibility

'Each year, nearly 50 million newborn children are not registered, barely a third of countries outside North America and Europe have the capacity to obtain usable mortality statistics, and half the countries in Africa and Southeast Asia record no cause of death data at all.'

(Source: Setel *et al.*, 2009, p. 1570)

Registration_System.aspx) is probably the best known. The SRS was initiated in 1964–65 on a pilot basis and then became fully operational five years later. From 3,722 sample units (villages and urban blocks) in 1969–70, by 2007 it had expanded to 7,597 sites across the country's states and union territories, covering about 1.4 million households and 7 million people. The SRS uses a dual record system, involving continuous enumeration of births and deaths by a resident part-time enumerator checked against an independent six-monthly retrospective survey by a full-time supervisor. In 1999 cause of death surveying (using *verbal autopsy* methods – see Box 2.2) was merged with the SRS. Bangladesh and Tanzania are other countries that use sample vital registration systems.

Demographic surveillance sites (DSS)

Another approach to obtaining mortality data used in a number of developing countries is the establishment of designated demographic surveillance sites. These sites cover a defined geographic area within which processes are set up to collect data on births and deaths, along with other health-related demographic, social and economic information, for the resident population of that area. As they normally relate to just a few areas, such data cannot be taken

---

BOX 2.2 Verbal autopsy cause of death assignment

For the many countries with poor or no vital registration and medical certification of death systems, so-called verbal autopsy (VA) has become the leading way of deriving information on the distribution of causes of death. Verbal autopsy is an indirect approach to determining the probable biomedical causes of a death through inter-viewing the person (household member, friend, caregiver) who best knew about the health and well-being of the deceased person and the events leading to the person's death. The data gathered in the field are then used to assign and code the cause of death. Verbal autopsy is very effective for identifying diseases with distinctive symp-toms, but not as reliable for those with less specific symptoms. In the past, different approaches to verbal autopsy (e.g. differing questionnaires, physician review versus diagnostic algorithms for determining cause of death from the interview material) and varying expertise of field interviewers and data coders have posed difficulties in comparing cause of death data between places and over time. The World Health Organization has recently produced a manual of verbal autopsy resources and guide-lines in an attempt to standardize VA data collection and processing (WHO, 2007c).

---

to reflect the national population accurately, but they nonetheless give useful insights. The actual surveillance process varies, from regular visits to households by local officials to annual household interview surveys. Verbal autopsy methods are usually employed to gain cause of death information. Thirty-seven demographic surveillance sites across nineteen developing countries (principally in Africa and Asia) are coordinated under the umbrella of the INSIGHT network (http://www.indepth-network.org).

While the usual developing country situation of only one, two or perhaps three quite small DSS sites in a country cannot provide nationally representative data, with enough appropriately chosen surveillance sites a DSS system can provide such data. China is an illustration of this with a comprehensive nationwide system of disease surveillance points (DSP). Recently revised and strengthened, the system operates in all parts of China and covers nearly 6 per cent of the population. On this scale the Chinese DSPs essentially constitute a deaths sample registration system. A mix of verbal autopsy and medical certification is used for determining cause of death. The ultimate plan is to merge the country's disease surveillance points and civil registration systems.

Demographic and health surveys

Sample household surveys are another option for obtaining data on the levels and causes of mortality in the absence of adequate civil registration systems. If the households are selected on a nationally representative basis, information useful for health planning can be obtained. In some cases mortality data has been collected from internal stand-alone country efforts; in other cases through international survey programmes, such as the Demographic and Health Surveys (DHS) project of the US Agency for International Development (USAID) (http://www.measuredhs.com) and the WHO's World Health Survey (http://who.int/healthinfo/survey/en/index.html).

While the data produced from internal stand-alone surveys are useful for the country concerned, the comparability built into the international DHS and WHO surveys are of greater global health value. These surveys have produced particularly useful information on child and maternal mortality. Some countries also glean data on child mortality from paired questions in their population censuses, asking women their number of liveborn children and the number still alive (or who have died). Countries without alternative sources of adult mortality estimates were encouraged by the United Nations Statistical Division to use the 2010 round of censuses also to gather data on this.

Classifying causes of death

Part of making sense of death is attributing causes, and medical history and medical anthropology show us many ways societies have done this over the ages. Indeed, numerous different cause of death belief and classificatory systems persist around the world today. For example, traditional belief systems in deaths being caused by such things as 'loss of soul', 'intrusion of disease spirits', 'sorcery' or 'curses' are found alongside Western medical diagnostic perspectives in many countries, not just developing nations.

For valid comparisons of cause of death patterns in different populations, however, it is essential for deaths to be categorized according to a standard internationally agreed classification. Otherwise, health analysts would be in a 'comparing apples with oranges' situation. The classificatory scheme that has been developed for this is the *International Statistical Classification of Diseases and Related Health Problems* (ICD), published by the World Health Organization. The ICD is organized around the aetiology and pathophysiology of diseases. Diseases are ordered into 'chapters', with the bulk of these chapters relating to particular organ systems (e.g. circulatory, respiratory, digestive, genitourinary). The other chapters cover such things as infectious and parasitic diseases, neoplasms, developmental diseases and injuries.

To keep up with advances in medical science, changes in diagnostic terminology and emerging disease/health problems, the ICD is periodically revised. The first version of the classification (ICD-1) came into operation in 1900 and was based on a pre-existing classification developed by a French physician, Louis Bertillon, in 1893. The current edition, ICD-10, came into use in 1994, although some countries are still employing ICD-9. Work is presently under way on preparing ICD-11, with publication planned for 2014 and implementation the following year.

Over its various revisions, the ICD has grown considerably in size, from under 200 cause of death categories in ICD-1 to 1655 (3 character) and 11,400 (4 character) categories in ICD-10. While revisions of the ICD are essential, they create statistical discontinuities between editions and make time-series analyses of some diseases difficult. For example, the change from ICD-9 to ICD-10 produced a large 'paper' increase in deaths caused by Alzheimer's disease and a large artificial decrease in deaths from pneumonia. Most developed countries with strong health statistics agencies carry out and publish statistical comparability studies of the new and most recent ICD editions to guide researchers and policy-makers in the examination of trends over time.

Underlying and multiple causes of death

Traditionally, cause of death statistical reporting and analyses have focused on what is termed the *underlying* cause of death. This is defined as the disease or condition considered to have initiated the sequence of events leading directly to a particular death. Death, however, is frequently a more complex process in which *multiple* causes play a role.

For example, an all too common occurrence in poor countries is for children to suffer from malnutrition and for this to lead to the children in their weakened state developing and succumbing to pneumonia. In this situation pneumonia is the *immediate* cause of death and malnutrition the *underlying* cause. Both conditions are obviously important for health planning, and cause of death statistics are more useful if the role of both is shown. In some cases the children may also have had other significant conditions that contributed to their deaths, but were not related to the malnutrition or pneumonia: for example, diabetes. Recording the presence of diabetes would further enhance the information value of the cause of death statistics of these children.

The relevance and value of multiple causes of death data is the same for developed nations. For instance, in most of those countries the leading underlying cause of death is ischaemic heart disease (IHD). Some people with this condition go on ultimately to die from heart failure. Identifying both causes in such cases – the *underlying* (i.e. IHD) and the *immediate* (i.e. heart failure) – adds value to the data. In turn, other conditions will often have made contributions to those persons' deaths, but will not be related to the coronary train of events: perhaps emphysema, diabetes, cancer or Alzheimer's disease. Ideally, those too should be recorded.

Multiple cause of death statistics that capture details of the underlying cause of death plus other significant conditions which led to or contributed to death (i.e. *associated* causes) thus provide a fuller and more useful picture of mortality patterns than singular underlying cause of death data. The Standard International Medical Certificate of Cause of Death (see Box 2.3) provides space for certifiers to record all relevant diseases and conditions present at the time of death. As noted above, though, most published mortality statistics and analyses to date have focused on underlying causes of death.

BOX 2.3 Standard International Medical Certificate of Cause of Death

Cause of death		Approximate interval between onset and death

I
Disease or condition directly
leading to death*

(a) . . . .
due to (or as a consequence of)

Antecedent causes
Morbid conditions, if any,
giving rise to the above
cause, stating the underlying
condition last

(b) . . . .
due to (or as a consequence of)

(c) . . . .
due to (or as a consequence of)

(d) . . . .

II
Other significant conditions
contributing to the death,
but not related to the disease
or condition causing it

. . . .

. . . .

*This does not mean the mode of dying, e.g. heart failure, respiratory failure. It means the disease, injury, or complication that caused death.

From our earlier comments on civil vital registration, it will be clear to all readers that the quality of mortality statistics varies greatly between countries and, in many cases, also within countries. Here we will expand on this issue. Data quality varies in two main ways – in completeness and in accuracy – although, of course, there are other important quality considerations: for example, the timeliness, comprehensiveness and comparability of statistics.

As noted earlier, millions of deaths (and births) around the world every year are never officially recorded. This makes measuring the level of mortality in many countries very difficult. The WHO and other international agencies attempt to adjust for incompleteness in calculating comparable country-specific mortality estimates, but much uncertainty remains about the 'true' death rates in many low- and middle-income nations. Table 2.1 illustrates this uncertainty, showing the very large inter-agency variation in life expectancy at birth estimates for 2007 for ten developing countries. Occasionally, the WHO gives estimated 95 per cent uncertainty intervals for some of its mortality indicator point estimates. These are a useful reminder of the flimsy evidence base of the mortality figures for many countries, but unfortunately they are published only intermittently.

The major accuracy shadow hanging over mortality data relates to cause of death statistics. Reliable figures on the cause of death structure within populations are essential for informed health policy-making and planning at all levels, but reality falls well short of this desideratum. By the WHO's evaluation, country information on causes of death is not available for most causes for seventy-eight of the organization's member states (Table 2.2).

Table 2.1 Differing estimates of life expectancy at birth, 2007: alternative agency databases

Country	World Health Organization	United Nations Population Division	UNICEF	World Bank	United States Census Bureau
	Life expectancy at birth (both sexes combined; years)				
Angola	53	47	42	43	38
Cote d'Ivoire	54	57	48	48	54
Grenada	68	75	69	69	65
Iraq	63	68	59	60	69
Lao People's Democratic Republic	61	65	64	64	56
Liberia	56	58	45	46	40
Namibia	59	60	52	53	49
Papua New Guinea	63	61	57	57	65
Rwanda	50	50	46	46	55
Sierra Leone	41	47	42	43	54

Sources: WHO, *World Health Statistics*; UNDESA-PD, *World Population Prospects*; UNICEF; World Bank, *World Development Indicators*; and United States Census Bureau websites, 2009

Table 2.2 Cause-specific mortality data – levels of evidence: (a) number of WHO member states; (b) population, 2004

(a) Number of member states

Region	Level of evidence*				
	Level 1 (Good)	Level 2	Level 3	Level 4 (Poor)	Total states (N)
Africa	–	4	2	47	53
Asia	2	22	4	19	47
Europe	12	27	–	2	41
Latin America and the Caribbean	1	30	–	2	33
North America	2	–	–	–	2
Oceania	1	7	–	8	16
Total states (N)	18	90	6	78	192

(b) Population (,000s)

Region	Level of evidence*				
	Level 1 (Good)	Level 2	Level 3	Level 4 (Poor)	Total population
Africa	–	120406	24498	755019	899923
Asia	132072	421833	2497353	837227	3888485
Europe	116284	613945	–	105	730334
Latin America and the Caribbean	11247	518624	–	15711	545582
North America	328799	–	–	–	328799
Oceania	4050	21119	–	6984	32153
Total population	592452	1695927	2521851	1615046	6425276

Note: * Technical definitions of the different levels of evidence are given in the 'Notes for Table' sheet of the source Excel file.

Source: WHO, 2009e

Where cause of death certification is attempted, diagnostic accuracy is a major problem, varying considerably among and within countries. In the less developed world sufficiently trained diagnostic personnel are generally lacking, making incorrect attribution of cause of death more likely. The proportion of ill-defined deaths also tends to be higher in such countries. However, although accuracy is generally more problematic in developing countries than richer nations, it would be a mistake to assume 100 per cent accuracy in certifying causes of death in the latter bloc. With a substantially higher average age at death in developed nations, many decedents in such countries are host to several serious degenerative conditions and it is not always easy to specify which was the genuine underlying cause of death correctly.

Translating the causes entered on death certificates to the ICD codes is another area where errors occur. A further significant problem is misspecification of age at death. In combination, these problems make international comparisons of total and cause-specific mortality between countries using raw data from the countries themselves difficult.

WHO mortality estimates

The World Health Organization encourages member states to submit data on the number of deaths and the causes annually – for review, adjustment where deemed necessary, and ultimately inclusion in the organization's 'Mortality Database' and publications. The data received are very patchy. A 2007 review reported that over the period 1996–2005 only 118 of the member countries sent in cause of death statistics and that the data could be described as of 'high quality' for only 31 countries. In the case of a further 24 countries the data were adjudged to be of 'medium–high' quality. These 55 countries accounted for only 20 per cent of the world's population. For 17 countries, including China and India, the data were deemed of 'limited use' due to being over a decade old, less than 50 per cent complete, in non-standard format, or giving only partial coverage (Mahapatra *et al.*, 2007).

Detailed underlying cause of death estimates for all member states are published on the WHO's 'Global Burden of Disease' website. While the estimates are useful, users of them need to be careful to keep in mind the very mixed quality of the data on which they are based. For many of the listed countries, the estimates are based on statistical modelling, not 'real' mortality data (good or bad) from the countries. A danger is that some users will ignore the WHO's accompanying explanatory notes and take the statistics to indicate that we accurately know the cause-specific mortality pattern of all countries. As will be clear from the above discussion, nothing could be further from the truth.

Sub-national mortality data

Most assessments of total and cause-specific mortality data quality are at the national level. But variations in completeness of coverage and accuracy of diagnosis and coding also occur at the sub-national level, particularly (but not exclusively) in developing countries. Not surprisingly, death registration and certification data are generally found to be better for urban than rural areas across the less developed world.

Also, data for poorer regions tend to be of lower quality than that for wealthier ones. In Brazil, for example, recent research found death registration much less complete and the proportion of ill-defined deaths significantly higher in the lower socio-economic northeastern and northern regions compared with the wealthier southern region (Franca *et al.*, 2008).

Morbidity

Mortality statistics clearly provide important indications of the health of populations, but not a full picture. To use the words of Kaplan (1990), they 'note the dead and ignore the living'. However, it is important to know the health problems (*morbidity*) people are living with as well as those they are dying from. Some of these health problems will be illnesses that ultimately show up as leading killers in cause of death statistics (e.g. heart disease, hypertension, cancers, HIV/AIDS), but there are also many low case-fatality conditions (e.g. musculoskeletal disorders, mental illnesses, eyesight problems, some injuries) that nonetheless seriously detract from people's quality of life and constitute a heavy load on healthcare services.

Morbidity data are obtained from a variety of sources. Leading ones include hospital inpatient records, doctor and other primary health care consultation records, disease registers, notifiable disease records, disease surveillance systems, and health surveys. Without the clear biologically defined endpoint that underlies death statistics morbidity is a more problematic dimension of health to operationalise and interpret. At what point can illness be said to exist? What proportion of conditions meeting the threshold for rating as illness end up in the health system and getting counted? How accurate are illness diagnoses? How can the duration and severity of illness be factored into morbidity accounting? In turn, the scope and quality of morbidity data, as for mortality, vary greatly from country to country, making valid international comparisons of the burden of illness difficult.

Healthcare utilization records

In countries where people have good access to hospitals and other healthcare services utilization records can provide useful information about the state of health of the populations. The global picture painted by utilization data is patchy, however. For example, the comparability of hospital admissions data showing the incidence of specific health conditions is compromised by national differences in the availability of hospital beds and medical staff, and differing access (geographic, financial, cultural) to those facilities. For instance, in health-facilities-deficient, low-income countries, the odds of people with coronary artery disease being diagnosed with that condition and then admitted to hospital for bypass surgery and subsequently showing up in formal hospital statistics are considerably poorer than fellow heart disease sufferers who happen to live in richer, better-resourced Western nations. Ditto in general the wider respective disease surveillance, recording and reporting capacities of rich and poor countries.

Health surveys

Most developed countries conduct national (and sometimes, regional) population health surveys as part of regular health monitoring and input to knowledge-based health policy development and planning. These surveys usually involve the collection of subjective health information (i.e. self-reporting by survey respondents) through structured questionnaires, though in some countries formal health examination survey programmes (e.g. measuring such things as blood pressure, height, weight, body dimensions, lung function, blood and urine samples) are also conducted. Some developing countries also conduct periodic health interview surveys, but many do not have the financial, administrative or professional capacity to do so. Because of different survey designs and reporting of results, direct comparison of national health interview survey findings is difficult.

The Demographic and Health Surveys project of the US Agency for International Development and the World Health Organization's World Health Survey (WHS), mentioned earlier in the 'Mortality' section of this chapter, are useful attempts to produce more comparable international morbidity data. These survey-generated data need to be used carefully, though, in particular the WHS tabulations which for most countries are based on relatively small sample sizes. The extent to which some of the WHS self-reported items genuinely indicate national 'health reality' is problematic. For example, Table 2.3 lists several high-mortality developing countries in which WHS respondents ostensibly reported better personal health levels than those in very low-mortality Sweden. The developing country variations also raise questions. What explains the Pakistan–India–Bangladesh gradient in self-rated health values when all three countries share very similar life expectancy levels? The sizeable differences in results for neighbouring Bangladesh and Myanmar are similarly surprising, given their reasonably comparable life expectancy and healthy life expectancy levels. The notion of what constitutes 'very good' and 'good' health clearly varies between populations.

The WHS results also contain interesting tabulations of self-reported health conditions. Again, though, questions hang over what to make of the data. Table 2.4 illustrates with figures on angina and depression for selected countries. The diagnosed angina levels for Chad and Malawi are far outside the normal age-specific biological expectation for that condition.

Table 2.3 Percentage of World Health Survey respondents rating their health as 'Very Good' or 'Good', by age, 2002–04; and national life expectancy and healthy life expectancy at birth, 2002

Age years	Sweden %	Malawi %	Burkina Faso %	Pakistan %	India %	Bangladesh %	Myanmar %
18–29	72.6	85.0	80.8	86.4	70.3	56.1	87.3
30–44	66.0	79.3	72.0	79.3	60.2	47.4	81.9
45–59	63.0	70.9	59.5	63.4	45.6	35.3	75.5
60–69	52.6	61.5	37.7	48.5	30.7	29.7	68.8
70–79	41.8	45.2	27.8	44.4	22.8	18.0	58.7
80+	36.0	32.8	11.1	31.6	20.4	14.6	49.7
Life expectancy at birth, 2002	80.4	40.2	41.7	61.4	61.0	62.6	58.9
Healthy life expectancy at birth, 2002	73.3	34.9	35.6	53.3	53.5	54.3	51.7

Sources: WHO, *The World Health Report* and *World Health Survey* websites

Table 2.4 Percentage of World Health Survey respondents indicating having received diagnoses of angina and depression in the last twelve months, by age, 2002–04

Age years	Angina			Depression	
	Chad %	Malawi %	Sweden %	Brazil %	Mexico %
18–29	17.2	10.4	0.2	14.4	3.1
30–44	20.0	15.4	0.1	18.4	5.0
45–59	25.5	17.2	4.6	24.7	6.7
60–69	28.5	19.2	8.4	24.6	6.3
70–79	29.7	17.2	19.3	20.6	7.0
80+	32.8	14.2	10.1	16.1	4.2

Source: WHO, *World Health Survey* website

Likewise, the Brazilian depression figures are significantly at odds with those for all other Latin American countries included in the WHS.

Disease registers

Population-based disease registers are a valuable source of information for certain areas of public health and epidemiological work. These registers are databases that attempt to collect information on all individuals with a particular disease in a geographically defined population. Registers have a lengthy history and have at various times been created and maintained for a wide range of diseases and conditions: for example, leprosy, tuberculosis, blindness, psychiatric illness, diabetes, cancer, coronary heart disease and HIV/AIDS. For some conditions, registration has been/is compulsory. With the registration of individuals involved, important ethical issues concerning patient name recording and confidentiality surround registers. Problems of completeness and comparability, however, limit the use of many registers for international disease monitoring.

Cancer has been the most productive field of disease register use in global health (Box 2.4), and in many countries it is mandated by law that all newly diagnosed cases are reported to the geographically relevant cancer registry. In 1966 the International Association of Cancer Registries (IACR; a non-governmental organization) was set up to help cancer registries in countries around the world improve data quality and comparability. A European Network of Cancer Registries (ENCR) was established with a similar charter for the European Union in 1989. The Cancer Information Section (CIS) of the WHO's International Agency for Research on Cancer is also involved in such work, including providing administrative facilities and a secretariat to the IACR and ENCR. Another of the CIS's core activities is data dissemination, producing the five-yearly *Cancer Incidence in Five Continents* series.

BOX 2.4 Cancer registry data and organizations

Cancer registries record details of new cancer cases (e.g. the site of the cancer, extent of the disease at diagnosis, age and sex of the individual affected, the individual's usual place of residence, etc.), information on treatment, and disease outcomes (e.g. five-year survivorship, mortality). Aggregated data are normally made available for population-based cancer monitoring and research.

- European Network of Cancer Registries: http://www.encr.com.fr/encr_about.htm
- Indian Cancer Society, Cancer Registry Division: http://www.indiancancer society.org/cancer-registry/cancer-registry.htm
- International Association of Cancer Registries: http://www.iacr.com.fr/iacr-top. htm
- International Agency for Research on Cancer: http://www.iarc.fr/en/about/index. php
- NSW Central Cancer Registry Statistical Reporting Module: http://www.cancer institute.org.au/cancer_inst/statistics/registry.html
- United Kingdom Association of Cancer Registries: http://82.110.76.19/
- US Centers for Disease Control and Prevention, National Program of Cancer Registries: http://www.cdc.gov/cabcer/npcr/about.htm

Notifiable (reportable) health condition statistics

Some health conditions are considered to be of particular public health importance and when cases occur are required by law to be reported to government health authorities. These are principally infectious diseases, but some non-infectious conditions (e.g. cancer, workplace injuries, motor vehicle accident injuries) also have mandatory reporting requirements in many countries.

Reported cases of a communicable disease may give an early warning of a looming major outbreak (e.g. a possible new influenza epidemic or pandemic) as well as allow continuous monitoring of the infectious disease landscape. However, the completeness of reporting unfortunately varies between jurisdictions (cities, states, provinces, countries). Also, completeness varies between health conditions, generally being fuller for more serious conditions than those perceived by the public and health diagnosticians to be less life threatening.

At the international level notification requirements of states are governed by the WHO's *International Health Regulations* (2005). This legal instrument replaced the former requirement for states automatically to notify cases of certain diseases (cholera, plague and yellow fever) to the WHO with a criteria-based decision instrument designed to identify potential 'public health emergencies of international concern' (PHEIC). (Details of the criteria and decision instrument are available at http://www.who.int/ihr/en.)

Internet-based data sources

An expanding morbidity data collecting and reporting avenue is the internet. Box 2.5 outlines four examples of such systems. ProMED-mail, launched in 1994, was the first initiative of this nature. Some systems are open access, others are restricted and require a subscription payment.

Population data

Raw figures on the number of deaths or morbidity episodes by themselves are simply 'counts' and are limited in what they tell about comparative health levels between different populations. India, for example, by dint of its extremely large population size has far more deaths each year (between 9 and 10 million) than any smaller developing country. The absolute magnitude of this annual toll is significant in the sense that any substantial improvement in overall global life expectancy or any other core health indicator is obviously going to require major health improvements in India. However, the 9–10 million count alone gives no idea where India stands in the international life expectancy rankings table. To establish that comparative perspective, the death figures for India and every other country need to be related to the respective 'populations at risk'. Reliable national and subnational population figures (i.e. overall totals and disaggregated by age and sex) are thus a vital component of health information systems.

Most developed nations obtain this necessary population data from regular high-quality population censuses, or in a few cases through population registers. The majority of developing countries also conduct population censuses, though the quality and regularity of these enumerations are more variable. The United Nations Statistical Division encourages all countries to conduct at least a decennial census and has provided professional assistance on census design, conduct and data processing to many developing countries' national statistical offices. No matter what degree of planning, all censuses suffer from errors: for example, undercount (or occasionally overcount) and misspecification of the age of individuals. Every two years the United Nations Population Division conducts a review of world population and

---

BOX 2.5 Examples of internet-based data sources

- ProMED-mail (Programme for Monitoring Emerging Diseases): http://www. promedmail.org. An open-access global electronic reporting system for outbreaks of emerging infectious diseases and acute exposures to toxins that affect human health. The website and email are used to provide up-to-date and reliable news about threats to human, animal and food plant health around the world, seven days a week. ProMED-mail is a programme of the International Society for Infectious Diseases.
- Global Public Health Intelligence Network (GPHIN): http://www.phac-aspc. gc.ca/media/nr-rp/2004/2004_gphin-rmispbk-eng.php. A web-based early-warning system run by the Public Health Agency of Canada that gathers preliminary reports of public health significance in seven languages on a real-time, 24/7 basis. GPHIN gathers and disseminates relevant information on disease outbreaks and other public health events (e.g. bio-terrorism and exposure to chemical and radioactive agents, natural disasters) by monitoring global media sources such as news wires and websites. Users of GPHIN pay a subscription fee.
- Google Flu Trends: http://www.google.org/flutrends. A philanthropic initiative by Google which uses aggregated Google search data to estimate flu activity in near real-time in twenty countries. Graphs showing flu intensity over twelve-month periods are provided. For some countries sub-national (e.g. provinces, states) graphs are also available. The website has open access. Flu Trends is part of Google's wider Predict and Prevent initiative (http://www.google.org/predict. html) to detect disease threats earlier and predict when and where future pandemics might strike.
- HealthMap: http://www.healthmap.org. HealthMap brings together a range of data sources to produce a unified and comprehensive view of the current global state of infectious diseases and their effect on human and animal health. The website integrates outbreak data of varying reliability, ranging from news/media sources (e.g. Google News), to curated personal accounts (e.g. ProMED-mail), to community contributions (e.g. eyewitness accounts), to validated official alerts (e.g. World Health Organization). Through an automated text-processing system, the data are aggregated by disease and displayed by location for access to the original alert. The HealthMap website has open access.

---

disseminates the resulting data on its website (http://esa.un.org/unpd/wpp/index.htm) and on CD-ROM. Estimated population totals (with accompanying age and sex disaggregations) for countries are also produced by the US Census Bureau and made available on its online international demographic database (http://www.census.gov/population/international/data/idb/informationGateway.php).

Demographic surveillance systems and health surveys normally also collect population at risk data in their operations. Like population censuses, they also generally record details of the social and economic characteristics of their reference populations to investigate differential mortality and morbidity patterns and the determinants of health.

Health indicators

The data sources outlined above are just that, sources of raw *data*. To transform the data from those sources into higher-order population health *information* a variety of measures have been developed by demographers, epidemiologists and statisticians. In this section we provide an introduction to the most commonly used of these measures. Three groups of measures are identified: first, measures of mortality; second, measures of morbidity; and third, what have become known as 'summary measures of population health' – measures that incorporate both mortality and morbidity data.

Mortality

Crude death rate

The simplest measure of overall mortality in a population is the *crude death rate* (CDR). This is simply the total number of deaths in a specified period (usually a year) divided by the average total population in that period (usually taken as the mid-period population), then multiplied by 1,000. (The use of the multiplier is to ensure the resulting CDR is a whole number, being expressed as per 1,000 population. For some rare health events, rates have to be multiplied by 100,000 or even 1 million to ensure whole numbers.)

The CDR is used quite frequently because it is simple to calculate, easily understood and not very data demanding. In some cases it is the only mortality measure the available data allow. However, it has a major weakness as a reliable indicator of health standards, taking no account of the different age and sex compositions of populations. For example, despite having markedly better health, Japan has a higher CDR than India (approximately 9 per 1,000 versus approximately 7 per 1,000 in 2007), due to its significantly older population and the greater risk of dying at higher ages.

Age-specific death rates

These rates measure the force of mortality at each age, thus overcoming the above weakness of the CDR. To calculate *age-specific death rates* (ASDRs), data on both deaths and population by age are necessary, the number of deaths of people in each age group over a defined period being divided by the average population in that age group. Again, the resulting rates are normally expressed per 1,000 population to avoid decimal fractions. With ASDRs, temporal and spatial comparisons of mortality at given ages can be made.

Because mortality also varies considerably by sex, ASDRs are frequently calculated separately for males and females. Sometimes age/sex-specific rates are also calculated separately for different racial groups in a population. In the United States, for example, much health data is made available separately for the white, black, Hispanic and Asian populations. While age- (and sex- and race-) specific rates allow 'like with like' mortality comparisons, handling the often very large amount of data involved can become burdensome and the volume of detail unnecessary.

Other age-focused mortality rates

Besides age-specific death rates, there are three other age-focused mortality indicators widely used in global health monitoring, research and planning: the infant mortality rate, the child mortality rate and the adult mortality rate.

The *infant mortality rate* (IMR) measures the number of deaths to infants under one year of age per 1,000 live births over a given period. Globally it is considered to be one of the key indicators of countries' levels of development and health conditions. It is also very useful for charting sub-national variations in health status (and socio-economic well-being) in developing countries. In the past it has also been widely used as a health indicator within developed nations, but in many of these the national rate and its internal social and geographical variations have now shrunk to levels making the measure less useful as a summary indicator of overall health and well-being.

The *child mortality rate* (CMR), also known as the *under-five mortality rate*, denotes the probability (per 1,000 live births) of a child dying before its fifth birthday. The largest component of the CMR is neonatal mortality, deaths in the first four weeks of life. Like the infant mortality rate, the CMR is widely used as a basic international population health indicator and is a standard variable in the WHO's annual *World Health Statistics* report. Reducing the CMR is one of the Millennium Development Goals.

The *adult mortality rate* (AMR) measures the probability of dying between the ages of fifteen and sixty years per 1,000 population. This is an important age bracket in which to monitor health as it covers the main working-age groups. The AMR is also one of the standard global health indicators included in *World Health Statistics*.

Standardized (adjusted) death rates

These are summary measures of mortality which adjust for compositional differences between populations that affect the probability of dying. Age is the most common compositional factor standardized for in health analyses. It is frequently also desirable to control for sex and sometimes race differences between populations. Data availability allowing, standardization can also be done for social variables that influence the risk of death (e.g. occupation, socio-economic status). When death rates are standardized for age (and other compositional attributes), populations with very similar crude death rates can emerge with significantly different standardized rates. Table 2.5 gives a clear illustration of this for cardiovascular disease mortality. Wherever possible, age and other compositional influences on mortality should be controlled for in temporal and geographical population health comparisons. Rates can be standardized in two ways – directly or indirectly. Calculation details for the two methods can be found in standard demographic texts.

Life expectancy

Life expectancy is another widely used measure in population health. Expectations of life can be calculated in two ways: *period* (or current) life expectancy and *cohort* (or generational) life expectancy. Life expectancy at birth (ELB) is the most commonly cited figure. However, expectancies can be calculated for any age.

Table 2.5 Crude and age-standardized death rates per 100,000 population (both sexes combined) for cardiovascular diseases in selected countries, 2004

Country	Crude death rate	Age-standardized death rate
Japan	249	103
Australia	248	136
China	246	279
Sri Lanka	249	301
Mongolia	254	475

Source: WHO, 2009e

Period life expectancy is the most commonly used measure. This indicates the average number of additional years a person of a given age could expect to live if the age-specific death rates for a given year (or few years) were to remain unchanged. No allowance is made for later actual or projected changes in mortality. Period life expectancy at birth in 2000, for example, would be calculated using the mortality rate for age zero in 2000, for age one in 2000, for age two in 2000, for age three in 2000, and so on. Period life expectancy at birth is seen as a good overall indicator ('snapshot') of current health status.

Cohort life expectancy, on the other hand, allows for actual or projected changes in mortality over a particular birth cohort's existence. For example, American males born in 1900 lived, on average, for 51.5 years, but at their time of birth had a life expectancy of only 46.4 years (Bell and Miller, 2005). Looking forward, cohort life expectancy at birth in 2000 would be worked out using the mortality rate for age zero in 2000, for age one in 2001, for age two in 2002, for age three in 2003, and so on. By allowing for changes in mortality, cohort life expectancy is a better indication of how long a person of a given age lived, or would be expected to live, than the period measure. The period life expectancy at birth for males in the United States in 2000 was 74.0 years, but a cohort figure of 81.1 years has been projected (US Social Security Administration, 2011). However, when cohort life expectancy calculations go beyond historical experience to incorporate assumed future mortality, a subjectivity factor is obviously introduced.

Age-specific death rates differ for males and females and therefore separate life expectancy estimates for the two sexes are usually calculated and reported. Separate estimates are sometimes also calculated by race and ethnicity. Unless explicitly stated otherwise, all life expectancy figures cited in this book are period measures.

The poor quality of death registration in many countries means that life expectancy figures, like other mortality measures, should be seen as point estimates within varying uncertainty intervals. The *World Health Report 2006* (WHO website) gave confidence intervals for its 2004 life expectancy (and some other mortality) estimates. For example, Afghanistan's period life expectancy at birth estimate (both sexes) of 42 years was calculated as falling within an uncertainty interval of 30 and 53 years, and many other poor nations are listed with intervals of 10 or more years. Developed nations with complete vital registration, on the other hand, were generally reported with uncertainty intervals of only 0–1 years.

Potential years of life lost

This is a measure of *premature* rather than total mortality, focusing on deaths that can be considered untimely. For instance, at the current average life expectancy level in developed countries, all deaths before age seventy-five might be considered premature and to involve a loss of potential years of life (PYLL). From this perspective, a person dying on his or her 40th birthday loses 35 potential years of life, one dying aged 70 loses 5 years, and so on. The measure thus applies differential values to death at each age, giving greater weight to deaths that occur to younger persons than those at older ages. Individual decedents' 'lost' years are summed to give the particular population's aggregate PYLL for the period concerned. This is usually done for both all-cause and cause-specific mortality. Through the age truncation and weighting procedures, the proportion of PYLL due to particular causes of death will vary compared to those causes as a proportion of all deaths. Deaths from accidents and suicide, for example, tend to contribute substantially more to PYLL than to total mortality.

Cause-specific death rates

Where data are available on the various causes of death in a population, rates for the individual causes can be calculated: for example, the death rate from cancer, from heart disease, from infectious diseases, and so on. Calculating these respective rates is important for identifying and prioritizing health problems. Cause-specific death rates can be crude, age/sex-specific, or age/sex standardized, depending on the need and data availability. Cause-specific rates are normally expressed as deaths per 100,000 population as the rates of occurrence for individual causes are generally low.

Maternal mortality ratio

This measure refers to the deaths of women from complications of pregnancy or childbirth, these deaths being expressed as a ratio per 100,000 live births. Reliable data for calculating the ratio are not available for many developing countries, but the global ratio is estimated at around 400 maternal deaths per 100,000 live births, with 99 per cent of cases in developing countries. The ratio is an important global health indicator as such deaths are for the greater part preventable. By combining the maternal mortality ratio with a population's fertility levels, the lifetime risk of dying from maternal causes can be estimated. Reducing the maternal mortality ratio is another of the health-related Millennium Development Goals.

Morbidity

Many of the types of measurement outlined above for mortality also apply to morbidity. Thus, depending on need and data availability, the frequency of disease and other health problems can be measured in crude, age/sex-specific and age/sex standardized fashion, just like mortality. Similarly, as with potential years of life lost through premature death, years of good health lost due to illness, injury or disability can be estimated. There are, however, also several distinctive features of measuring morbidity. These are outlined briefly below.

Prevalence and incidence

The frequency of a disease (or injury or other health-related condition) in a population can be measured in two basic ways: the number of people in a defined population with the disease at a given point in time (*prevalence*) and the number of new cases of the disease in that population over a given time period (*incidence*). Mortality, by contrast, obviously just involves incidence.

To calculate a prevalence rate, the number of persons in a population with a disease is related to the total population at the specified time. The rate may be calculated in crude form and expressed as a percentage (or per some other appropriate 10^n factor), or in age/sex-specific or age/sex-standardized fashion. Prevalence rates thus show the magnitude of a given health problem and are important in planning services and allocating resources. However, as they include persons who may have contracted the disease many years ago, they are not so useful in aetiological (causal) studies.

Incidence rates, on the other hand, relate the number of new cases of a disease over a specified period to the population at risk of contracting the disease. The population at risk is usually taken as the mid-period population. Theoretically, persons who have already got the disease should be excluded from the at-risk population, but that is often impossible. Incidence data are valuable in investigations of disease aetiology and epidemic diffusion and control.

Case fatality rate

A follow-up measure to disease incidence is the *case fatality rate*. This is the proportion of persons contracting a disease who die from that disease. For example, most people who contract ebola die of the infection, whereas only a very small proportion of cases of normal seasonal influenza perish. The case fatality rate is partly a measure of the virulence ('killing power') of a disease, but can also reflect other factors, such as differences in available healthcare. For instance, a higher proportion of HIV/AIDS sufferers in sub-Saharan Africa die from the disease than do sufferers in developed Western nations due to lower access to antiretroviral medicines.

Summary measures of population health

In the discussion of mortality indicators we described several as 'summary' measures of health (e.g. life expectancy at birth, the age/sex-standardized death rate, the infant mortality rate). That is a fair descriptor for them in the sense they sum up a lot about health standards in a given population in a single figure. They do not tell the whole story, however, as they say nothing about the morbidity side of health.

One of the important statistical developments in measuring health in recent years has been the development of a suite of health measures that overcome that limitation by simultaneously incorporating information on both mortality and morbidity into a single number. The term 'summary' has increasingly been formally applied to these combined measures under the umbrella title 'Summary Measures of Population Health' (SMPH).

There are two broad categories of SMPH: health *expectancies* and health *gaps*. The most commonly used are outlined below.

Health expectancies

These measures modify standard mortality-based life expectancy figures to estimate how long a person could expect to live in various health states. They are hence, in a sense, measures of quality of life as well as quantity of life. Two of the most commonly used health expectancy measures are *health-adjusted life expectancy* (sometimes called *healthy life expectancy*) and *disability-free life expectancy*.

Health-adjusted life expectancy (HALE) estimates the average number of years that a person of a given age can expect to live in 'full health'. Morbidity data from health surveys and other sources weighted by severity of the health problem are used to estimate the years likely to be spent in ill-health. HALE is calculated by subtracting the years in less than full health from the life expectancy of persons of that age. National HALE at birth estimates are regularly published by the WHO. (The measure was introduced by the WHO in the *World Health Report 2000* as *disability-adjusted life expectancy* (DALE), but changed to health-adjusted life expectancy (HALE) the following year.)

Disability-free life expectancy (DFLE) is a similar expectancy measure, but in this case, as the name indicates, based on health loss from disability. DFLE estimates thus indicate the average number of years a person of a given age is expected to live free of disability if current patterns of mortality and disability continue to apply. Other indicator names are sometimes used: for example, the European Union uses a DFLE indicator called *healthy life years* (HLY).

Health gaps

Gap measures are based on a specified health norm or goal (e.g. life expectation at birth of eighty years) and quantify the difference between that goal and the actual health of a population. The most widely used gap measure is *disability-adjusted life years* (DALYs). This is defined as the years of life lost to premature mortality (YLL) plus equivalent years of healthy life lost due to poor health or a disability (YLD). The morbidity component (YLD) is weighted for the duration and severity of the health condition. One DALY is equal to one lost year of healthy life. The concept of DALYs was introduced by the World Bank in its 1993 *World Development Report* and has since been adopted by the WHO as the standard measure of the burden of disease in populations. The reference health 'ideal' used by the WHO is life expectancy at birth of 80.0 years for males and 82.5 years for females. By calculating disease/condition-specific DALYs, the contribution of individual diseases/conditions to the total disease burden can be determined and health planning guided accordingly. The DALY measure has been criticized by some for its 'value choices', specifically the use of non-uniform age weights and the valuations of some non-fatal health outcomes in the calculations.

Discussion topics

1   The World Health Organization defines health as 'a state of complete physical, mental and social well-being, and not merely the absence of disease or infirmity'. How adequate and useful do you consider that definition to be?
2   How good are the population health statistics for your country in terms of coverage and timeliness?

3   The determinants of population health

Virtually all readers of this book will be aware that numerous factors influence the health of populations and could probably come up with a list of some of those factors without too much difficulty. Some important influences would likely get nominated on most readers' lists – e.g. the extent of poverty, housing quality, access to health services, diet – while other factors would be less widely identified. In this chapter we attempt to bring together the major determinants of population health in two related conceptual models, one highlighting the *multi-level* nature of determinants, the other their *stage* in the disease or disability process.

A comprehensive conceptual understanding of what produces good and bad population health is critical. Without such a guiding framework health policy is more or less formulated in a vacuum and chosen interventionary actions risk being ineffective or, even worse, counter-productive.

The specific conceptualization followed by health policy-makers and planners is also important, determining the type of health 'solutions' chosen. For example, in the eyes of many health researchers and decision-makers, poor health in developed nations basically comes down to bad lifestyle choices (e.g. smoking, excessive alcohol, overeating, inadequate exercise), and health improvement efforts should therefore focus on these areas. There is no argument that lifestyle factors have an important influence on health. But many so-called lifestyle 'choices' are rooted in the broad social and economic structural contexts and personal circumstances within which people live and are not in any genuine sense free choices. Without taking the effect of these structural contexts and personal circumstances into consideration, lifestyle-focused health promotion can very easily become a 'blame the victim' exercise and produce less than desired health gains.

What determines population health?

Two key appreciations are essential to understanding population health: first (returning to this chapter's opening sentence), the production of good and bad health involves many factors; second, the complex relationships (interactions) between factors. While the particular mix of determinants varies from health problem to health problem, the two underlying features of *multicausality* and *interaction* are almost invariably present.

A range of conceptual models of population health can be found in the literature. The various frameworks unsurprisingly share many common features, but they also have their own distinctive elements and emphases. Five of the most widely cited frameworks are:

- The *epidemiological triad (triangle)* model. This is the traditional model of disease causation in epidemiology, explaining the occurrence of disease as the result of interactions between three factors – agent, host and environment. Changes in disease incidence are seen as occurring due to changes in the factors and their relationships. (See Box 3.1.)

BOX 3.1   The epidemiological triad (triangle)

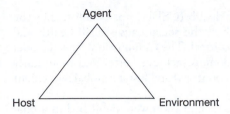

This agent–host–environment model was originally developed to explain infectious disease causation, with the agent component referring to infectious micro-organisms (e.g. bacteria, viruses, protozoa, parasites, fungi). With the growing importance of non-infectious conditions, the notion of disease agent has subsequently been widened to include physical, chemical and (psycho-)social causes of disease. An agent has to be present for a particular disease to occur, but in itself is not sufficient to trigger the disease. For example, many people are exposed to the bacterium that causes tuberculosis (*Mycobacterium tuberculosis*), but they do not all develop active TB. The host has to be susceptible to a disease (e.g. to be in a poor nutritional state or to have an impaired immune system, for example from having HIV), and the environment (i.e. extrinsic factors – disease vectors, climate, population crowding, sanitation, etc.) needs to bring together the agent and host. Many diseases have more than one agent. Changes in any one of the three components – e.g. changing agent virulence or altered population mixing or changing climatic conditions – will cause the rate of occurrence of the disease to change.

(Reading: Mausner and Kramer, 1985; Rockett, 1999)

- The so-called *health field model/twenty-first-century field model*, which brings together what are termed global factors (community and social environment, physical environment, family and individual environment), the healthcare system and the notions of primary, secondary and tertiary disease prevention (see Box 3.3) (Evans and Stoddart, 1994; Ratzan *et al.*, 2000).
- A detailed *globalization and health* framework formulated by Woodward and WHO colleagues (2001).
- The WHO Global Burden of Disease *comparative quantification of health risks* framework of physiological, behavioural, environmental and socio-economic risk factors (Murray *et al.*, 2003; WHO, 2009a).
- The *social determinants* framework developed for the WHO Commission on Social Determinants of Health (CSDH, 2008). (See Box 3.2.)

A multi-level model

All five frameworks offer valuable perspectives for understanding global health patterns and the model we advance here draws upon each of them, plus other health research. We, however, adopt a *geographical scale-based* organizing framework, arguing that the forces driving global health differentials can usefully be categorized into four levels – global, regional (international), national and sub-national. Completing the model, both shaped by and mediating these forces, are individual level health determinants (Figure 3.1).

BOX 3.2   WHO Commission on Social Determinants of Health

The Commission on Social Determinants of Health (CSDH) was established by the World Health Organization in 2005 to address the social causes of ill-health and health inequities (i.e. avoidable health inequalities). The Commission's specific brief was to assemble evidence on what can be done to achieve better and more fairly distributed health (both between and within countries) and foster a global movement to achieve it.

The findings and recommendations of the Commission were published in a final report titled *Closing the Gap in a Generation*, launched in August 2008. (This report and other documentation related to the Commission can be accessed on the WHO website http://www.who.int/social_determinants/en/.)

Coming out of its investigations, the Commission made three overarching recommendations (principles for action):

1   Improve daily living conditions.
2   Tackle the inequitable distribution of power, money and resources.
3   Measure and understand the problem and assess the impact of action.

Under each overarching recommendation, the Commission made a range of specific recommendations. For example, under 'Improve daily living conditions' there were twenty-one recommendations dealing with: equity from the start; healthy places, healthy people; fair employment and decent work; social protection across the life-course; and universal healthcare.

The Commission stated that if the actions it recommended were pursued, much could be done towards closing the health gap in a generation. To this end, three numerical health equity targets involving increasing life expectancy at birth and reducing adult mortality and the under-five mortality rate between 2000 and 2040 were proposed. The WHO was urged to develop these targets and to take the lead in achieving them.

While the Commission's report has been widely endorsed, it has nonetheless also been criticized. Stevens (2009, p. 298), for instance, argues 'it presumes its conclusions and is highly selective with its evidence, giving it a lot in common with political propaganda'.

The notion of forces operating at different geographical scales is certainly not new. For example, different-level influences are identified in Woodward *et al.*'s (2001) globalization and health model, and likewise in extensions of that model by Labonté and Torgerson (2005). The recent final report of the WHO Commission on Social Determinants of Disease does the same (CSDH, 2008). The specification and characterization of geographical scales here, though, are more explicit and encompassing.

Although identified and discussed below separately, the four sets of forces – global, regional, national and sub-national – are closely interrelated, both with each other and in many of their resultant influences on health outcomes. In general influences flow down the hierarchy – for example, global forces having regional, national and sub-national impacts; national policies influencing local areas; and so on. But flows up the hierarchy also occur: for example, intranational political discord can spill over borders and influence political

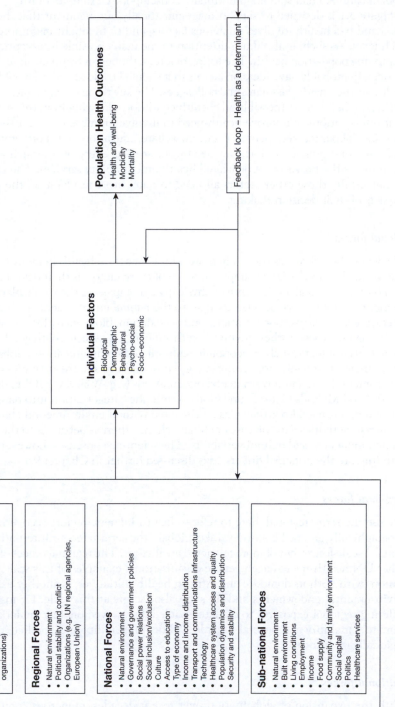

Global Forces
- Natural environmental patterns and changes (e.g. climate change, land degradation, biodiversity loss, ocean acidification)
- Human environment (e.g. globalization, population increase, urbanization, international organizations)

Regional Forces
- Natural environment
- Political stability and conflict
- Organizations (e.g. UN regional agencies, European Union)

National Forces
- Natural environment
- Governance and government policies
- Social power relations
- Social inclusion/exclusion
- Culture
- Access to education
- Type of economy
- Income and income distribution
- Transport and communications infrastructure
- Technology
- Healthcare system access and quality
- Population dynamics and distribution
- Security and stability

Sub-national Forces
- Natural environment
- Built environment
- Living conditions
- Employment
- Income
- Food supply
- Community and family environment
- Social capital
- Politics
- Healthcare services

Individual Factors
- Biological
- Demographic
- Behavioural
- Psycho-social
- Socio-economic

Population Health Outcomes
- Health and well-being
- Morbidity
- Mortality

Feedback loop – Health as a determinant

Figure 3.1 The determinants of health

instability and conflict at the higher regional and global levels with, again, flow-on effects to population health. The longstanding Israeli–Palestinian conflict and the civil wars in Somalia and Afghanistan are unfortunate contemporary examples of this.

Figure 3.1 is designed to support diagrammatically our argument that the production of good and bad health involves numerous factors, and to highlight major forces operative at each level. As such, it also draws attention to the many possible interventionary points for improving population health. The listing of forces, though, is by no means exhaustive. Every reader will probably have ideas on factors that should be added and we would encourage you to discuss these with classmates and colleagues. The key thing to appreciate is the interactive multicausality of most (possibly all) health conditions. Flowing from this is the implication that interventions to improve health need to involve far more than just the health sector. Housing, labour market, income, taxation, welfare, education, transport, environmental and other sectoral policies and actions need to be seen as every bit as much a part of health planning as the provision of dedicated health and disability services. The corollary of that is that ideally those other sectors all need to take into consideration the possible health impacts of their decision-making.

Global forces

We define these forces as those whose workings impact on health in many countries around the world. The *worldwide* geographical scope of these factors is their defining feature. Some are absolutely 'global' in the sense of physically encompassing the whole planet (e.g. climate change). Many involve adverse changes to the *natural* environment, such as rising atmospheric greenhouse gas concentration, land degradation, biodiversity loss, ocean acidification, declining fish stocks. Others involve health-influencing aspects (both good and bad) of the *human* environment, such as economic, cultural and communications globalization, population increase, urbanization, rising energy consumption, and the activities of international governmental and non-governmental organizations (e.g. WHO, UNICEF, the World Bank, the Bill and Melinda Gates Foundation). While the categorization into natural and human is convenient, it is also artificial as all the cited natural environmental changes are driven by human activities. (In the case of climate change there is debate as to the relative role of human influences and natural variability. The scientific consensus, however, is that human activities are the principal drivers, as is discussed further in Chapter 9.)

Regional forces

We use the term 'regional' here to refer to health-influencing forces covering a number of geographically grouped countries. Like 'global', the term refers to international- (transnational-) scale forces, but of more restricted areal scope. The regional offices of the WHO and other UN health-related agencies are organizational examples of this scale. The European Union, with both its domestic and African health initiatives, is another example. Natural environmental endowments and risks are also factors at this scale: for instance, through differing regional exposures to climate-enabled disease vectors (e.g. malarial mosquitoes), climate variability and natural hazards. Political instability and conflict can also operate regionally on health.

National forces

With the expansion of globalization over recent decades, numerous commentators have touted the demise of nation states as important players on the international stage. Such claims are generally very premature, though, and in the case of health particularly so. Global economic (and cultural, political, communications, etc.) structures and processes are certainly a defining part of the current world, but national forces remain very powerful determinants of health. While needing to avoid invoking environmental determinism, a country's natural environmental features are clearly important to health. National cultural traditions regarding gender status and roles and ethno-racial relations are similarly important. Where countries fit on the 'welfarist' to 'free market' socio-political continuum likewise has major implications for their population health, through the effects of progressive or regressive taxation regimes, differing degrees of income inequality and the presence or absence of welfare and health 'safety nets'. In short, as Figure 3.1 shows, virtually all dimensions of nation states have implications for the health of their populations. Some of these dimensions are obviously influenced by outside forces, but national elements still remain. For example, heavily indebted developing countries may be forced to reduce public spending on health due to domestic austerity pressures imposed by IMF and World Bank structural adjustment programmes, but the governments of those countries still have to decide where to prioritize health expenditure relative to other sectors, such as defence, public employment, prestige infrastructure projects, etc.

Sub-national forces

Sub-national-level determinants of health range from factors associated with the broad internal regional (geographic and/or political) divisions of countries down to the local community living environment. Hints of intranational regional influences are implied in elements of the 'National Forces' box of Figure 3.1 (e.g. access to education and healthcare, population distribution), but conceptually we think it best to distinguish a complete sub-national scale.

The living conditions, employment opportunities, healthcare services and other features of places within countries that influence health in large measure flow from power structures and decision-making higher in our framework: for example, a multinational automobile manufacturer's decision to close down selected offshore operations; a central government's decision how and where to allocate healthcare funds; national environmental health regulations. But other sub-national forces are endogenous to the areas concerned – for example, micro-climatic and wind-circulation patterns influencing the concentration/dispersion of local/regional atmospheric pollution, population pressures forcing settlement in hazardous locations, high/low levels of community social capital, state/provincial government policies, geographic remoteness, poor soils for food production, etc.

Individual factors

The global, regional, national and sub-national forces we have been discussing come together in varying mixes around the world as the diverse settings on which the planet's seven billion inhabitants play out their lives. Whether those lives are long and healthy or short and plagued by poor health is heavily influenced by the settings in which individuals and groups find themselves. For those unfortunate in the lottery of birth to be born into severe poverty in a very lowly developed country, overall life and health prospects are grim. Conversely, those born into a prosperous Western nation have very good healthy life expectancy odds.

However, a particular mix of forces does not guarantee a given health outcome. Individual attributes (biological, socio-economic, psycho-social) and behaviours (e.g. diet, physical activity, cigarette smoking, alcohol consumption, drug taking) mediate between the contextual forces and experienced health. Persons with higher incomes and educations, for instance, almost invariably do better than average health wise, in whichever country (or part thereof) they live. Education conveys health advantage through both enhancing people's health literacy and improving their employment and income prospects, while income is critical in determining their nutrition, housing quality and access to healthcare. Likewise, healthy behaviours, such as undertaking regular exercise, not smoking and avoiding excessive alcohol consumption, will generally enhance health prospects in even the most disadvantaged countries and communities. We discuss these issues in more detail in Chapter 7.

We should reiterate here, though, the point made earlier in the chapter: that is, many so-called lifestyle behavioural 'choices' are rooted in the broad social and economic structural contexts and personal circumstances within which people live and are not in any genuine sense *free* choices. To give a simple example, regular physical exercise may not be a real option for some people due to their particular working or family commitments, income constraints, or the built environment in which they live. Similarly, persons in areas with few or no opportunities for schooling are not well equipped to make informed health decisions. In turn, persuasive marketing campaigns by alcohol and cigarette manufacturers in tandem with powerful social peer pressures make smoking and excessive drinking not so easily avoidable for many people as might first be thought.

Intergenerational influences are also important. For instance, for children brought up in households in which the parents smoke, smoking can appear the norm. In similar fashion, adult tendencies towards unhealthy eating, inadequate exercise and the like are often established in early childhood and adolescence through poor parenting. Positive parenting is thus an essential element of successful population health promotion.

Figure 3.2 outlines the major personal risk factors and interrelationships considered to lie behind ischaemic heart disease (IHD). Complex multicausality, as shown here, is typical of

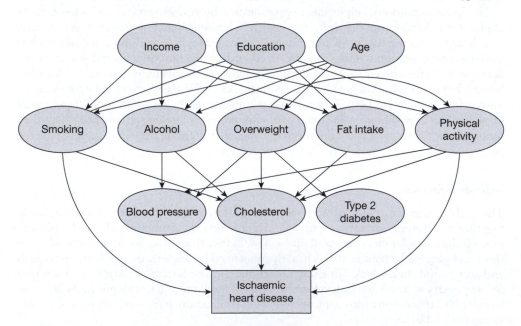

Figure 3.2 The causal chain: personal risk factors for ischaemic heart disease

Note: Not all interactive pathways are indicated.
Source: WHO (2009a), Fig. 1, p. 2

most leading non-communicable diseases. To complete the causal chain, the contextual natural and human environmental forces (global, regional, national, sub-national) need to be added – e.g. the built environment, work environments, food availability and supply chains, food and environmental health regulations, food outlets and pricing, food advertising, food cultures, health promotion resources, community health literacy, community income levels, exposure to air pollution, climatic factors, etc.

Feedback effects: health as the driver

With the discussion above of individual factors, our conceptual model of the determinants of population health is completed. One further set of forces and outcomes remains to be noted, though: that is, the reverse influence of population health outcomes on the various contextual and individual determinants – health *feedback* effects.

Both good and bad population health outcomes have these flow-on effects, making health, in the language of statistics, both a dependent (*effect*) and independent (*cause*) variable. High mortality and morbidity among young working-age adults, for instance, will deplete the workforce of potentially productive members and retard economic development. HIV/ AIDS in sub-Saharan Africa is a classic example, in the worst-affected countries seriously reducing the labour supply, government tax revenues and growth of gross domestic product (GDP). The pressure of people sick with HIV or AIDS consumes much government funding that in other circumstances would have gone to other sectors. Education is also badly affected, through the illness and deaths of large numbers of teachers. Major impacts are also felt at the individual and household levels. The loss of income earners to AIDS exacerbates poverty levels, with the deaths of parents consigning many children to precarious lives as orphans. Malaria is another example of a disease that has serious economic and social feedback effects for both population groups and individuals.

Hanging over the world's people is the possible ultimate adverse health feedback loop of a deadly global influenza pandemic. In the case of such an event, all aspects of life and all relations between nations – political, economic, social, cultural, demographic, etc. – would be affected. The 2003 SARS outbreak that rapidly spread from Guangdong Province in China to over thirty countries around the world gave a limited insight into the ramifications of such a pandemic.

The above examples all focus on adverse health feedback effects. There is also, of course, the positive side, whereby gains in population health, beyond improving the length and quality of life for individuals, have important wider non-health benefits – for example, a larger and more productive workforce, a greater attraction of the country to foreign investment and tourism, greater social stability, improved political viability and enhanced national and international security. Improving population health is thus an important pathway to achieving broader economic, social and political development.

Positioning the determinants of health

A useful additional way of thinking about health determinants is in terms of their position (*stage*) in the production of good and bad health. What are the underlying root causes of health inequality between population groups? What factors come into play later in the causal chain? Viewing determinants in this manner in turn clarifies the various points at which policy and intervention efforts can be directed and the health returns likely to flow from different actions.

From this stage perspective, three discrete but closely interrelated sets of determinants can be identified: *upstream, midstream* and *downstream* influences on health (see Figure 3.3).

Upstream determinants are macro-level factors, such as globalization, government policies, labour markets, business environments, income structures, educational systems, societal power relationships, cultural contexts and the like. These factors are distant (i.e. upstream) from the ultimate emergence of illness and disease but produce the social and economic inequalities between and within nations which underly differing population health fortunes. Poverty, social gradients, racism, gender discrimination, social exclusion, etc. established by these macro factors are the fundamental originating causes of poor health.

Shaped by the upstream context, further down the pathway to actual health status are midstream determinants – health behaviours, psycho-social factors such as stress, self-esteem, isolation and marginalization and social support, and the healthcare system (e.g. access, quality, utilization).

Finally, there are downstream physiological and biological determinants. Figure 3.4 illustrates this model with reference to low birthweight-related infant mortality, a major health problem in many less developed countries.

Efforts to improve health can be directed at all positions in the 'causal stream'. This aligns with the long-established notion in public health and epidemiology of *levels of prevention* (see Box 3.3). Upstream interventions addressing the root causes of poor health offer the greatest potential population-wide gains, but are difficult and frequently slow to engineer successfully. Poverty, for example, which underlies more deaths around the world than any other single factor, is so deeply entrenched by powerful international and national (self-) interests that progress to release its deadening hand is glacial. Likewise, the deadly sex discrimination against females in several Asian cultures cannot be turned around overnight, nor the marginalization and discrimination suffered by many indigenous peoples, nor the

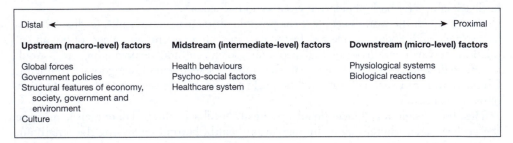

Figure 3.3 Upstream, midstream and downstream determinants of health: general model

Source: After Turrell *et al.*, 1999

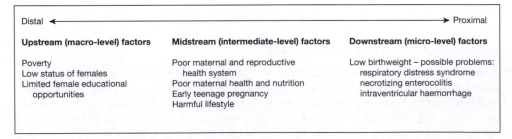

Figure 3.4 Upstream, midstream and downstream determinants of health: low birthweight-related infant mortality in less developed countries

Note: Not all determinants are listed.

limited educational opportunities available to children in many poor countries. For substantial permanent gains in global population health, however, international- and societal-level changes in these areas are essential.

Midstream interventions are generally easier to implement and while they do not address the fundamental social, economic, political and environmental determinants, they can deliver significant results. Health promotion campaigns aimed at reducing risky health behaviours (e.g. to stop smoking, to undertake more exercise, to avoid unprotected sex) are examples of this level. The WHO's Expanded Programme on Immunization (EPI) against major childhood killers (e.g. measles, polio, tetanus) and the use of insecticide-treated bed nets for protection against malarial mosquitos are other examples. However, upstream poverty reduction remains the fundamental necessary intervention for solving many of these health problems: to remove the need for poor women in developing countries to engage in prostitution and expose themselves to the risk of HIV/AIDS; to enable households in malaria zones to be able to afford better malaria protection; to improve financial access to maternal, reproductive and childhood health services in poor countries.

Downstream interventions focus on physiological and biological functioning problems, repairing or managing the damage and avoiding premature loss of life. Common examples for leading global health problems include: drugs and surgery for atherosclerosis, surgery, radiotherapy and chemotherapy for cancer, medication for hypertension, oral rehydration and zinc supplement therapy for childhood diarrhoea, highly active antiretroviral therapy (HAART) for HIV/AIDS, artemisinin-based combination therapies (ACTs) for treating malaria, tablets and/or insulin for managing diabetes, medication and psychotherapy for mental disorders and neonatal intensive-care units for low birthweight babies. Many of these health conditions are preventable or manageable upstream and midstream, but ultimately

---

BOX 3.3 Levels of disease and injury prevention

Three levels of prevention – *primary*, *secondary* and *tertiary* – are generally recognized by public health specialists and epidemiologists.

Primary prevention refers to measures taken to stop a disease (or injury) from occurring. These focus on upstream and midstream determinants of health. Upstream examples are government policies and actions to reduce poverty, air pollution regulations, workplace safety legislation, driving laws and the like. Midstream examples are such actions as immunization programmes, healthy living (e.g. smoking cessation, increasing exercise, dietary improvement, safe driving) promotional campaigns and fall-proofing the homes of frail elderly persons.

Secondary prevention covers actions to detect and diagnose disease in its early stages, thereby limiting its severity and improving the likelihood of successful treatment. Population screening programmes (e.g. mammograms for breast cancer, pap smears for cervical cancer, cholesterol and blood pressure checks) are examples.

Tertiary prevention refers to attempts to prevent the progression of established disease or injury, reduce disease-related complications and (as far as possible) restore function. The conditions concerned may be acute (e.g. severe gastrointestinal disease, malaria) or chronic (e.g. diabetes, HIV/AIDS, coronary artery disease, schizophrenia) and involve surgical, drug, behavioural or other treatment. Whether some preventive actions are best considered secondary or tertiary is not always certain.

need to be addressed at this downstream point. However, the capacity for such downstream interventions obviously varies greatly between countries.

Policies and actions to improve global population health need to target all three sets of determinants – upstream, midstream and downstream. Equally apparent from the above discussion should be the realization that improving population health involves far more than the strictly defined 'health sector'. All aspects of government, society and environment are, in essence, health-related. Policies and interventions need to reflect that fact.

Discussion topics

1   Are there any other factors you would add to the 'determinants of health' model portrayed in Figure 3.1?
2   How valid do you consider Stevens's (2009) claim that the WHO report (CSDH, 2008) on the social determinants of health is biased?

Part II

Global health and health transition – past and present – places and groups

4   Global health

Where we are and how we got there

Introduction

In 1800, little more than 200 years ago, global average life expectancy at birth (as can best be estimated) was around 28–29 years. Over the course of the following century this figure inched up to 32 years (Riley, 2005a). Since then, however, the level has risen dramatically, more than doubling to give a child born today an average expectation of life of 68 years. (This is the estimate for 2009 given in WHO, 2011a.) Interpolating United Nations estimates (UNDESA-PD, *World Population Prospects* website) gives a 2010 global average of 69 years.) This rolling back of mortality is one of the most monumental (arguably *the* most monumental) revolutions in human development, holding diverse major implications at all scales – for individuals, for societies and for the overall global community.

The gains of this health revolution have not been evenly shared, however: the lottery of birth and death deals very different outcomes around the globe (Figure 4.1). For the child lucky enough to be born in a high-income country, average life expectancy (both sexes combined) today is 80 years (83 for girls, 77 for boys). By contrast, the average life for the child if born in the low-income nations of the world is only 57 years (59 for girls, 55 for boys). Life expectancy in the most favoured nations (Japan and San Marino, 83 years) is 36 years greater than that of the lowest-rating country (Malawi, 47 years) (2009 statistics in WHO, 2011a). At the sub-national level even greater highs and lows are found (see Chapter 5). In terms of healthy life expectancy (HALE), the WHO estimated national averages (for 2007) range from a high of 76 years for Japan down to a low of 35 years for Sierra Leone. The estimated years of healthy life 'lost' from total life expectancy at birth globally was 13.2 per cent. Across the WHO's six regions, equivalent 'lost' healthy years ranged from 9.5 per cent in Europe and the Western Pacific to 13.5 per cent in Africa. While variable data availability and quality give many national HALE estimates a sizeable uncertainty interval, they nonetheless paint another unequivocal picture of global health inequality and the chasm between the world's most and least fortunate inhabitants.

Beneath these aggregate life expectancy indicators of health are to be found a range of health profiles ('disease-scapes'). There are some countries in which infectious diseases predominate, others in which non-communicable diseases are the main killers, and other, intermediate, countries where both infectious and non-communicable conditions (the *double burden*) pose heavy burdens of disease (see Table 4.1). These profiles reflect various stages in what is called epidemiological/health transition (see Box 4.1). While the focus of this book is on the contemporary and likely future epidemiological/health scenes, this transition process can be dated back many millennia. In turn, it should be seen as one strand of a suite of interconnected other transitions (see Figure 4.2) – in fertility, age structure, nutrition, urbanization, technology, and social and economic development.

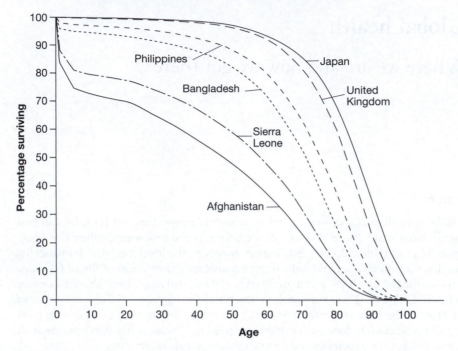

Figure 4.1 Survival curves for persons born in selected countries, 2008
Source: WHO, *Life Tables for WHO Member States* website

Table 4.1 Major causes of death, World and WHO income groups, estimates for 2008

Cause	World ($e_0 = 68$) (HALE = 59) %	High-income countries ($e_0 = 80$) (HALE = 70) %	Middle-income countries ($e_0 = 68$) (HALE = 61) %	Low-income countries ($e_0 = 57$) (HALE = 49) %
Communicable, maternal, perinatal and nutritional conditions	27.5	6.6	25.1	57.6
Infectious and parasitic diseases	15.3	2.1	14.0	33.9
Respiratory infections	6.2	3.9	5.5	11.5
Perinatal conditions	4.6	0.4	4.6	8.6
Non-communicable diseases	63.5	87.2	65.2	33.3
Malignant neoplasms	13.3	26.5	12.2	5.0
Neuropsychiatric disorders	2.3	6.3	1.6	1.4
Cardiovascular diseases	30.5	36.5	32.6	15.8
Respiratory diseases	7.4	5.8	8.7	3.7
Injuries	9.0	6.2	9.7	9.1

Note: e_0 = life expectancy at birth (years), 2008.
Sources: WHO, *Global Burden of Disease* and *World Health Statistics* reports websites

BOX 4.1   Epidemiological/health transition

The term 'epidemiologic(al) transition' refers to the shift in the major causes of death from infectious diseases (e.g. tuberculosis, smallpox, cholera, diarrhoea and enteritis, plague, pneumonia, measles) and famine to chronic, degenerative ailments (e.g. heart disease, stroke, cancers, diabetes, chronic obstructive pulmonary disease) associated with the long-term decline in mortality from high to low levels. The term was coined by Abdel Omran (1971), but the notion of such a transition can be found in earlier demographic and international health writings.

In his foundation statement on the transition, Omran argued the shift in diseases involved three major successive stages: the age of pestilence and famine; the age of receding epidemics; and the age of degenerative and man-made diseases. Three basic models of epidemiological transition were identified: the classical (Western) model; an accelerated model; and a contemporary (or delayed) model. In turn, three major categories of disease determinants were outlined: ecobiological; socio-economic, political and cultural; and medical and public health.

The validity and universality of epidemiological transition as a concept in general and Omran's theory in particular have been widely debated across a range of disciplines. Aspects that have attracted particular attention have been his impression of smooth, uninterrupted advancement (linear progression) through the transition, the seeming end-state accorded the third stage and its implied vanquishing of infectious disease, the relative importance of different disease determinants, the limited attention given to morbidity, and the broad social and geographic brush of the model.

The term 'health transition' was subsequently introduced to widen the focus from just death and illness to health in its full positive as well as negative sense and to the cultural, social and behavioural determinants of changing health (Caldwell *et al.*, 1990).

(Reading: Omran, 1971; McCracken and Phillips, 2009)

The pathways and patterns of epidemiological/health transition display both commonalities and diversities. Likewise, while it is common to think of and hope for continual improvement in the human condition, there is no preordained inevitability about universal future global health improvement and epidemiological evolution.

In this chapter we pick up many of these issues. Several will in turn be further pursued in later chapters. The organizing structure we have adopted is essentially one of changes in human health over time, with the focus being on the dramatic changes of the modern era. Space constraints limit both the width and depth of our discussion, but we hope the chapter conveys some idea of the great health journey humankind has completed to date.

Health transitions: past and present

Palaeolithic hunters and gatherers

Although we can only speculate about the diseases that affected our Palaeolithic ancestors, contemporary hunter–gatherer societies give some ideas as to likely human–environment disease interactions and patterns. Palaeolithic skeletons also provide clues. The low population density, geographic mobility and likely food resources of those times allow further deductions about probable disease patterns.

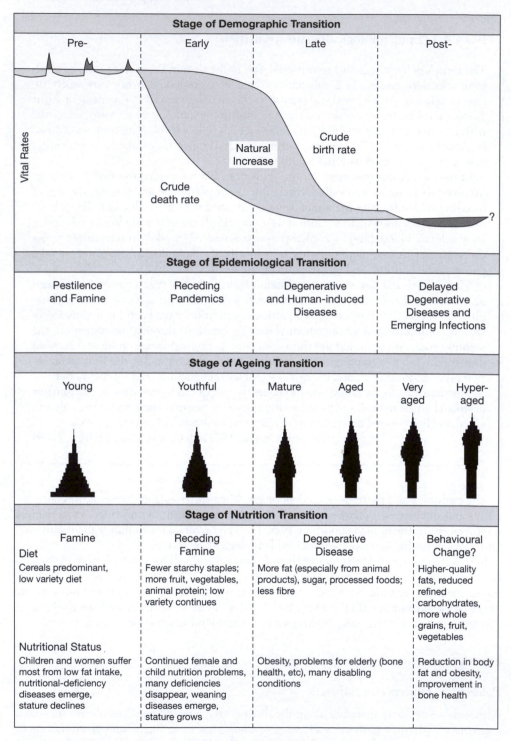

Figure 4.2 The demographic, epidemiological, ageing and nutrition transitions

Source: McCracken and Phillips, 2009

Zoonoses (infections transmitted from animals) would almost certainly have been major sources of disease, coming from both wild animal reservoirs and probably semi-domesticated dogs. Diseases possibly received in this manner could have included rabies, brucellosis, anthrax, salmonellosis, plague, Chaga's disease, leptosprosis, rickettsiosis and tularaemia. Gangrene and tetanus from anaerobic bacteria would have been other likely causes of death, along with mosquito-spread encephalitis, tsetse fly-vectored trypanosomiasis (sleeping sickness), tick-borne viral diseases and chronic infections, such as herpes and yaws. Several researchers have suggested staphylococcal and streptococcal infections may also have been major killers. Over and above infection, violent deaths through war and homicide were also probably important. Periodic famine, either directly through starvation, or indirectly by lowering immunity levels to infections, likely also contributed.

The relatively small size of hunter–gatherer bands, their geographic mobility and overall sparse population density meant deadly communicable diseases such as smallpox, influenza, measles and mumps did not plague Palaeolithic populations. These diseases need larger and more concentrated populations to support continuous transmission. Likewise, the small population numbers and mobility would have given protection against the 'crowd' diseases (e.g. cholera and typhoid) associated with concentrated build-up of refuse and human faecal matter and pollution of water sources.

Exactly how healthy Palaeolithic peoples were remains uncertain. Some researchers convey the image of 'brutish and short' lives. Others, in the words of Caldwell and Caldwell (2003, pp. 158, 156), paint a picture of 'the golden age of "Paleolithic man"' in which it sometimes seems they 'might be almost immortal'. The flow-on from this debate is whether the subsequent Neolithic period was a healthier era or initially a time of health deterioration. No resolution of this debate is possible here, but, as outlined above, although free from many killer diseases, our hunter–gatherer ancestors faced no shortage of conditions making for high morbidity and shortish lives. The limited skeletal evidence suggests a life expectancy of around 20–25 years (McMichael, 2001), but estimates into the low to mid-thirties have also been published.

Emergence of agriculture and fixed settlements – a Neolithic mortality crisis or not?

Beginning around 10,000 years ago, human life started to change from hunting and gathering to a more settled, domesticated plant- and animal-based existence. This change, known as the Neolithic Revolution, emerged in Mesopotamia (today's Iraq) and then later, independently, in other parts of the Old World, and also in Mesoamerica and South America. The label 'revolution' suggests sudden change, but the actual move to agriculture and sedentary village settlement was a lengthy and involved process. Alongside and connected with this change in economy and population distribution came a similarly gradual change in health and disease patterns.

The move to agriculture and fixed settlements had both good and bad implications for the well-being of their inhabitants. On the positive side, settled farming would have offered food security advantages in the form of stored surplus grain and root crop supplies, plus meat, milk and eggs from the newly domesticated animals. Some argue, however, that these nutritional advantages were countered by diets becoming less varied (i.e. heavily reliant on crops) and the dangers of food poisoning associated with stored reserves. The permanent housing of the villages would have been beneficial in providing shelter and warmth, but at the same time would have provided a habitat for disease-transmitting vermin (e.g. rodents, ticks, fleas, flies).

Sedentarism had two particularly serious health consequences for the villagers. First, the increased numbers of people living close together, in tandem with inadequate sanitary practices, resulted in dangerous build-ups of refuse and human faecal material, contaminating water supplies and other parts of the new living environment. In this compromised environment gastrointestinal infections would have flourished. Second, the domesticated animals (cattle, sheep, pigs, goats, dogs, poultry, etc.) essentially cohabited with the farming households, the close contact leading to many pathogens crossing the species divide. Measles, mumps, chickenpox, influenza and smallpox are among the many infectious diseases that jumped species during this agricultural revolution. In the past tuberculosis (TB) has also usually been cited as having crossed species (from cattle), but recent examination of ancient DNA suggests human TB evolved *before* bovine TB.

The clearing of land for cultivation and herding and the development and operation of irrigation systems would have been other aspects of Neolithic agrarian life increasing exposure to disease agents (e.g. malaria and schistosomiasis).

What these various disease threats collectively translated into in terms of Neolithic life expectancy is uncertain. The conventional wisdom is that mortality rose and accordingly life expectancy fell with the Neolithic Revolution, based on the many new threatening infectious diseases discussed above. A detailed review by Caldwell and Caldwell (2003), however, shows that this conclusion needs further examination. What can be said, though, is that the Neolithic saw the ushering in of a new disease-scape that was to remain dominant until the non-communicable disease transition of the late nineteenth and twentieth centuries. Also, the incipient steps towards urbanism of the new agricultural villages were to translate thousands of years later into towns and cities and an increasingly urban global health environment.

Historic disease transfers

Today most people are aware of how disease originating in one location can rapidly spread around the world in a dangerous illustration of the global nature of health. The most dramatic recent illustration of this is HIV/AIDS, which from African origins rapidly became a global epidemic over the last two decades of the twentieth century.

Continental- and inter-continental-scale disease transfers are a key strand of the story of the evolution of human disease-scapes. Wherever humans have travelled their diseases have always been close companions and in turn have often been passed on in the contact with distant communities. Sometimes such transfers have been 'exchanges', with the different population groups swapping their main infections. The impact of these transfers/exchanges in many cases has been monumental, shaping (and sometimes completely destroying) civilizations, with the consequences of many of these interactions continuing to this day.

Malaria is an example *par excellence*, dating back as an unwelcome ecological companion of humans to the very earliest times of prehistory in Africa. From its hearth in West and Central Africa, the disease spread northwards and westwards 10,000–5,000 years ago to Mesopotamia, Egypt, South and Southeast Asia, and then subsequently to China and other parts of Asia. Trading contacts saw the disease later establish itself around the Mediterranean 2,500–2,000 years ago and then into northern Europe 1,000–500 years ago. The deadly *Plasmodium falciparum* variety of the disease then jumped to the New World via West African slaves transported to the Caribbean and Central America by European colonizers in the early sixteenth century. There is debate about whether the other varieties of the disease – *P. vivax* and *P. malariae* – were also introduced to the Americas by Europeans or were already present in Amerindians, perhaps brought from Southeast Asia by early trans-Pacific voyagers or acquired through species jump of simian *Plasmodium*. Today's malaria zones are the legacy of these historic migrations.

Military and trading contacts between Eurasian civilizations were the source of many historic disease transfers/exchanges. The most devastating such outbreak was the mid-fourteenth-century Black Death (bubonic plague) pandemic which is estimated to have killed between a quarter and a third of the total population of Europe. This catastrophic outbreak is believed to have originated in China in the 1330s, moved along the Silk Road and other trade routes to reach Constantinople (today's Istanbul) in 1347 and then advanced through Western and Northern Europe over the next three years. The plague also spread widely in China, causing millions of deaths. The Middle East was affected, too. The massive death toll shook all aspects of life in Europe – society, economy, politics and religion – with many present-day historians tracing the end of feudalism, the roots of capitalism and the impetus for the Protestant Reformation of the sixteenth century to the Black Death. In turn, in Asia the Black Death severely weakened the powerful Mongol Empire through population loss and the decline of trade, a development which was to help the subsequent rise of Western Europe as a world power.

Other major examples of historic Eurasian disease transfers were smallpox and cholera. Smallpox is thought to have emerged in human populations about 12,000 years ago. The mummified body of Pharaoh Ramses V of Egypt, who died in the mid-twelfth century BC, has a pustular rash that many take to be the earliest physical evidence of the disease. However, smallpox has not been proven unequivocally from the body. It is believed that traders transported the disease from ancient Egypt to India in the first millennium BC, from where it spread into China in the first century AD, and then on to Japan in the sixth century. Exactly when the disease spread to Europe is unknown, but it is increasingly believed that the Antonine Plague that ravaged the Roman Empire between AD 165 and 180 was small-pox, brought back by soldiers returning from the Near East. The even earlier devastating Plague of Athens (430–427 BC) is considered by some scholars to have been smallpox, too. Whatever the exact date of entry to Europe, the disease had become endemic by the Middle Ages and plagued the region's populations up to the early nineteenth century. Edward Jenner's 1796 experiment proving that vaccination with cowpox gave immunity to smallpox ultimately provided the critical breakthrough against the virus and the start of a fight that eventually saw the World Health Assembly in 1980 declare the world to be free of naturally occurring smallpox, making it the only human disease ever to be completely eradicated.

Cholera is another dramatic case of wide-scale disease transfer. Long established on the Indian sub-continent, the disease spread to Europe and North America via land and sea trade routes in several lethal pandemic waves during the nineteenth century. The poor housing, personal hygiene and sanitation conditions in the rapidly growing industrial cities of Western Europe, Russia and the United States of that time proved fertile beds for the *Vibrio cholerae* bacterium to flourish and for millions to lose their lives. Improvements in the disposal of human excreta and the provision of safe water supplies eventually saw the disease recede as a major health threat in Europe and North America, but it is still a serious problem in South Asia and at times in other developing countries.

The most complex and famous historic disease transfer was the so-called 'Columbian Exchange' – the spread of infectious diseases from the Old World to the New (and the possible reverse conveyance of New World pathogens to the Old World) by Columbus and other European explorers and colonists; and, later, African slaves. Old World diseases carried to the Americas included smallpox, measles, bubonic plague, typhus, malaria, yellow fever, influenza, chickenpox, typhoid, diphtheria, mumps and whooping cough. Native Americans had no immunity to any of these diseases and on coming into contact with them succumbed in massive numbers. Smallpox, in particular, wrought a devastating toll throughout the Americas and is generally seen as an important factor in Hernán Cortés' and Francisco Pizarro's respective easy conquests of the large Aztec (Mexico) and Inca (Peru) empires with very small military forces. All told, it is estimated that 80–95 per cent of the Amerindian population was wiped out in the century and a half following Columbus's arrival in the Caribbean in 1492, with some regions losing their total populations. This massive depopulation from infectious disease stands as one of the largest demographic disasters in human history.

The Columbian Exchange was a very uneven process, as disease flow in the reverse direction – from New World to Old – was, at worst, limited. The pre-contact Native American populations had relatively few infectious diseases to spread to Europeans as they had domesticated fewer animals than Eurasian societies and hence had not experienced as much across-species disease transfer. The most contentious aspect of disease flow from West to East concerns venereal syphilis (*Treponema pallidum* subspecies *pallidum*). A syphilis epidemic spread across Europe soon after Columbus's first voyage to the Americas and is taken by many historians as proof of the disease having been brought to the continent by the returning Columbus and his crew. There was certainly syphilis in the New World, and Columbus and his men could have acquired it through sexual contact with the natives of Hispaniola. Others have argued that syphilis had been present in Europe well before Columbus's voyage, but had not been specifically identified due to the existence of other diseases (e.g. leprosy) with similar symptoms. However, recent detailed molecular genetic research supports the Columbian New World theory of syphilis's origin.

The same process of European epidemiological invasion and indigenous depopulation was later repeated in other parts of the world – Australia, New Zealand, the Pacific islands, Southern Africa, etc. In Australia, for instance, a severe epidemic devastated the Aboriginal population of the Sydney region in early 1789, little over a year after the start of European settlement. The immigrant white population was virtually untouched. Smallpox is generally taken to have been the disease involved, but chickenpox has also been suggested. Over the following decades, venereal syphilis, gonorrhea, tuberculosis, influenza, measles and other Old World infections were added to the Aboriginal disease-scape, contributing to a major decline from pre-white settlement population numbers. Throughout the Pacific, explorers and trading vessels brought infections in train. (Islanders frequently labelled foreign vessels 'disease boats'.) Captain James Cook, for example, introduced tuberculosis to Hawaii in his 1778 visit. The same visit also resulted in a rapid spread of venereal disease across the whole Hawaiian archipelago. In Fiji in 1875 between a quarter and a third of the population died from measles over six months in an epidemic seeded by a few cases contracted in New South Wales and transported back to the islands. As these examples show, Old World pathogens found the virgin soil of non-immune native populations welcoming ground.

Urbanization

Since Neolithic times, one of the main developments in human organization has been the growth of concentrated settlements. Beginning with the first small agricultural villages of 10,000 years ago, this trend has evolved to today's situation in which a majority of the world's people (51 per cent) live in urban areas. By comparison, in 1800 the figure was 3 per cent; in 1900, 14 per cent; and in 1950, 30 per cent.

This urban transformation has been a major force behind demographic and health transition and we can confidently predict this will continue. Inevitably, the future global health environment will be increasingly urban. Here we briefly outline some of the key health outcomes of urban development over time. The focus is historical. Contemporary and future urbanism and health will be given greater attention later.

For the majority of human history, urban residence has been epidemiologically dangerous. As previously outlined, the Neolithic populations that made the first moves to sedentary village living exposed themselves to numerous health risks. Two were particularly important: first, geographically fixed living and inadequate sanitation capabilities meant dangerous localized build-ups of human faecal material and the threat of contaminated water supplies; second, there was the danger of contracting infections from their co-resident domesticated herd animals.

Over the subsequent millennia, as genuine towns and, later, cities emerged, the second threat diminished, but the first remained a constant of urban life right through to the twentieth century. Cities were demographic 'sinkholes', their frightful living conditions regularly consuming more of their inhabitants than were being produced through births. For example, life expectancy at birth in London in the first half of the seventeenth century was in the low twenties (years), whereas the figure for England and Wales as a whole was 35–36 years. Infant and child mortality was particularly heavy. According to John Graunt's (1662) life table for the city's population, 60 per cent of individuals died before sixteen years of age. Cities could keep growing only through ongoing migration from the countryside. Crowded living, atrocious sanitation and poor nutrition in combination made an ideal environment for person-to-person and 'filth'-type infections to flourish – plague, tuberculosis, smallpox, dysentery, typhus, typhoid, cholera, pneumonia and various others. As best as we can estimate, a causes of death stocktake in Europe at the end of the eighteenth century would have shown smallpox and tuberculosis to be the leading adult killers and diarrhoeal illnesses, smallpox, respiratory infections and childhood diseases accounting for most children. In its early stages, the Industrial Revolution of the late eighteenth and nineteenth centuries worsened living and working conditions in many Western world cities. The nineteenth-century cholera outbreaks in Europe and the United States were particular 'beneficiaries' of these conditions.

Today, with greatly improved living standards and normally an advantage in access to health services, city residents generally enjoy better health than their rural counterparts. But that is only a development of the past century. As recently as 1900, urban dwellers in Europe, North America and Australia typically bore a life expectancy at birth 'urban penalty' of four–five years (sometimes more), compared to their rural counterparts. That is not to say urban residence today does not still hold certain health disadvantages. Urban populations, for example, tend to have greater exposure to industrial and motor vehicle air pollution and consequent risk of related respiratory problems.

Global health at the turn of the twentieth century

As stated in the introduction to this chapter, global life expectancy at birth entering the twentieth century was about thirty-two years. Like today, though, this global average masked wide regional differences in health fortunes. In China and India, for example, the figure is thought to have been no more than the mid-twenties, little different from the level of the Palaeolithic hunters and gatherers of 10,000 years earlier. At the other end of the spectrum were a number of countries whose people enjoyed life expectancies of fifty years or more – Denmark, Netherlands, Norway, Sweden, Australia, New Zealand and Canada. Women (non-Maori) in New Zealand had already surpassed sixty years.

In most of Western Europe, North America and Australasia, health transition (i.e. persistent gains in survival) was entrenched. Virtually all these gains were traceable to falling death rates from infectious diseases. Exactly why these rates fell at this time, however, remains a matter of debate. There is a popular tendency to ascribe rising longevity to improved medical care, but, apart from smallpox vaccinations, medical improvements in the narrow sense played little part in these nineteenth-century developments (McKeown, 1976). The key role is usually ascribed by researchers to better nutrition due to innovations in agricultural production and distribution and rising incomes making food more affordable. Improved diets were not the whole story, though, and indeed in some cases the evidence for the food supply–mortality relationship is weak. Medical intervention in the wider public health sense (e.g. sanitary reform, food safety regulations), although generally slow in translation from legislation to widespread practice, probably has not received the credit it deserves.

Most readers will be aware that one of the basic features of contemporary global health is a positive relationship between countries' economic development and life expectancy: that is, inhabitants of poor nations on average have shorter lives than people in rich countries. While absolute life expectancy values then were far different from today, the same basic national wealth–health association existed in 1900. The values and trend line for twenty-eight countries for which reasonable estimates of both 1900 GDP per capita and life expectancy are available is shown in Figure 4.3, revealing a mildly curvilinear relationship with an r^2 (GDP per head transformed to natural logarithms) of 0.58. For then, as today, per capita GDP (while not a flawless indicator) was a summary surrogate of personal incomes, availability of healthcare, living standards and other aspects of material well-being that impact on health.

Deaths in the poorer countries were almost entirely due to infectious diseases and nutritional deficiencies – diarrhoeal diseases, respiratory illnesses, neonatal infections, malnutrition and the like. In the more developed countries, meanwhile, infectious disease mortality, as noted above, was falling, but pathogens of one sort or another nonetheless still dominated cause of death profiles. The United States figures for the time, presented in Figure 4.4 and Table 4.2, can be taken as broadly representative of developed country cause of death patterns of the day. Down the cause of death rankings, however, signs of a new epidemiological future were slowly emerging, with increasing proportions of deaths occurring to heart disease, cancer and stroke as more people survived childhood and through to older ages and the different disease risks of those ages. The accompanying survival chart for Sweden

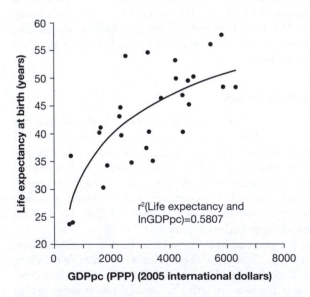

Figure 4.3 Life expectancy at birth and GDP per capita, 1900

Sources: Kinsella, 1992; Riley, 2005c; University of California, Berkeley and Max Planck Institute for Demographic Research, *The Human Mortality Database* and Gapminder websites

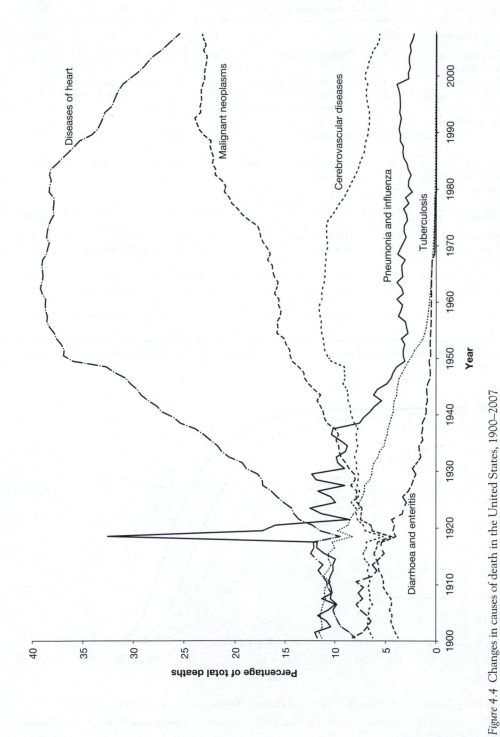

Figure 4.4 Changes in causes of death in the United States, 1900–2007

Sources: United States Centers for Disease Control and Prevention website: http://www.cdc.gov/nchs/data/dvs/lead1900_98.pdf and http://www.cdc.gov/NCHS/data/nvsr/nvsr58/nvsr58_19.pdf

Table 4.2 Epidemiological transition in the United States and Mexico

Cause of death	%	Cause of death	%	Cause of death	%
(a) United States	*1900*		*1950*		*2007*
Pneumonia and influenza	11.8	Diseases of heart	36.9	Diseases of heart	25.4
Tuberculosis	11.3	Malignant neoplasms	14.5	Malignant neoplasms	23.2
Diarrhoea, enteritis, and ulceration of the intestines	8.3	Vascular lesions affecting central nervous system (stroke)	10.8	Cerebrovascular diseases (stroke)	5.6
Diseases of the heart	8.0	Accidents	6.3	Chronic lower respiratory disease	5.3
Intracranial lesions of vascular origin (stroke)	6.2	Certain diseases of early infancy	4.2	Accidents (unintentional injuries)	5.1
(b) Mexico	*1955–57*		*1980*		*2008*
Gastroenteritis	17.5	Heart diseases	11.6	Heart diseases	17.3
Influenza and pneumonia	15.5	Accidents	11.0	Malignant neoplasms (cancer)	12.7
Childhood diseases	10.4	Influenza and pneumonia	8.8	Diabetes mellitus	12.8
Heart diseases	7.1	Enteritis and other diarrhoeal diseases	8.6	Cerebrovascular disease (stroke)	6.1
Malaria	5.1	Malignant tumours (cancer)	6.1	Accidents (unintentional injuries)	6.0

Sources: United States Centers for Disease Control and Prevention and WHO, *Global Burden of Disease* websites; Frenk *et al.*, 1989

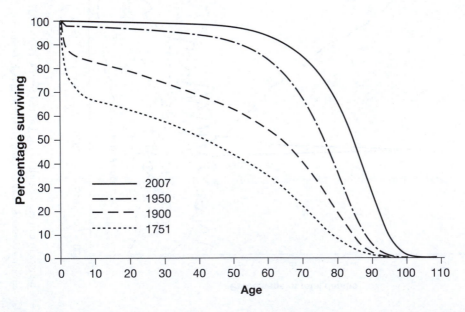

Figure 4.5 Changing survival curves for persons born in Sweden, 1751, 1900, 1950 and 2007

Source: University of California, Berkeley and Max Planck Institute for Demographic Research, *The Human Mortality Database* website

(Figure 4.5) illustrates the broad more developed world experience, although the onset, pace and magnitude of the survival transition varied. In the Swedish case, the proportion of persons surviving to 50 rose from 44 per cent in 1751 to 62 per cent in 1900.

Twentieth and twenty-first centuries: health revolution

As the twentieth century dawned, people around the globe could have had no idea of the enormous unprecedented improvements in population health that were to be gained during its course and on into the following century – average life expectancy for a newborn baby jumping from the estimated 32 years of 1900 to 68 years in 2010. Presumably there would have been the natural human hopes for health improvement – of losing fewer children in infancy and childhood, of a lower likelihood of marriages being broken by early death, of living substantially longer and healthier lives – but the pace and magnitude of the gains that would be achieved would certainly have been inconceivable to all but the most optimistic. Against this backdrop of large overall gains in global health, however, there have also been major setbacks and unequal progress.

1900–50

Rapid gains in longevity occurred in most Western nations in the first half of the century. In the space of those few decades, gains of 15–25 years life expectancy at birth were widely achieved in developed nations around the globe. As in the nineteenth century, falling infectious disease death rates were the main factor. Figure 4.4 demonstrates this decline of the major old infectious killers for the United States. Also as in the nineteenth century, most of this decline in the Western nations had little to do with technical medicine (i.e. vaccines or antibiotics) as the bulk of the reduction in mortality from infections occurred before the introduction of effective antimicrobial measures. For example, sulphonamides (sulpha drugs) became available only in the late 1930s; penicillin was not widely available for civilian use until the mid-1940s; and streptomycin not until a few years after that.

Although medical vaccines and therapies came into play only at the tail end of the Western world's 'old' infectious disease era, medical science played an important part in the way that it informed public and individual health practices. Validation of the 'germ theory of disease' (i.e. that microorganisms are the cause of many diseases) in the late nineteenth century through the work of Louis Pasteur, Robert Koch and other medical researchers led to new understandings and approaches to improving population health. Legislation and public works to improve water supplies, sewage and garbage disposal and food hygiene now had a firm scientific foundation. Public health officials also used the new microbiological knowledge in campaigns to improve the personal health behaviours of individuals, such as washing hands before cooking and eating, cleaning cooking equipment, protecting food from flies and other insects, sterilizing bottles and milk, improving ventilation in homes, and isolating family members infected with contagious diseases. Broad social and economic improvements affecting food availability and quality, housing standards and general education also helped.

Through these public health and broad macro-social/economic developments, aided in the late 1930s and 1940s by antibiotics, a totally new epidemiological landscape had emerged in these more developed nations by mid-century, their former infectious-disease-dominated cause of death profiles having given way to one in which chronic degenerative conditions predominated. Whereas pneumonia, tuberculosis and diarrhoea/enteritis had led their cause of death tables in 1900, now, with the threat of communicable diseases dramatically reduced and more people accordingly surviving to older ages, a new triumvirate of heart disease, cancers and cerebrovascular disease (stroke) was firmly entrenched. The United States data in Table 4.2 are illustrative of the transition. By 1950, average life expectancy in these more developed countries had risen to just under 65 years. In a few (Norway, Netherlands, Sweden, Iceland, Denmark), it had even attained or surpassed the biblical 'three score and ten' years.

Outside Europe, North America and Australasia there was little substantial improvement in life expectancy levels until the 1920s and 1930s. (There were a few exceptions to this – notably Argentina and Japan.) Improvement became somewhat more widespread in the 1940s, but for the majority of the world's peoples significant reductions in infectious disease mortality and resultant gains in longevity were not to come until the second half of the century. By the United Nations' estimation (UNDESA-PD, 2011), average life expectancy at birth for the less developed regions in 1950 was only 41.0 years, and in the so-called least developed countries even lower at 36.3 years. The global average was 46.5 years. Figure 4.6 displays the global breakdown of those figures. Figure 4.7 shows the temporal progression of the health transition, charting when countries attained a life expectancy at birth of 50 years. The Mexico 1955–57 panel in Table 4.2 broadly illustrates the developing world diseasescape at mid-century.

1950 to the present

This period has seen unprecedented gains made in human health. By 2010, around twenty countries had national life expectancy levels of 80 years or more (Figure 4.8). Globally, average life expectancy for a newborn baby rose twenty-two years during the course of the six decades to 2010, compared with around fourteen years over the first half of the century. Not surprisingly, given their earlier larger gains, the more developed nations have registered smaller increases than developing world countries, an average of thirteen years as against twenty-six years. As the apparent current upper limits on average life expectancy are approached, gains become intrinsically harder to come by biologically. Despite the unprecedented global gains, however, the period has not been one of universal, continuous advancement. Periods of life expectancy reversal have been experienced at times by some countries due to varying mixes of political, social, economic and epidemiological upheaval. Key distinguishing features of this era have also been the roles played by medical advances in the form of effective vaccines, drugs, diagnostic measures, surgery and intensive care, major international public health programmes and non-governmental health-funding players.

With communicable diseases essentially under control, the chronic and degenerative diseases of adulthood have been increasingly centre stage in the developed industrial nations. In the two decades or so after the Second World War, many of these countries experienced rising death rates from heart disease and stroke, giving rise to widespread talk of a 'cardiovascular disease epidemic'. High cigarette smoking rates, diets rich in fats, sugars and salt, and increasingly sedentary lifestyles were key contributing factors. In the United States, for example, by the mid-1950s one in every two deaths was due to heart disease or stroke. This situation continued through to the early 1970s before starting to decline. Since 1970, the age-adjusted heart and cerebrovascular disease death rates have fallen by two-thirds and three-quarters, respectively. Similar patterns have been documented in numerous other developed countries. These huge declines are generally credited to a combination of medical advances (e.g. improved diagnosis and treatment of cardiovascular conditions, better preventive medications, more cardiovascular specialists, increased heart attack and stroke care facilities) and individual behavioural changes (e.g. dietary changes, decline in cigarette smoking, actions to reduce hypertension). In the past, heart disease has generally

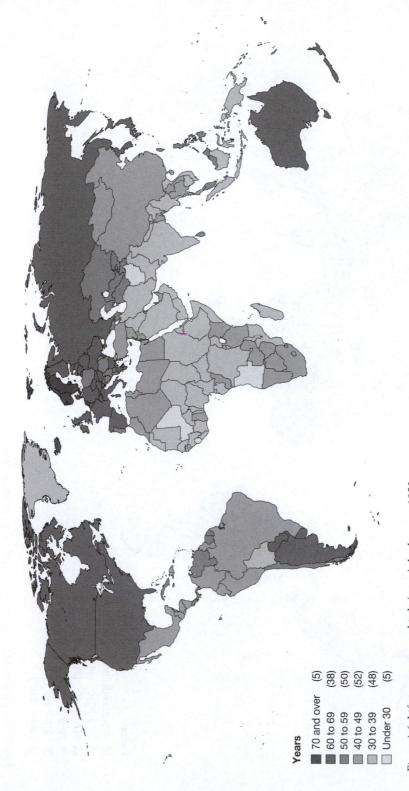

Years

- 70 and over (5)
- 60 to 69 (38)
- 50 to 59 (50)
- 40 to 49 (52)
- 30 to 39 (48)
- Under 30 (5)

Figure 4.6 Life expectancy at birth (years), both sexes, 1950

Source: UNDESA-PD, 2011

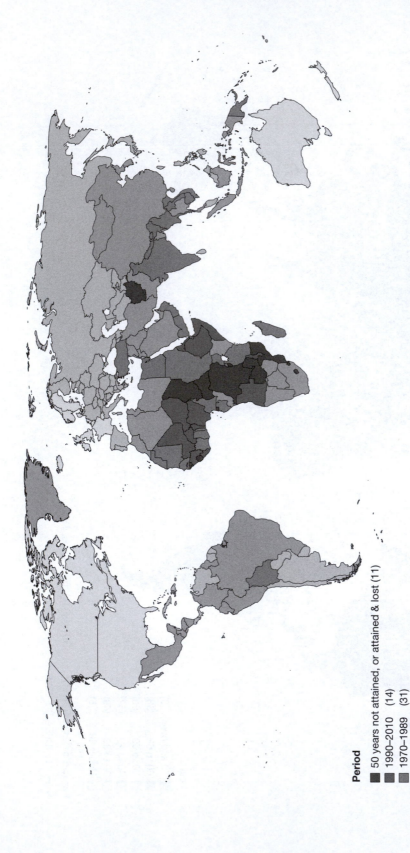

Period

■ 50 years not attained, or attained & lost (11)
■ 1990–2010 (14)
■ 1970–1989 (31)
■ 1950–1969 (49)
□ 1910–1949 (79)
□ Before 1910 (14)

Figure 4.7 Period that life expectancy at birth of 50 years was attained

Sources: UNDESA-PD, 2011; Kinsella, 1992; Riley, 2005c; University of California, Berkeley and Max Planck Institute for Demographic Research, *The Human Mortality Database* and Gapminder websites

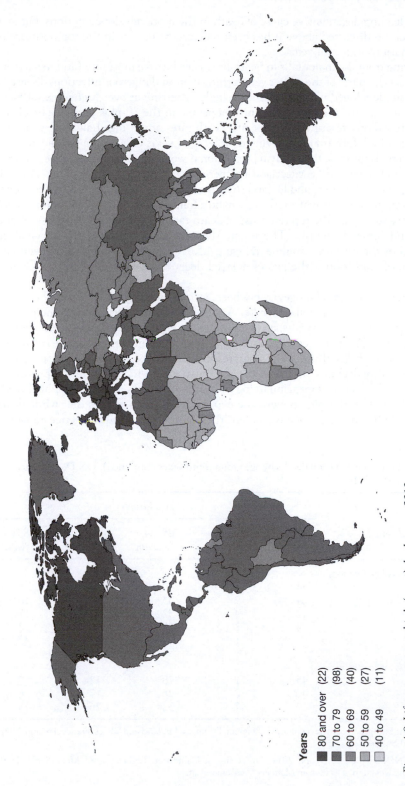

Figure 4.8 Life expectancy at birth (years), both sexes, 2010

Source: UNDESA-PD, 2011

Years

80 and over	(22)
70 to 79	(98)
60 to 69	(40)
50 to 59	(27)
40 to 49	(11)

been the leading degenerative cause of death in the more developed nations, but as a result of the declines discussed above it has been replaced by cancer in the top position in many of these nations in recent years.

Following from the major falls in heart disease and stroke mortality (and to a lesser extent some cancers), on top of the earlier vanquishing of most dangerous infectious diseases, deaths in the more developed nations are increasingly occurring at ever-higher ages. Over 40 per cent of deaths in those countries are now of people in the 80-plus years age bracket (Table 4.3) and based on present age/sex-specific death rates on average half of newborn children in them can look forward to surviving to at least 80 years of age. In a significant number of individual such nations, the survival proportion is well above this average – e.g. San Marino (72 per cent), Japan and Switzerland (68 per cent), Monaco (67 per cent), Australia and Italy (66 per cent), France and Iceland (65 per cent), Sweden and Spain (64 per cent). This pattern of increasing survival, on the one hand a human success story, has unfortunately seen a new entry surge into the top ten cause of death rankings in many countries – Alzheimer's disease and other dementias. The progressive *rectangularization* of the survival curve is illustrated by the Swedish example in Figure 4.5. These developments have been labelled a new stage of transition – the age of delayed degenerative disease (Olshansky and Ault, 1986).

Whether the increased longevity has been accompanied by more years of healthy life has become a topic of considerable debate. Are the extended years of life principally years of good health, or simply extra years of poor health, as postulated by Verbrugge (1984) in a classic paper? The two scenarios have respectively become known as the *compression* and *expansion of morbidity* theses. The compression thesis, the optimistic perspective, argues that as mortality declines, ill-health and disability will be increasingly compressed into the later years of life due to improving living standards and medical and public health advances (Fries, 1980). The alternative view, the expansion scenario, argues that while death rates from many chronic diseases have fallen, their incidence and prevalence remain largely

Table 4.3 Percentage of total deaths by age group (both sexes combined), UN Development Regions, 1850–2010

Regions and period	Age Group				
	0–4 % deaths	5–24 % deaths	25–64 % deaths	65–79 % deaths	80+ % deaths
UN more developed regions					
1850*	34	13	30	17	6
1900*	24	9	33	24	10
1950–55	12	4	32	34	17
1975–80	4	2	25	40	28
2005–10	1	1	24	33	42
UN less developed regions					
1950–55	45	11	28	12	3
1975–80	40	10	26	17	6
2005–10	20	7	32	26	15

Note: * Eight European countries combined (Belgium, Denmark, England and Wales, France, Iceland, Netherlands, Norway and Sweden).

Sources: UNDESA-PD, 2009 and 2011; University of California, Berkeley, and Max Planck Institute for Demographic Research, *The Human Mortality Database* website

unchanged, leaving increasing numbers of unhealthy survivors. Unfortunately, detailed data internationally are often too scanty to give definitive support to either scenario, although HALE Project data from Europe suggest that, while European populations are ageing, the proportions of older persons with disability are decreasing. Recent US research based on twenty years of data from the National Long-Term Care Survey has reported disability rates among older Americans have also declined substantially (Redfoot and Houser, 2010). Overall, evidence therefore seems to be mounting for the compression thesis, though there is continuing debate about methodological issues and data interpretation.

At the end of the Second World War in 1945, most less developed nations were firmly rooted at the base stage of epidemiological transition, with infectious diseases heavily dominating their populations' health profiles and overall mortality high. In parts of Latin America and a few colonial territories around the world there had been successes against some infectious disease risks, but for the bulk of the developing world's peoples life and death were very much about communicable disease and high morbidity and mortality.

During the war, both the Allies and Axis powers invested considerable effort in devising ways to protect their troops from infectious disease (e.g. dealing with human excreta, cleaning up water supplies, eradicating disease vectors, developing vaccines and antibiotics) and treating those who were wounded or fell ill. After the war, this health knowledge and technology was transferred to the wider global community and brought immediate sub-stantial reductions in mortality wherever it was applied. Average life expectancy at birth in the less developed regions rose by six years in the 1950s and eight years over the following decade, although a third of the latter increase was a 'China effect'. Subsequent medical, scientific and technological research has progressively added to the population health armoury, making virtually all major infectious diseases in the developing world (with the exception of HIV/AIDS) now theoretically medically preventable and/or treatable. For example, infant and child survival have benefited enormously from the development of a string of prophylactic vaccines: polio (oral vaccine), measles and mumps in the 1960s; rubella, chickenpox, pneumonia and meningitis in the 1970s; *Haemophilus influenzae* type b (Hib) in 1985; and rotavirus in 1998. The introduction of oral rehydration therapy (ORT) in the early 1970s and, in the past few years, zinc supplement therapy to fight the developing world scourge of diarrhoeal diseases has also saved millions of lives. Better nutrition, improved basic living standards, rising educational levels and improvements (albeit not uni-versal) in women's status have been important complements to modern medicine. However, after the 'easy' health gains of the 1950s and 1960s, life expectancy increases since then have become more gradual. Indeed, a few developing countries are still struggling to attain a life expectancy at birth of at least 50 years (Figure 4.7). High infant and child mortality remain a heavy brake on longevity. In around fifty developing countries over 5 per cent of children born die before their first birthday and several per cent more before they reach age 5.

An important strategic part of health progress in the developing world over this period has been the implementation of various targeted disease elimination programmes. One of the first was launched in 1959, when the World Health Assembly passed a resolution to eradicate smallpox globally. By 1967, vaccination had brought annual cases down from 50 million to 10–15 million per year. An intensified immunization and case detection campaign was then implemented and the last known natural case of smallpox was finally reported (in Somalia) in 1977. Three years later the World Health Assembly formally announced the disease as having been eradicated globally. Malaria, polio, measles and several other infectious diseases have also been internationally targeted in this way. Renewed energy has been put into the fight against malaria in recent years with the disease's inclusion in the Millennium Development Goals (MDG Target 6.C) and the United Nations' endorsement of the Global Malaria Action Plan in 2008. Malaria was also targeted earlier, in the 1950s and 1960s, but complacency set in after initial impressive gains, control efforts were relaxed and the pathogen resurged. The Millennium Development Goals also target tuberculosis (MDG Target 6.C) and HIV/AIDS (MDG Targets 6.A and 6.B), with eradication and treatment plans in place for both diseases (the WHO's Stop TB Strategy and Global Plan to Stop TB; the Joint United Nations Programme on HIV/AIDS; and the World Bank's Global HIV/AIDS Programme of Action). Several programmes have focused on infant and childhood mortality as many of the leading causes of death at those ages are readily preventable or treatable. Major initiatives in this area have been the World Health Organization's Expanded Programme on Immunization (launched in 1974), the Global Alliance for Vaccines and Immunization (created in 1999), the World Health Organization/UNICEF Integrated Management of Childhood Illness strategy (initiated in the mid-1990s), and the inclusion of child mortality reduction as Millennium Development Goal 4.

Health in the developing world from 1950 onwards also benefited from the initiation of national family planning programmes. While the primary focus of these programmes was to bring about fertility decline, they also had health benefits, in particular for women and children. With less frequent childbearing and wider birth intervals, women were less exposed to maternal health risks and better able to give care to the children they did have. In fact, from originally starting out as stand-alone, purely fertility-reducing initiatives, family planning programmes came to be ever more integrated with maternal and child healthcare activities. General economic and social development also contributed to falling birth rates. The relationship between fertility decline and health also worked in the reverse direction. As infant and child mortality declined, couples could see that the 'replacement' and 'insurance' births that had been necessary for earlier generations in high-child-loss times to achieve a desired number of surviving children were no longer essential. Between 1950 and 2010 the average total fertility rate for the developing world fell from 6.2 to 2.6 children per women. In parallel fashion, the infant mortality rate dropped by around 75 per cent.

An increasingly important contributor to improving population health in less developed nations over the past two decades has been non-governmental philanthropic funding. Private funding of global/international health programmes goes back considerably further than this, but it is over this more recent time frame that it has become especially influential. Major contributors include the Bill and Melinda Gates Foundation, the Ford Foundation and the Rockefeller Foundation. The Gates Foundation (http://www.gatesfoundation.org/global-healthPages/overview.aspx), for example, has made available billions of dollars in grants for a range of targeted global health problems – among them, increasing access to vaccines in developing countries; reducing HIV/AIDS, malaria, pneumonia, tuberculosis, tropical parasitic diseases, malnutrition, diarrhoeal infections, and maternal, neonatal and child mortality; improving girls' education; tobacco control; and clean water and sanitation projects. The Gates Foundation's grants support both proven health improvement tools and research and development of new interventions. In recent years, the Ford Foundation (http://www.fordfoundation.org/issues/sexuality-and-reproductive-health-and-rights) has targeted the area of sexuality and reproductive health and rights, while the Rockefeller Foundation (http://www.rockefellerfoundation.org/who-we-are/our-focus/global-health) has been working on making health systems in developing countries more accessible and affordable and improving the monitoring, detection and response to infectious diseases to reduce the risk of pandemics developing.

The United Nations' 2010 stocktake of world demographic prospects showed all nations to have higher levels of life expectancy than they had at the start of the post-Second World War era, with, as previously stated, the more developed regions averaging an increase of around thirteen years and the less developed ones about twenty-six years over the six decades. These clearly rate as substantial improvements in life prospects for humankind in both blocs of nations. However, the gains were not geographically evenly distributed in either bloc. In the worst cases, health levels actually deteriorated for varying periods, sending earlier hard-earned life expectancy gains into reverse. Also tempering satisfaction with the gains is the fact that much readily preventable mortality and morbidity still remains to be conquered. This is obviously particularly true of poorer nations, but it holds for developed nations as well.

Life expectancy reversals

The classic statements of demographic and epidemiological transition theory (Notestein, 1945; Omran, 1971) convey the impression of seemingly uninterrupted human health improvement and cause of death change. The last several decades, however, have shown there is nothing guaranteed about humankind enjoying progressively longer lives. A range of crises have seen previously won life expectancy gains eroded in a number of populations and, in cases, a reversion to a more infectious-disease-dominated cause of death regime.

The African HIV/AIDS epidemic has been the most dramatic illustration. Zimbabwe's life expectancy at birth, for instance, is estimated by the United Nations to have fallen from around 62 years in the late 1980s to 43 in 2003; in Botswana, Swaziland and Lesotho, around 15 years life expectancy were shaved off; and in Zambia and South Africa around 10 years (UNDESA-PD, 2011). A corollary of the AIDS epidemic has been a resurgence of tuberculosis morbidity and mortality following the increased prevalence of immune system impairment.

Significant life expectancy decline also occurred in several of the former Soviet Union republics, where economic uncertainty, social disruption and political upheaval following the dissolution of the USSR in 1991 and rapid transition to capitalism caused death rates, especially among young and middle-aged males, to soar. Causes of death associated with heavy alcohol consumption were particularly involved. It is often overlooked that there were also periods of life expectancy decline before this, from the mid-1960s through the 1970s and then in the tumultuous two or three years before the final break-up of the Union.

Armed conflict, both internal and international, has driven life expectancy down in other cases. For example, in Cambodia, the direct and indirect mortality of the Vietnam War and then the Khmer Rouge (1975–79) era saw life expectancy drop by over ten years; in East Timor in the 1970s, the last years of Portuguese colonial rule and the subsequent Indonesian invasion and occupation inflicted a toll of almost seven years lost life expectancy; while in Iraq there was an estimated loss of around two years after the 2003 United States-led invasion and subsequent explosion of internal ethno-religious violence. The 1990s Rwandan Civil War and Genocide and Sierra Leone Civil War are further instances. Small declines also occurred in Sri Lanka at various times during its thirty years of civil war. To these cases can be added countries where armed conflict has not reversed life expectancy but has held back much health progress that could otherwise have been expected. Angola, the Democratic Republic of the Congo, Mozambique, Ethiopia and Sudan are all states that have suffered heavily in this way.

Other reversals have occurred but do not show up in overall national averages. For example, while life expectancy statistics for the United States population as a whole show steady increase over recent decades, levels have declined among some inner-city young black male populations with the emergence of a deadly epidemiological cocktail of unemployment, violence, accidents, illicit drug taking and HIV infection and resultant rising *social pathology* mortality.

Health and economic development

Earlier in the chapter attention was drawn to what might be called the (unfortunate) 'basic rule' of global health: namely, that people in poor countries generally have shorter lives than their contemporaries in rich nations. As was shown, this relationship is not new. We reported (Figure 4.3) how around 60 per cent of the variation in life expectancy for twenty-eight countries around 1900 was statistically accounted for by their national income (GDP per capita natural logarithm) levels. Similar analyses for 1950, 1980 and 2009 give essentially the same results (r^2 for 1950 = 0.58; 1980 = 0.69; 2009 = 0.65). (Logarithmic (ln) models were selected to handle the curvilinear nature of the relationships. A small number of countries with highly extreme per capita GDP values were excluded in the 1950, 1980 and 2009 analyses.) Figure 4.9 plots the data trendlines for the four dates.

These analyses have important implications. The r^2 values confirm that national income is an important influence on health, but, equally importantly, they show it is not the only determinant. The graphed trendlines meanwhile show that the life expectancy of people in each income category (measured in constant dollar terms) has steadily moved higher over the 100-plus-year time period. That is, a given income is associated with better health at each later date, again indicating other factors are involved. The curvilinear form of the trendlines also indicates that the gains in life expectancy from increasing per capita GDP become less after an inflection point around $5,000. The 2009 trendline in Figure 4.9, for example, shows that increasing per capita GDP from $1,000 to $5,000 corresponds to a gain of 10.7 years' life expectancy, whereas doubling income from $5,000 to $10,000 equates with a gain of only 4.6 years.

Consideration of selected countries reinforces the point. For their level of per capita national income, some countries are 'poor performers' on life expectancy, while others are

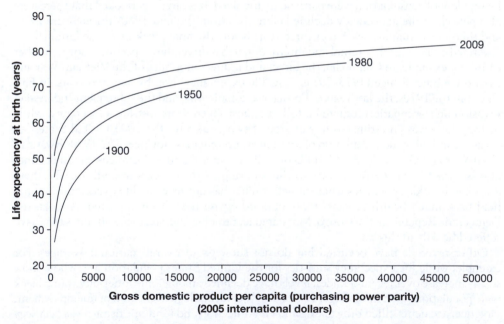

Figure 4.9 Life expectancy at birth and GDP per capita, 1900, 1950, 1980 and 2009

Sources: Kinsella, 1992; Riley, 2005c; University of California, Berkeley and Max Planck Institute for Demographic Research, *The Human Mortality Database* and Gapminder websites

the opposite, having higher life expectancies than would be predicted. For example, the West African nation of Equatorial Guinea has a high GDP per capita by developing world standards, but a very low life expectancy (approximately 51 years). The high income level derives from the country's large oil and gas revenues, but those benefits have not flowed down to the material well-being and health of the general population. The neighbouring state of Gabon is a similar case – nationally wealthy from oil but the bulk of the population remaining poor and lagging on health progress. In the 1960s and 1970s, oil-rich Saudi Arabia was the same. At the other pole are countries in which health has attained very good levels without high or rapidly rising incomes, such as Sri Lanka, Cuba, Chile, Costa Rica and Vietnam. The strategic keys to success in these countries have been emphases on improving public health (e.g. sanitation, child vaccination campaigns, basic reproductive health services) and socially oriented development (e.g. education, improving women's status).

Pairwise comparisons of some countries are a useful way to round out this topic. Take, for example, Indonesia and the Republic of the Congo. The two states have very similar GDP per capita figures (2005 international dollars), but Indonesia has almost a twenty-year life expectancy advantage. Likewise, Nepal and Burkina Faso match up closely in terms of per capita GDP, but the Nepalese enjoy a fourteen–fifteen-year advantage. The comparison list could go on – Vietnam and India; Eritrea and Guinea Bissau; Laos and Nigeria. Each pairing clearly shows that a certain national income level does not necessarily equate with a particular life expectancy. In other words, other factors are involved.

Contrary to what many readers might expect, there has also been little association ($r^2 = 0.01$) globally between economic growth and life expectancy change over recent decades (see Figure 4.10). The same is true when just the less developed countries are examined, though in the case of the more developed nations there has been a moderate association ($r^2 = 0.23$). The important point, however, is that significant improvements in health can be achieved without high incomes or rapid economic growth.

Health and income inequality

A topic of considerable debate in population health research over the past two decades has been whether, in addition to *absolute* income effects, health status is influenced by the distribution of income within societies (i.e. *relative* income). There is an intuitive logic to the idea that unequal income distribution negatively affects population health levels. Where a heavily disproportionate share of income (and wealth) is held by a small segment of the population, the economic capability of the remainder of the population to look after their health is compromised, particularly in very low-income, less developed nations. In rich industrialized nations, on the other hand, income inequality is argued to affect health through psycho-social pathways, with persons at the lower end of very unequal income distributions feeling, by dint of their position, unfairly disadvantaged, distrustful, stressed and lacking a sense of control over life. These feelings are seen as frequently leading to poor health behaviours, such as tobacco smoking, excessive alcohol intake, illicit drug taking, poor nutrition and inadequate physical exercise (Wilkinson and Pickett, 2009).

The negative income inequality–poor health hypothesis has become influential in research interpreting health inequalities and guiding policies to improve population health, both between and within countries. However, it has also received considerable criticism because of the lack of high-quality income distribution data for many nations, the small number of countries included in some analyses, and the lack of control at times for possible confounding factors (e.g. educational attainment, gender in/equality) (Judge *et al.*, 1998; Mackenbach, 2002). Also, while some examples may be cited of countries where a low

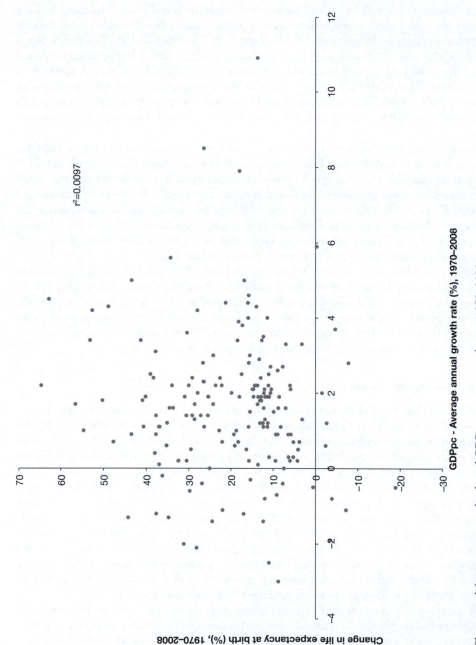

r^2=0.0097

GDPpc - Average annual growth rate (%), 1970–2008

Change in life expectancy at birth (%), 1970–2008

Figure 4.10 Change in life expectancy at birth and GDP per capita growth rate, 1970–2008

Source: WHO, *World Health Statistics* reports website

degree of income inequality seems to have been an important part of health progress beyond what national income per head would have led one to expect (e.g. Cuba, Vietnam, Sri Lanka), the wider empirical evidence is mixed. Much of the research has focused on wealthier nations and results have varied according to which countries have been included.

Our own tests of the hypothesis that income inequality has an independent effect on international population health, after controlling for per capita national income, similarly provide mixed results. For the purposes of this book, we assembled a data set combining three types of variables – health status, *absolute* income (gross national income per capita – PPP international dollars), and *relative* income (the Gini index of income inequality and the ratio of the income share of the richest 20 per cent to the poorest 20 per cent). Four health measures were selected: life expectancy at birth, the infant mortality rate, the child (under 5 years of age) mortality rate, and the adult mortality rate. The health and national income data were for 2008 while the income inequality figures were for the latest survey year. There were 142 countries for which the Gini index could be used and 124 in the case of the 20/20 ratio. Analyses were carried out for the respective 'all countries' data sets and then separately for the World Bank's low-, medium- and high-income group countries, the United Nations' least, less and more developed groupings, and the OECD group of countries. Partial correlations were calculated to test whether the income inequality measures significantly added to the explanation of the health differences between countries over and above average per capita national income.

Statistically significant contributions by income inequality were found in the following cases:

- Adult mortality (all countries) and the ratio of the richest to poorest 20 per cent (partial correlation = 0.220).
- Adult mortality (World Bank's middle-income countries) and the ratio of the richest to poorest 20 per cent (partial correlation = 0.319).
- Adult mortality (United Nations' less developed countries) and the ratio of the richest to poorest 20 per cent (partial correlation = 0.222).
- Life expectancy at birth (United Nations' least developed countries) and the ratio of the richest to poorest 20 per cent (partial correlation = -0.429).
- Adult mortality (United Nations' least developed countries) and the ratio of the richest to poorest 20 per cent (partial correlation = 0.430).
- Infant mortality (OECD countries) and the Gini index and the ratio of the richest to poorest 20 per cent (partial correlations = 0.556 and 0.630).
- Child mortality (OECD countries) and the Gini index and the ratio of the richest to poorest 20 per cent (partial correlations = 0.593 and 0.662). (In these analyses, infant and child mortality both correlated more highly with the income inequality variables than with GNI per capita.)

The results thus give some support to the income inequality hypothesis, but equally show no universal such effect. Also, other uncontrolled-for confounding factors may be involved in the above results.

The issue of income inequality and health will be returned to in the next chapter, in the context of *within*-country health differences.

Global health . . . widening the explanatory net

In the preceding two sections we have focused on the roles of national income and income inequality in determining health levels around the world. Income characteristics are clearly important, but they are not the whole story. The 'unexplained variation' in the reported statistical analyses along with the various cited examples of 'aberrant' cases (i.e. countries with better or worse health than would be expected on purely economic grounds) make this point. Of course, this also accords with the multiple determinants of health model set out in Chapter 3.

Table 4.4 portrays a little of this complexity, showing the statistical relationships between various measures of health and a wider range of hypothesized explanatory variables. The set of social, economic and infrastructure variables assembled by no means captures anything like the full array of factors that influence global health. Also, the explanatory variables are intercorrelated to varying degrees. National capacities for expenditure on health, for instance, are obviously strongly influenced by level of economic development. However, the variables do widen the perspective. Both the simple bivariate correlations (r) of each variable with each health indicator and multiple regression (R^2) results are presented. All revealed relationships are in the direction previous health research and *a priori* reasoning would suggest.

Perhaps the most interesting results shown in the table relate to the adult literacy variable, indicating the significance of social development as well as economic development for health. Money invested in raising literacy levels is one of the most productive policy options for lifting health levels, working in both direct and indirect ways. Also interesting is the drag effect on health of rapid population growth.

Table 4.4 Correlations (r and R^2) of selected health indicators with social, economic and infrastructure variables, WHO member states, late 2000s

	Health indicators			
Variables	*Life expectancy at birth (years) 2008* (r)	*Infant mortality rate 2008* (r)	*Under-5 mortality rate 2008* (r)	*Adult mortality rate 2008* (r)
Bivariate correlations				
1 Physicians per 10,000 population, 2000–09	0.677	−0.652	−0.624	−0.593
2 Hospital beds per 10,000 population, 2000–09	0.485	−0.523	−0.509	−0.386
3 Per capita total expenditure on health (PPP int.$), 2007	0.639	−0.534	−0.486	−0.553
4 Population annual growth rate (%), 1998–2008	−0.429	0.527	0.525	0.294
5 Adult literacy rate (%), 2000–08	0.689	−0.776	−0.787	−0.512
6 Gross national income per capita (PPP int.$), 2008	0.684	−0.597	−0.543	−0.598
7 Income Gini coefficient, 2000–10	−0.332	0.291	0.259	0.346
Stepwise regression models (N = 105 countries)				
R^2	0.613	0.735	0.728	0.375
Significant variables (in order of entry)	5,3	5,4,6,2	5,4,6,2	6,5

Sources: WHO, *World Health Statistics* reports and United Nations, *Human Development* reports websites

The global health divide: convergence or divergence?

There have clearly been remarkable worldwide improvements in mortality since the middle of last century and many strands of that improvement have been covered in the preceding sections of this chapter. However, have these improvements added up to a significant narrowing of the gulf in death rates among countries? Are the world's peoples moving closer towards sharing increasingly similar life expectancies, or does the global health divide remain intransigent?

To some extent, the answers to these questions depend on the approach taken to measuring the differences in mortality between countries. Using a population-weighted dispersion measure of mortality (DMM), Moser *et al.* (2005) report that from 1950 until the late 1980s there was global convergence of life expectancy at birth, but then a shift to divergence. Their DMM analysis of infant mortality, on the other hand, indicated continued convergence since 1950. Goesling and Firebaugh (2004, p. 136) report similar findings for life expectancy: 'between-country inequality declined from 1980 to about 1992, but then increased from 1992 to 2000 in a significant reversal of the long-term trend'.

However, from the point of view of (a) decadal percentage improvement in life expectancy, (b) the absolute size of the more developed–less developed world life expectancy gap, and (c) the changing ratio of average developing world life expectancy at birth to that of the more developed nations, notable convergence has occurred. To illustrate, over each of the six decades since 1950, the percentage improvement in average life expectancy at birth in less developed regions has exceeded that of the more developed regions; from an absolute life expectancy disadvantage of twenty-five years in 1950, the less developed regions now suffer an eleven-year disadvantage; and nowadays newborn children in the developing world have an average life expectancy 85 per cent of that of more developed world infants, compared with 61 per cent in 1950. Despite the improving relative position of the developing regions, though, a substantial, morally indefensible gap in life chances between that world and developed nations clearly remains to be bridged.

Epidemiological profiles

A key theme running through this chapter has been the notion of ongoing epidemiological/health transition – that is, the evolving cause of death and illness profiles of human populations over time and space. As has been shown, in broad-brush terms the transition has been from a (pre)historic infectious disease-dominated era to a world increasingly characterized by chronic, degenerative-type disease morbidity and mortality. Countries around the world are at various points on this epidemiological path, as illustrated in Figure 4.11. The data are 2008 estimates for member states of the World Health Organization and the cause of death categories are as defined by the WHO. Three basic groups of countries can be identified – *early* (N = 38), *mid* (N = 33) and *late* (N = 122) transition. As in any grouping exercise, the allocation of some border cases can be queried, but the broad tripartite division gives a useful summary view.

In all the early transition countries around six or more of every ten deaths are from communicable, maternal, perinatal and nutritional conditions. All of these countries bar two (Afghanistan and East Timor) are sub-Saharan African nations, and in several of them HIV/AIDS is a major contributor to the death statistics. The non-communicable disease toll in these countries ranges between one-sixth to one-third of deaths, with injuries accounting for the remainder. This profile is an early, emerging version of the *double burden* of disease (see the discussion of mid transition states below). An often-overlooked fact is that while the overall non-communicable disease deaths percentage is low in these countries in cases,

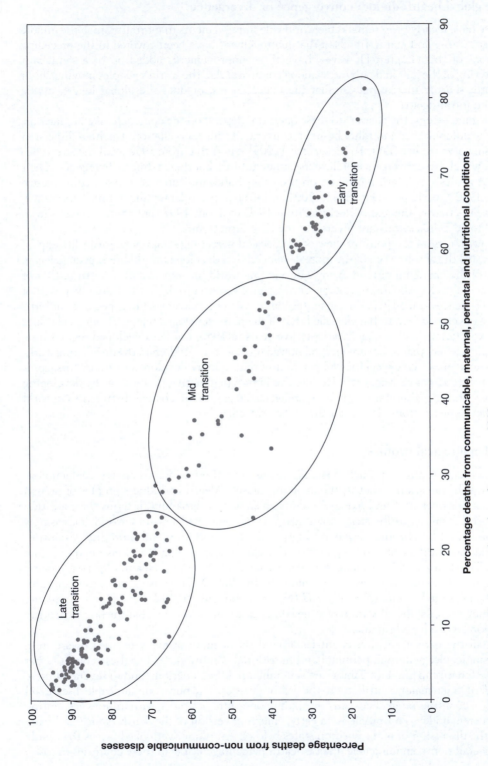

Figure 4.11 Causes of death and stage in epidemiological transition, 2008

Source: WHO, *Global Burden of Disease* website

their age-standardized death rates from degenerative conditions are higher than in many more developed countries. For example, 21 of the top (worst) quintile of age-standardized death rates from cerebrovascular disease among the 193 WHO member states in 2008 were poor, early transition countries, 16 in the top quintile for chronic obstructive pulmonary disease and liver cancer were likewise, and 14 in the case of diabetes mellitus. These 'unexpectedly' high death rates can be largely traced to inadequate degenerative disease prevention, diagnosis and treatment resources.

In the mid transition bloc, the importance of communicable, maternal, perinatal and nutritional conditions is weaker, ranging from just over half down to a quarter of all deaths. Counterbalancing this, degenerative disorders assume more importance. With the exception of Gabon, Namibia, Peru and Algeria, these are all low- or low–middle-income nations (World Bank List of Economies, December 2010). As alluded to above, countries in this middle group bear, to varying degrees, a *double burden* of disease – that is, coexisting old-style (infectious) and new-style (degenerative) health problems. Ultimately, everyone must die of something, and with the rolling back of infectious killers an increase in the proportionate importance of degenerative disease mortality is thus inevitable. However, death rates of the latter are often unnecessarily elevated in developing countries due to the increasing adoption of fat-, sugar- and salt-rich Western diets and frequently high levels of tobacco smoking. Inadequate health services are also a key factor in many of these nations. Richer groups and locations in these countries tend to be characterized by 'modern' disease profiles, while poorer groups and places often suffer more from old-style diseases. This epidemiological *polarization* poses difficult questions for the countries in terms of health resourcing priorities. A further problem is that the expanding mortality from degenerative diseases in the developing world on average occurs at significantly younger ages than in rich developed nations. The estimated median ages of persons dying from non-communicable diseases (all types combined) in low- and middle-income countries, for example, are respectively fifteen years and nine years lower than the comparable median in high-income nations. Table 4.5 details the gaps for selected specific causes of death. The limited prevention, diagnostic and treatment services for cancer, heart disease, COPD and other degenerative disorders in much of the developing world are major factors behind these disparities. In the case of cancer, for instance, around fifteen African nations and several countries in Asia do not have a single radiation therapy machine (IAEA, 2003).

In the final group (late transition), the bulk of deaths are from non-communicable conditions, as infections are no longer major killers (less than 25 per cent of deaths). The countries in this group are a mix of rich developed nations and more economically and/or socially advanced developing states.

Table 4.5 Median age at death from selected non-communicable causes of death, by WHO income group, estimates for 2008

Causes of death	High-income countries Median age (years)	Middle-income countries Median age (years)	Low-income countries Median age (years)
Total non-communicable diseases	80	71	65
Malignant neoplasms	74	64	58
Diabetes mellitus	78	70	67
Cardiovascular diseases	82	74	69
Respiratory diseases	81	75	66

Source: WHO, *Global Burden of Disease* website

Table 4.6 Leading causes of death, selected WHO member states at different stages of epidemiological transition, estimates for 2008

Early transition

Angola (e_0 = 46)	% of Deaths	Chad (e_0 = 46)	% of Deaths	Sierra Leone (e_0 = 49)	% of Deaths
Lower respiratory infections	14.6	Malaria	13.7	Malaria	15.9
Diarrhoeal diseases	14.0	Lower respiratory infections	13.5	Lower respiratory infections	12.9
Malaria	6.5	Diarrhoeal diseases	12.3	Diarrhoeal diseases	10.4
HIV/AIDS	4.8	HIV/AIDS	6.7	Tuberculosis	8.6
Prematurity and low birthweight	3.8	Tuberculosis	3.9	Prematurity and low birthweight	4.4

Mid transition

Cambodia (e_0 = 62)	% of Deaths	Pakistan (e_0 = 63)	% of Deaths	Yemen (e_0 = 64)	% of Deaths
Lower respiratory infections	12.9	Ischaemic heart disease	13.3	Ischaemic heart disease	11.8
Tuberculosis	9.5	Lower respiratory infections	12.6	Lower respiratory infections	11.5
Ischaemic heart disease	7.5	Diarrhoeal diseases	7.6	Diarrhoeal diseases	9.5
Cerebrovascular disease	5.7	Cerebrovascular disease	6.9	Prematurity and low birthweight	5.9
Hypertensive heart disease	3.4	Tuberculosis	4.8	Road traffic accidents	4.3

Late transition

Canada (e_0 = 81)	% of Deaths	South Korea (e_0 = 80)	% of Deaths	Sweden (e_0 = 81)	% of Deaths
Ischaemic heart disease	17.9	Cerebrovascular disease	15.2	Ischaemic heart disease	19.0
Trachea, bronchus, lung cancers	7.7	Ischaemic heart disease	8.1	Cerebrovascular disease	9.4
Cerebrovascular disease	6.6	Trachea, bronchus, lung cancers	6.5	Alzheimer's and other dementias	7.0
Alzheimer's and other dementias	5.1	Diabetes mellitus	5.4	Trachea, bronchus, lung cancers	4.0
Chronic obstructive pulmonary disease	4.3	Stomach cancer	5.0	Colon and rectum cancers	3.3

Note: e_0 = life expectancy at birth (years), 2008.
Source: WHO, Global Burden of Disease website

While the broad 'stage of transition' groupings of Figure 4.11 are useful, it is important to dig beneath them. Countries that have similar epidemiological profiles in this coarse typology may differ in important ways when a finer-grained cause of death classification is used. Tables 4.6–4.8 illustrate this point. In Table 4.6 the chosen countries clearly show the heavy infectious disease dominance of early-stage transition, the infectious and degenerative disease mix of mid-stage transition, and the predominantly degenerative disease pattern of late-stage transition populations. But treating Cambodia and Pakistan (Table 4.6, middle panel), for example, as epidemiological clones would miss important distinctive elements of their respective infectious disease profiles. Likewise, in the late-transition examples (Table 4.6, bottom panel), South Korea does not show the ischaemic heart disease dominance found in Canada and Sweden, cerebrovascular disease (stroke) instead being its leading cause of death. Other late-transition variability is illustrated in Table 4.7, where six ostensibly demographically alike European nations (i.e. sharing similar life expectancies, median ages and proportions aged 65 and over) show no common cause of death mix can be assumed. Table 4.8, detailing selected national cancer profiles, demonstrates the same point at a finer

Table 4.7 Epidemiological variability between selected European countries with similar life expectancy and age structures, 2008

Country	Malignant neoplasms (Cancer) (C00–C97)* % deaths	Ischaemic heart disease (I20–I25) plus other heart diseases (I30–I33, I39–I52)* % deaths	Cerebrovascular diseases (Stroke) (I60–I69)* % deaths	Life expectancy (years)	Median age (years)	Persons aged 65+ (%)
Slovenia	31	22	11	79	41	16
Netherlands	30	18	7	80	40	15
France	28	16	6	81	40	17
Austria	26	28	7	80	41	17
Greece	25	27	15	80	41	18
Portugal	23	13	14	79	40	18

Note: * ICD-10 codes.
Sources: Eurostat Database and WHO, *World Health Statistics* reports websites

Table 4.8 Differing national cancer profiles, estimates for 2008

Country	Percentage of all deaths from cancers	Cancer site (percentage of cancer deaths)					
		Oesophagus	Stomach	Colon and rectum	Liver	Trachea, bronchus, lung	Breast
South Korea	30	2	17	10	16	22	2
Denmark	30	3	3	15	2	24	9
China	21	11	18	6	19	23	2
Serbia	21	1	6	13	4	24	8
Guatemala	11	1	22	3	15	6	3
Jordan	11	1	4	11	2	9	12

Source: WHO, *Global Burden of Disease* website

scale again. It is common in the population health literature (and we ourselves do it in places in this book) to treat cancer deaths as a collective entity and for countries with a similar proportion of deaths from cancer to be treated as epidemiologically akin. However, the three paired examples presented in Table 4.8 show this can mask what may be large proportional differences between cancer sites with significance for prevention and care programmes.

Adding morbidity to epidemiological profiles

In Chapter 2, we drew attention to the need to incorporate morbidity as well as mortality into assessments and comparisons of population health and introduced various so-called 'summary measures of population health' – measures which combine information on both mortality and morbidity into a single number. As noted there, one of the most useful and widely used such indicators is the DALY (disability-adjusted life year), which is calculated as the years of life lost to premature mortality plus equivalent years of healthy life lost due to poor health or a disability. One DALY is equal to one lost year of healthy life.

Table 4.9 presents summary WHO statistics of causes of death and DALYs for high-, middle- and low-income countries in 2008. The cause of death figures will engender little surprise given data and discussion earlier in this chapter. However, the DALY listings reveal a number of conditions that make important contributions to global, regional, national and local disease burdens, but which do not stand out in cause of death tabulations. Neuropsychiatric disorders, for example, account for only around 2.2 per cent of global deaths each year, but constitute an estimated 14.0 per cent of DALYs. In the high-income bloc of countries, these disorders contribute a quarter of the total disease burden. Even in low-income countries these conditions account for a tenth of the disease burden. Injuries are another area of health that show up in a more substantial light when DALY figures rather than just total (i.e. all ages) deaths are considered.

The relativities also work the other way. For example, cardiovascular diseases are estimated to cause 30 per cent of global deaths, but only about 10 per cent of the world's disease burden. Similarly cancer's global disease burden is substantially smaller than its relative contribution to mortality. The differences between total death and DALY disease standings flow from the DALY calculation only including premature deaths, giving early premature deaths heavier weighting than deaths later in life, and likewise weighting morbidity of early onset and long duration and severity most heavily. As noted in Chapter 2, the DALY measure is open to some criticism, but it does offer a useful, more conceptually complete picture of population health than mortality alone and, data allowing, should be incorporated in standard population health assessments, priority setting and resource allocation.

Alternative epidemiological profiles: the 'real causes' of death and ill-health

The causes of death and DALYs discussed throughout this chapter are based on the World Health Organization's *International Classification of Diseases* (ICD), which was outlined in Chapter 2. This is the conventional way of categorizing, labelling and analysing health disorders. By this schema heart disease, cancer, cerebrovascular disease, chronic obstructive pulmonary disease, pneumonia, tuberculosis, diarrhoeal diseases (e.g. shigellosis, typhoid, rotaviral enteritis, cholera), HIV/AIDS, malaria, etc. are what cause death and the loss of years of healthy life through illness or disability.

These terms describe pathological outcomes and end-states, but it can be argued those pathologies are not what really kill us. Rather, the real (actual) causes of death are the factors that lead to these pathologies. This takes us back to the conceptual discussion of

Table 4.9 Major causes of death and DALYs, World and WHO income groups, 2008

Cause	World %	High-income countries %	Middle-income countries %	Low-income countries %
Deaths				
Communicable, maternal, perinatal and nutritional conditions	27.2	6.4	14.0	46.9
Infectious and parasitic diseases	14.3	2.0	7.2	25.3
Respiratory infections	6.5	3.8	3.5	10.3
Perinatal conditions	5.0	0.4	2.6	8.8
Non-communicable diseases	63.2	87.5	75.2	43.5
Malignant neoplasms	13.8	26.6	16.4	7.0
Neuropsychiatric disorders	2.2	5.7	1.7	1.7
Cardiovascular diseases	30.4	37.1	37.6	21.3
Respiratory diseases	7.5	5.8	10.0	5.7
Injuries	9.6	6.1	10.8	9.6
DALYs				
Communicable, maternal, perinatal and nutritional conditions	36.0	5.7	19.7	52.0
Infectious and parasitic diseases	18.0	2.3	9.4	26.5
Respiratory infections	5.6	1.1	2.5	8.4
Perinatal conditions	8.0	1.2	4.9	11.3
Non-communicable diseases	51.4	85.6	65.0	36.7
Malignant neoplasms	5.7	14.8	7.8	2.8
Neuropsychiatric disorders	14.0	26.2	17.3	9.8
Cardiovascular diseases	10.5	14.5	13.6	7.6
Respiratory diseases	4.3	6.0	5.5	3.1
Injuries	12.6	8.7	15.3	11.3

Note: These cause of death statistics by income groups differ from the figures for 2008 presented in Table 4.1. The statistics in this table (Table 4.9) were calculated earlier (released in October 2008) and use an earlier United Nations *World Population Prospects* database. The statistics in Table 4.1 were released in May 2011. The country listings in the income groups used in Tables 4.1 and 4.9 are not identical.

Source: WHO, *Global Burden of Disease* website

the determinants of population health in Chapter 3 and the notion of *midstream* and *upstream* factors influencing the ultimate *downstream* biological production of good and bad health. For example, many deaths from heart disease, lung cancer and COPD are really due to tobacco smoking. The death certificate and ICD designations of heart disease, lung cancer and COPD are simply the end-state pathological conditions that brought life to an end.

In a 1993 study, McGinnis and Foege made a pioneering quantitative estimation of the actual causes of death in the United States, drawing on seventeen years of published health risk research to guide their calculations. The three leading causes identified were tobacco, diet/activity patterns and alcohol. Several further US studies along the same lines have since been done, as well as some in other countries.

Similar research has been conducted at the international level, mainly under the auspices of the World Health Organization. Much of this work was brought together in a recent major publication titled *Global Health Risks* (WHO, 2009a). This volume reports quantitative estimates of the comparative health risks of twenty-four physiological, behavioural, environmental and economic factors. Collectively, the twenty-four risk factors were estimated to be responsible for 44 per cent of global deaths and 33 per cent of DALYs. One-third of global deaths were accounted for by the ten leading risk factors and a quarter of all deaths by just five factors. The five leading global risks for mortality were identified as: high blood pressure; tobacco use; high blood glucose; physical inactivity; and overweight and obesity. For the burden of disease (measured by DALYs), the leading five were: childhood underweight; unsafe sex; alcohol use; unsafe water, sanitation and hygiene; and high blood pressure. One message coming from this research is how reducing exposure to a relatively small number of risk factors would significantly lift global life expectancy. For example, the WHO researchers attribute around five years of life expectancy loss to just the five leading risks and close to seven years to the leading ten risk factors.

Table 4.10 summarizes the estimated five leading risk factors causing deaths and DALYs by income groupings of countries. Developing intervention strategies to address the various sets of risks is essential for improving global health.

However, these risks are themselves underlain by other factors. For example, in all three country groupings lifestyle/behavioural risks play major roles. At first glance the road to better global health therefore might just seem to be to convince people to change their lifestyles and behaviours. This is the territory of classic health promotion – to convince people to stop smoking, to consume less alcohol, to eat more healthily, to exercise more, to

Table 4.10 Five leading risk factor causes of death and DALYs, by WHO income group, WHO member states, estimates for 2004

Deaths

High-income countries	% of deaths	Middle-income countries	% of deaths	Low-income countries	% of deaths
Tobacco use	17.9	High blood pressure	17.2	Childhood underweight	7.8
High blood pressure	16.8	Tobacco use	10.8	High blood pressure	7.5
Overweight and obesity	8.4	Overweight and obesity	6.7	Unsafe sex	6.6
Physical inactivity	7.7	Physical inactivity	6.6	Unsafe water, sanitation, hygiene	6.1
High blood glucose	7.0	Alcohol use	6.4	High blood glucose	4.9

DALYs

High-income countries	% of DALYs	Middle-income countries	% of DALYs	Low-income countries	% of DALYs
Tobacco use	10.7	Alcohol use	7.6	Childhood underweight	9.9
Alcohol use	6.7	High blood pressure	5.5	Unsafe water, sanitation, hygiene	6.3
Overweight and obesity	6.5	Tobacco use	5.5	Unsafe sex	6.2
High blood pressure	6.1	Overweight and obesity	3.6	Suboptimal breastfeeding	4.1
High blood glucose	4.9	High blood glucose	3.4	Indoor smoke from solid fuels	4.0

Note: The World Bank income groups in this table contain different countries from those in Tables 4.1 and 4.5, which are based on more recently defined groupings.

Source: WHO, 2009a

avoid unsafe sex, etc. But deeper, structural forces (upstream factors) underlie many risky behaviours. To take the unsafe sex risk factor in low-income countries as an example, simply informing women and men of the dangers of unprotected sex and making condoms available will only improve health so far. More fundamental strategies aimed at such things as reducing poverty and improving the status of women are the deeper keys to success. The 'real' causes of death and ill-health are thus in reality these forces – poverty, inequality, unequal power relations, structured discrimination and marginalization, poor governance, and the like.

Concluding notes – continuing and emerging challenges to global health

As will hopefully be clear from reading this chapter, the human health journey has come a remarkably long way. Equally, however, there is a long way to go before full human health potentials are realized and a just and equitable global population health achieved.

At present the major 'unfinished business' in global health is bridging the gap between the health expectancies of rich and poor nations. As shown, the gap has been narrowing, but there is still a considerable distance to go before newborn children in developing countries share the same health and longevity prospects as their fortunate counterparts in the rich developed nations. Under this overall 'unfinished business' umbrella is an array of specific challenges: reducing existing infectious disease threats; improving maternal and reproductive health; reducing infant and child mortality; preventing avoidable degenerative disease; reducing sub-national (e.g. geographic, social, ethnic) disparities in health; overcoming indigenous health disadvantage; eliminating gender- and age-based health problems and inequalities; attacking unhealthy lifestyles and behaviours; and various others.

At the same time, there are substantial unfolding new challenges in global health. Especially significant ones include: emerging and re-emerging infectious diseases; the health threats of climate and other environmental change; global population ageing; the emerging obesity 'epidemic'; the growing mental health burden of disease; bioterrorism and other geopolitical health threats. In the remaining chapters of the book, we examine these and other old and new challenges.

Discussion topics

1 To what extent would you say the main health problems in your country are a result of the population's personal health behaviour failings, or to deeper societal and global factors?
2 Do you believe globalization is primarily 'good' or 'bad' for global population health?

5 Global health

Sub-national inequalities

Introduction

The focus in Chapter 4 was on health inequalities at the nation-state and regional levels: that is, health differences *between* countries and groupings of countries. The various health statistics reported (e.g. life expectancy levels, infant mortality rates, cause of death percentages, hospital bed/population and physician/population ratios, per capita health expenditures, etc.) were aggregate national and regional averages. Underlying these averages, however, are sub-national variations, disparities in health status, healthcare resources and the use of health service *within* countries. The array and magnitude of such inequalities vary from nation to nation, but no country is free of them. The major cleavage lines are socio-economic status, ethnicity and race, sex and gender, and geographical location. Frequently, the dimensions of inequality overlap. Ethnic/racial disparities, for example, often also involve socio-economic and gender-based layers. Similarly, geographic inequalities in health often incorporate both place and socio-economic elements.

If the two basic goals of global health – improving the health of all peoples and eliminating health inequities (Box 5.1) – are to be achieved, it is important to pay attention to health heterogeneity *within* countries as well as *between* countries. The internal heterogeneity is, by definition, what combines to produce a country's aggregate health profile and hence is critical to understanding the national situation and to guiding policy and programme development. Unfortunately, the availability and quality of sub-national health data is limited for many countries around the world, particularly low-income developing nations. The data situation is especially weak in relation to socio-economic, ethnic/racial and sex/gender health disparities. Geographic differences tend to be somewhat better documented.

National health statistics indicating improving population health can hide the fact that not all segments of the population may be equally sharing that progress and that some groups may indeed be experiencing deteriorating health status. The following are just a few of many possible examples:

- Philippines: over the period 1980–2006 average national life expectancy at birth increased by around eight years, but in two provinces (Tawi-Tawi and Sulu) it declined (Gualvez, 2010).
- United States: while national life expectancy climbed by two years between 1983 and 1999, in a substantial number of counties mortality actually increased, especially for women (Ezzati *et al.*, 2008).
- India: the national maternal mortality ratio (per 100,000 live births) fell by over 15 per cent between 2001–03 and 2004–06, but in Haryana State it increased by 15 per cent and in Punjab by 8 per cent (Central Bureau of Health Intelligence – India, 2010).

- Guyana, Swaziland, Tonga: between 2000 and 2009 overall national life expectancy at birth rose. In each case the male level increased, but that for females declined. In Armenia, Georgia and Niue, meanwhile, male life expectancy was reported as falling, while that of females rose (WHO, 2011a).
- Cambodia, Haiti, Togo, Yemen: under-5 mortality declined in all four countries during the early 2000s, but in each case the percentage decline for the poorest quintile was substantially less than that of the richest quintile and the poor/rich rate ratio widened (WHO, *World Health Statistics* website).

Knowing how health is differentially distributed within a country is the desirable base on which to develop population health policies and interventionary strategies. If health disadvantage can be identified as being highly concentrated in a particular population group or areas, interventions can be targeted to that group or those areas (i.e. a *selectivist* approach). Alternatively, where data show across-the-board poor health a *universalist* approach, whereby all segments of the population are targeted, is more appropriate. Some dimensions of health inequality (e.g. economic, educational) often show a gradient pattern, health outcomes steadily worsening with progressively lower position on the dimension concerned. In such cases just targeting persons in the bottom ('worst-off') group misses significant health disadvantage further up the 'ladder' and a mix of universalist and selectivist approaches may be the best strategy. Van de Poel *et al.* (2008) show the relevance of socio-economic inequality patterns for setting health policies and programmes to reduce childhood malnutrition in developing countries. Geographic patterning is also significant. In India, for example, childhood malnutrition is a serious country-wide problem. However, four states (Uttar Pradesh, Madhya Pradesh, Bihar and Rajasthan) account for 43 per cent of all underweight children (Gragnolati *et al.*, 2005). This geography suggests a combination of country-wide and spatially targeted action.

Ideally data on internal health inequalities should be available on a regular, ongoing basis, enabling the effects of policies and programmes to achieve greater equity to be assessed and, where appropriate, modified. Unfortunately, however, as noted above, many less developed nations do not have these data resources, making effective health planning, monitoring and evaluation more difficult. However, USAID's Demographic and Health Survey (DHS) programme, the WHO's World Health Survey, the Global Equity Gauge Alliance (GEGA) initiative (http://www.gega.org.za) and other population health data-gathering efforts are improving the situation.

BOX 5.1 Health inequalities and health inequities

Population health analysts distinguish between health *inequalities* and health *inequities*.

Health inequality is the generic term for the differences (disparities, variations) in the health of individuals and groups between and within countries – for example, life expectancy variations between WHO member states; infant mortality differences between the constituent states/provinces/counties, income/wealth quintiles, ethnic groups, and age and sex groups of countries; maternal health differences by level of education, etc.

These inequalities can be expressed in absolute or relative terms.

continued

Absolute:

- Life expectancy at birth around the world in 2009 ranged from 83 years in Japan and San Marino to 47 years in Malawi.
- Between 1989–91 and 2002–04 the infant mortality rate gap between blacks and whites in the United States fell from +9.9 to +8.0 deaths per 1,000 live births.

Relative:

- Malawi's life expectancy at birth level is only 57 per cent of Japan's.
- In the periods 1989–91 and 2002–04 the infant mortality rate of blacks in the United States was 2.4 times that of whites.

Health *inequities* are viewed as those inequalities in health which are unnecessary and avoidable and involve some form of injustice. Identifying inequities thus involves normative judgement: what is avoidable (preventable) and what is unjust (unfair)?

Differences in health stemming from natural, biological variations (e.g. the higher risk of heart disease or stroke in the elderly than in young adults; genetic disorders) or freely chosen health-damaging behaviour, for example, would not generally be seen as inequities. But morbidity and mortality due to poor living and working conditions, or because of unequal access to education, healthcare services or safe water supplies would be, as they are both avoidable and unjust.

Not all cases are clear cut, though. Advances in medical science (e.g. stem cell technology, genomics) change the notion of what is avoidable and unavoidable. Likewise, what is freely chosen behaviour is not always clear. Is tobacco smoking genuinely freely chosen behaviour, or is it socially conditioned and patterned? Similarly, heavy alcohol or fast-food consumption?

(Reading: Whitehead, 1990)

Dimensions of health inequality within countries

Socio-economic status

(Note: in the epidemiological and public health literature, alternate terms, such as 'social class' and 'socio-economic position', are sometimes used in place of 'socio-economic status'.) Just as the socio-economic standing of countries plays an important role in determining international health status, the socio-economic status of individuals and groups critically influences health variations within countries. Socio-economic status has three primary dimensions – income (and wealth), education and occupation. These dimensions influence health in multiple ways, some direct, others indirect. They also overlap and interact, making it difficult to disentangle causal pathways and establish the impact of any single factor. The health effects of socio-economic status factors are often also mediated by other influences (e.g. internal politics, geographic location, age, family composition). Despite these complexities, policies and programmes targeted at mitigating the effects of socio-economic status on health offer the greatest potential health gains in most countries.

Income and wealth

Income and wealth differences are major determinants of health disparities within countries, working in various ways. Most obvious are the *direct* impacts through influencing the material standards of living that in turn affect health status (e.g. housing quality, nutritional level attainable) and the capacity to purchase healthcare. Advocates of the relative income–health hypothesis (introduced in Chapter 4) argue that low income also operates more *indirectly*, producing feelings of relative deprivation, alienation and stress that ultimately translate biologically into poor health. However, the latter socio-psychological mechanisms remain a matter of conjecture and debate.

Establishing income's impact on health is made difficult by the variable's relationship with the other two major dimensions of socio-economic status – education and occupation. A documented relationship between low income and poor health, for instance, may in part be a marker of harsh working conditions rather than solely an income effect. Likewise, low income may reflect low education and perhaps poor health knowledge and consequent risky behaviours.

There is a tendency in income/wealth–health analyses and policy interventions to focus on *poverty* and health: that is, the bottom end of the income/wealth hierarchy. This is perhaps understandable as improving the health of the poorest people in society is an obvious important goal. But inequality in health is not confined to the 'poor' versus the 'non-poor' (Wilkinson and Marmot, 2003). More frequently there is a social gradient of health, with health tending to worsen with progression down the income/wealth (and educational and occupational) ladder. By just focusing on those at the bottom of the ladder, much avoidable ill-health will be missed. Figure 5.1 illustrates this, showing the wealth gradient of childhood (under-5 years) mortality in Nigeria, Bolivia and Indonesia with data from recent DHS surveys. The accompanying Figure 5.2 summarizes the poorest–richest divide on the same mortality indicator across sixty-three countries. The average poor/rich rate ratio across the set of countries is 2.0.

While the strong positive relationship between income/wealth and health within countries is one of the most repeatedly reported, it is not absolutely universal. One exception that has attracted considerable attention is the so-called 'Hispanic mortality paradox' in the United States – that is, despite having lower average incomes and educational levels and higher poverty rates, Hispanics live longer than non-Hispanic white Americans (Arias, 2010). In the past it has been suggested that the difference was a data artefact, but recent research has rejected that. An alternative hypothesis is the 'healthy migrant effect': that the Hispanics who immigrate to the United States are among the healthiest of their home country populations. It has also been suggested that the immigrants bring with them a healthier diet and lifestyle (e.g. less fattening food, lower cigarette-smoking prevalence). Strong cultural and family ties in the Hispanic community have also been hypothesized as beneficial factors. The paradox, however, is not a totally across-the-board pattern. Hispanics have higher death rates than non-Hispanic whites from diabetes, chronic liver disease and cirrhosis, homicide and HIV.

Besides health status, health knowledge and healthcare access, utilization and quality also vary by income and wealth. For the poor in most countries, access to health services is problematic. The availability of services is frequently limited and cost considerations are often a major barrier. The Demographic and Health Surveys (DHS) programme has produced useful data on many of these issues for a wide sweep of developing countries. With respect to health knowledge (literacy), for example, the 2005–06 India DHS survey found only one-quarter of women in the lowest wealth quintile reported having heard of AIDS. In the middle quintile the proportion was 60 per cent and in the richest quintile it was 92 per

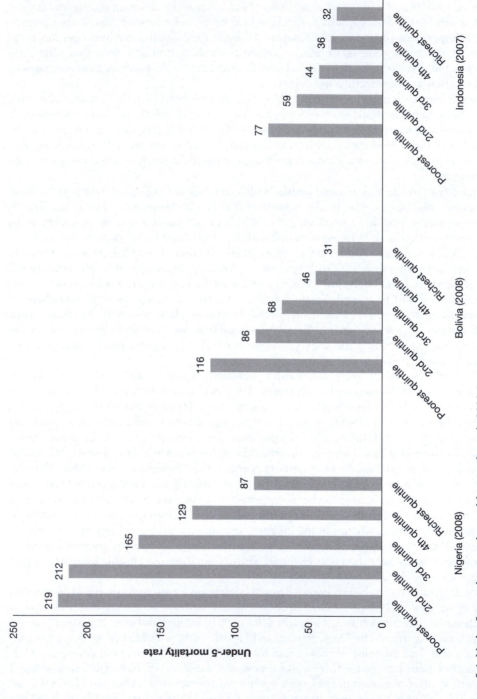

Figure 5.1 Under-5 mortality rates by wealth quintile, early 2000s*

Note: * Data relate to the decade preceding the survey.
Source: Demographic and Health Surveys website

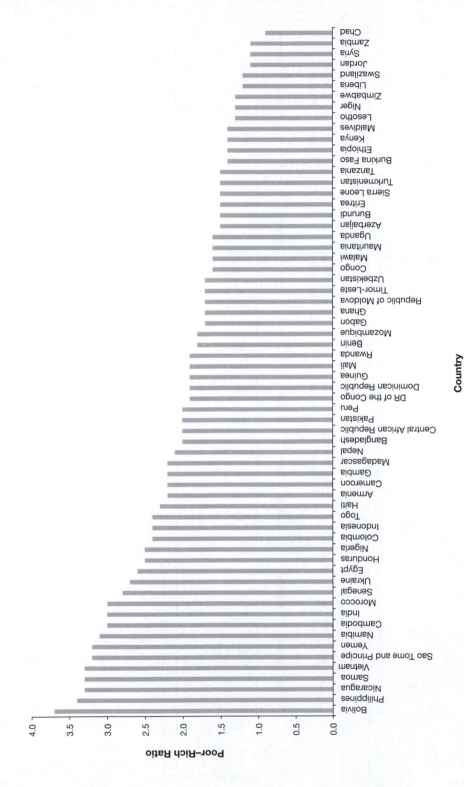

Figure 5.2 Under-5 mortality rate, ratio of rate in poorest quintile to rate in richest quintile, early 2000s*

Note: * Data relate to the decade preceding the survey.
Source: WHO, 2011a

Table 5.1 Percentage of women reporting serious problems in accessing healthcare: Bolivia, Egypt, Philippines, 2008

						Problem								
Wealth quintile	Getting money for treatment %			Distance to health facility %			Concern no provider available %			Concern no female provider available %		
	Bolivia	Egypt	Philippines	Bolivia	Egypt	Philippines	Bolivia	Egypt	Philippines	Bolivia	Egypt	Philippines
Lowest	82	70	74	76	29	58	80	72	54	61	51	30
Second	72	56	65	57	22	34	77	69	46	57	45	22
Third	66	47	60	51	18	26	75	67	36	55	40	17
Fourth	56	36	48	46	12	17	74	62	33	51	37	13
Highest	36	16	38	33	7	13	63	47	23	39	30	10

Source: Demographic and Health Surveys website

cent. In the case of tuberculosis (TB), a problem across all of India, nearly all women in the highest quintile had heard of the disease, but in the poorest group only three-quarters had. Awareness that TB spread through the air by coughing and sneezing was reported by seven out of ten people in the richest quintile, but by under 40 per cent of those in the poorest.

Accessing healthcare can involve multiple major problems – the distance to facilities, getting to services, being able to meet the cost of treatment, the availability of (culturally desired) providers, etc. All of these considerations invariably press most heavily on the poor (see Table 5.1).

The majority of key negative health behaviours (e.g. cigarette smoking, heavy alcohol use, drug taking) display similar economic gradients – in both developing and developed countries. Figure 5.3 illustrates with reference to cigarette smoking in India and the United States.

Educational attainment

Individuals and groups with high educational levels generally have better health than those with limited or no formal education. Like income, people's educational levels influence their health in a number of ways – again via both direct and indirect pathways. The direct influences are through health knowledge ('literacy'), attitudes and behaviour. In the case of health knowledge, schooling contributes in two ways. First, aspects of health usually form part of the core primary and secondary teaching curricula in most educational systems and a body of basic health knowledge on things such as the importance of hygiene and good nutrition, infectious diseases, threats to health and the like is acquired and (hopefully) attitudinal and behavioural foundations for healthy living laid. Second, there are the generic capabilities (e.g. reading, writing, evaluating, discussing) that education develops in people and enables them to acquire and understand health information and instructions, recognize personal and family ill-health symptoms, and have the ability and confidence to negotiate health systems.

In addition to these pathways, education influences health indirectly through its ties with income and occupation. While different levels of education do not rigidly translate to given types of occupations and income, higher-educated individuals are generally better placed to gain higher-status jobs and financial returns and, in turn, better health. For developing world countries, expanding educational participation and duration, particularly for girls, is probably the best long-term investment in health improvement that can be made. Better-educated young women are in turn better placed to enter the formal workforce and make higher contributions to their nations' economies. Figures 5.3–5.5 give several illustrations of how strongly health varies by educational attainment.

Occupations

Significant health differences between occupational groups are found in all countries. In part these reflect the direct influences on health of workplace hazards. Depending on their particular work environment, workers may be exposed to:

- physical hazards – e.g. heat, noise, radiation, dust, vibration;
- mechanical hazards – e.g. unsafe structures, unshielded machinery;
- chemical hazards – e.g. pesticides, solvents, gases, acids, metals;
- biological hazards – e.g. bacteria, parasites, viruses;
- psycho-social hazards – e.g. stress, monotony, workforce bullying, excessively long working hours; and
- regulatory hazards – e.g. inadequate safety standards, poor enforcement frameworks.

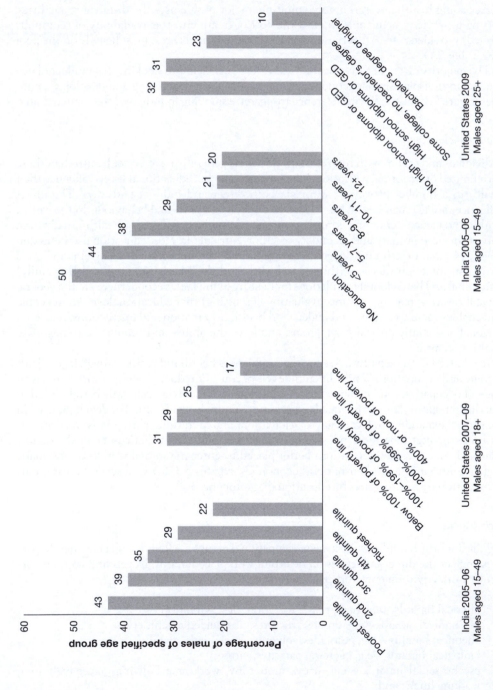

Figure 5.3 Current cigarette smoking by economic status and educational attainment, adult males, India and the United States, early 2000s

Sources: Demographic and Health Surveys website; NCHS, 2011

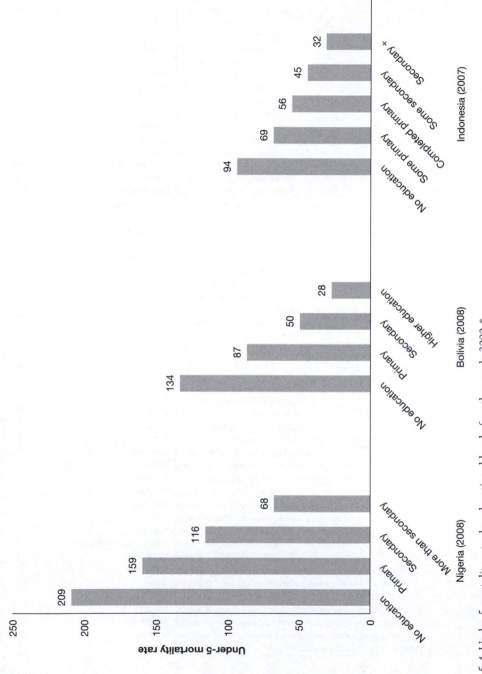

Figure 5.4 Under-5 mortality rates by educational level of mother, early 2000s*

Note: * Data relate to the decade preceding the survey.
Source: Demographic and Health Surveys website

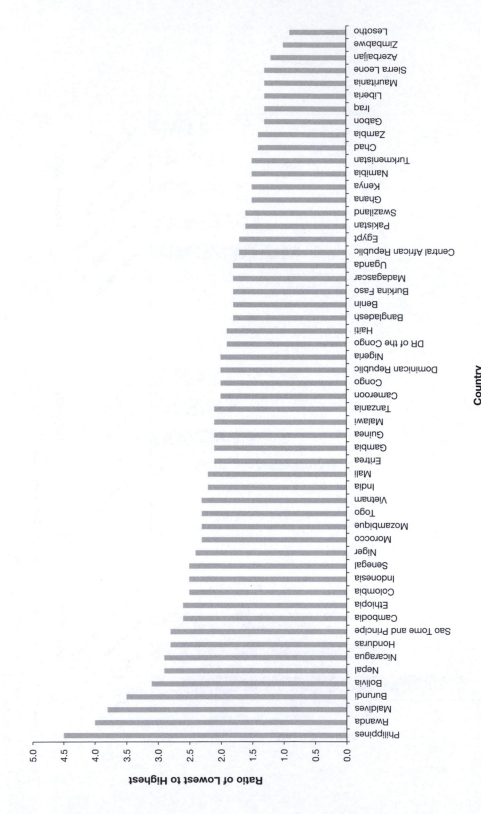

Figure 5.5 Under-5 mortality rate, ratio of rate for mothers with the lowest educational level to rate for mothers with the highest educational level, early 2000s*

Note: Lowest level is 'no education'; highest level is 'secondary education or above'; * Data relate to the decade preceding the survey.
Source: WHO, 2011a

Accentuating the impact of workplace hazards is that exposure to them is usually in confined spaces. For example, everyday living exposes virtually everyone to various types of chemicals and metals (e.g. pesticide residues on food, benzene-based products, chemicals in plastics, aluminium, lead, asbestos), but workers in industries producing or using such products generally have more intense and extended exposures. Generally workers in agriculture–fishing–forestry, mining, transportation and construction suffer the highest occupational injury death rates. In the United States, for example, deaths per 100,000 employed workers in those four industries in 2008 were respectively 30.4, 18.1, 14.9 and 9.7 (NCHS, 2011). In China, coal mining stands out, causing 85 per cent of all occupational injuries and diseases. In 2003 the industry was associated with 558,000 reported cases of pneumoconiosis (a lung disease caused by chronic inhalation of inorganic dust) with mortality rate of more than 30 per cent (WHO and China State Council DRC, 2005).

In most cases, however, the greater part of inequalities in mortality between occupation groups is reflective of the respective workers' educational and income levels, rather than risks associated with the jobs *per se*. The on-average shorter lives of unskilled manual workers compared to professional persons, for example, are more due to their generally lower education and wages than direct health-threatening dangers of their jobs. Occupational mortality differentials are thus principally socio-economic markers, though the direct loss of life through workplace injury or disease clearly remains a concern.

Life expectancy and other mortality indicators generally improve from low to high occupational status, though the steepness of the inequalities 'ladder' varies from country to country. Figure 5.6 illustrates the patterns for males in England and Wales for 1982–86 and 2002–06. Some argue the gradient reflects, besides occupational status, the degree of job control workers in the different occupational classes have (Wilkinson and Marmot, 2003). Ideally, occupational mortality inequalities should be disaggregated by causes of death and routinely monitored for trends to guide health planning. Data along these lines from the Australian Institute of Health and Welfare (2005) show differing manual/non-manual mortality gaps for males (aged 20–59) by cause and over time. For example, the disadvantage of male manual workers is especially marked for drug dependence, lung cancer, cirrhosis of the liver, pneumonia and influenza, and motor vehicle traffic accident mortality, and for some causes (e.g. lung cancer, ischaemic heart disease, diabetes) the relative disadvantage has been increasing.

In the case of morbidity, occupational group differences are again socio-economic markers, but much also flows from the workplace environment. Occupations involving heavy physical work, for instance, tend to have high injury rates. Australian data for 2005–06 serve as an illustration: the occupation groups with the highest injury rates were intermediate production and transport workers, tradespeople and related workers, and labourers and related workers. These three occupations accounted for 45 per cent of all injured workers, yet represented only 29 per cent of all employed persons. Many occupations within these groups involve physical work. By contrast, advanced clerical and service workers and professionals recorded the lowest injury rates (Australian Bureau of Statistics, 2007).

In developing countries many occupations carry high morbidity risks. Agriculture, the mainstay for the bulk of the economically active population in most such countries, involves exposure to a variety of health threats, such as pesticide poisoning, water-borne and water-associated diseases in irrigated areas (e.g. schistosomiasis, malaria, Japanese encephalitis, dengue), zoonotic infections from farm animals (e.g. avian and swine influenza). In many cases all family members – men, women and children – are involved in agriculture, inflating the associated disease burden. The poverty and poor living conditions of many rural dwellers accentuates these health problems.

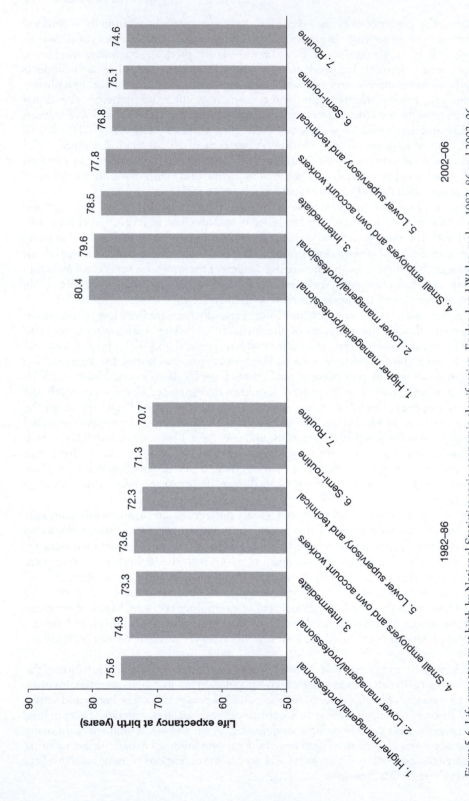

Figure 5.6 Life expectancy at birth by National Statistics socio-economic classification, England and Wales, males, 1982–86 and 2002–06

Source: United Kingdom Office for National Statistics, 2011

Other occupational sectors also carry disease-specific risks. Mining, as mentioned above with respect to China, produces a heavy toll in lung disease (e.g. silicosis, coal workers' pneumoconiosis) and injuries in many countries. With improved safety infrastructure, worker training and personal protective equipment (e.g. dust masks, respirators) much of this toll could be readily eliminated. The expanding manufacturing sector in the developing world also presents employees with many serious health risks. In general, industrial occupational health and safety considerations are accorded less attention than in more developed countries. Regulations are in place in some countries but often are not enforced. Depending on the industry involved, workers frequently face dangerous chemical exposures, heat and noise stress, toxic dust inhalation, unsafe machinery, forced lengthy working hours, poor workplace ergonomics and abusive factory floor labour management, but those desperate for work have little option other than to accept whatever conditions exist. With the search for lower production costs, many developed world corporations have set up factories (or subcontracted with local suppliers) in the developing world with workplace conditions that would not be legally permissible in their home countries. One particularly reprehensible aspect is the exploitative, sweatshop use of child labour in many countries. Apart from commonly causing physical and psychological damage, child labour hinders children's education and hence later life prospects. By the same token, neither sweatshops nor child workforces are totally foreign to contemporary developed nations.

Sex and gender

Health differences between males and females are a fundamental feature of all populations. Women live longer than men almost everywhere, but this is not, as might be expected, matched by better health throughout their lives. Some researchers argue that there is a clear sex morbidity–mortality paradox – worse female health but better survival. That generalization does not always hold up, however. The World Health Organization's estimates of YLD (years of lost healthy life) in Table 5.2, for example, suggest varying male/female morbidity relativities across ages and regions. National health surveys and related publications show the same. Tables in *Health, United States, 2010* (NCHS, 2011), for example, indicate American women to have higher cancer prevalence, eyesight problems and recent psychological distress statistics than males, but lower prevalence of heart disease, diabetes (physician diagnosed and undiagnosed) and overweight/obesity. The annual *Health Survey for England* (UK Department of Health website) shows similar variety, with males registering with better health on some indicators and worse health on others. Women around the world, however, almost universally experience higher morbidity than males from disabling depressive (unipolar) and anxiety disorders.

The different health fortunes and challenges of males and females have two bases – *sex* and *gender*. The two terms are frequently used interchangeably, but they are conceptually distinct and it is important to appreciate the distinction. Sex refers to the biological and physiological characteristics that distinguish males and females, such as chromosomal make-up, hormones and reproductive organs. Gender refers to the socially and culturally constructed roles that men and women play in society and the (power) relations between them. In other words, sex is the biological group into which people are born while gender refers to what it means in a given society to be labelled as male or female. While core biology is fixed, the roles and expectations of men and women can and do change over time and place. Both sex (*nature*) and gender (*nurture*) are important for health. They may work independently, but more often in tandem.

Sex clearly has an important impact on health. Death in pregnancy or childbirth is confined to females by physiology. Likewise, diseases of the reproductive system are obviously

Table 5.2 Estimated years of life lost to poor health by age and sex: World, Africa, Europe, 2004

Age group (years)	World		African Region*		European Region*	
	Males	*Females*	*Males*	*Females*	*Males*	*Females*
	Rates per 1,000		*Rates per 1,000*		*Rates per 1,000*	
0–4	130	136	194	194	80	76
5–14	50	49	68	58	38	34
15–29	94	114	109	163	90	89
30–44	88	91	116	133	78	77
45–59	103	100	125	123	79	82
60–69	111	115	124	136	87	87
70–79	92	95	107	121	83	84
80+	75	86	93	112	70	82

Note: * WHO region.
Source: WHO, *Global Burden of Disease* website

sex-specific: for example, cervical, ovarian and uterine cancer in the case of women, and prostate and testicular cancer for men. Some research suggests female hormonal status is a major factor in women's superior ability to survive cancer (Micheli *et al.*, 2009). Overall, biology is believed to convey a one–two-year life expectancy advantage on women.

The biological fact that women die of cervical cancer or men of prostate cancer does not in itself constitute a health inequity. The situation becomes inequitable when some of the deaths from those conditions could have been prevented but were not. Some of the reasons for such deaths will be the socio-economic factors discussed above – e.g. poverty, low education – but gender normally also plays a role. In many developing countries, the health of female household members is not rated as highly as that of males and so preventive and curative healthcare may be withheld from them. Or cultural values may prescribe that females only consult female health professionals and there may be no such people available for consultation. Cultural norms of maleness, meanwhile, may see men reluctant to seek medical help for perceived 'embarrassing' male physiology health problems. Often these gender factors are intertwined with the socio-economic ones.

Gender influences, however, are not confined to male- and female-specific health conditions. The socio-cultural roles and expectations associated with being a woman or a man influence all types of health and health behaviour. It is important to emphasize that this is true for both women and men. However, in terms of the burden of illness and premature loss of life in most countries gender is more costly and *unfair* for women than men. Relatively few men die or suffer ill-health from female-driven discriminatory societal power relations, but the reverse is not true. While the situation varies from country to country and culture to culture, the bulk of the world's females live in societies where they hold a lower social status than males and their health is accordingly compromised. The attitudinal data on wife beating presented in Table 5.3 are a confronting illustration.

Female subordination to men is most pronounced in the developing world, but is by no means restricted to those countries. While surveys in developed countries would not likely produce responses of the order shown in Table 5.3, significant numbers of women in them are subjected to domestic violence, discussed further in Chapter 10 (WHO, 2002, 2005; UNFPA, 2009). Also, in some multicultural Western nations, male-dominated cultural values, norms and behaviours with negative implications for female health have been transplanted by immigrants from the developing world to their new countries of residence (Barrett and Mulugeta, 2010; Gill and Mitra-Kahn, 2009; Remennick, 2006).

Table 5.3 Percentage of women/men aged 15–49 who agree a husband is justified in beating his wife for specified reason(s), early 2000s

Country	Women %*	Men %*
Bangladesh(2007)	36	36
India (2005–06)	54	51
Timor–Leste (2009–10)	86	81
Uzbekistan (2002)	70	59
Ethiopia (2005)	81	52
Ghana (2008)	37	21
Nigeria (2008)	43	30
Zambia (2007)	62	48
Samoa (2009)	61	46

Note: *Percentage who agree with at least one specified reason (e.g. burns the food, argues with him, goes out without telling him, neglects the children, refuses to have sexual intercourse with him).

Source: Demographic and Health Surveys website

In some Asian nations with strong culturally based son preference traditions (e.g. India, China, South Korea), female disadvantage begins even before birth. With the advent of sex determination technology (e.g. chorionic villus sampling, ultrasonography, amniocentesis), female foeticide (abortion) has become widespread. Female infanticide is also practised (see Box 5.2). Surviving girl children are meanwhile frequently neglected nutritionally and discriminated against in access to healthcare and education. Early life disadvantages for girls in turn often lead to later health problems for them (and their children) as adults.

In some cases the natural biological advantage of girls and women is overwhelmed by discrimination and disadvantage to the extent that female infant and child, and sometimes adult, mortality is as high or higher than that of males. In India, for example, in 2009 female infant mortality exceeded that of males in 26 of the 35 states and union territories. For the country as a whole, the female rate was 52 (per 1,000 live births) as against 49 for males. Life expectancy at birth statistics for 2002–06, meanwhile, showed that three states – Bihar, Madhya Pradesh and Uttar Pradesh – had a male longevity advantage (Central Bureau of Health Intelligence – India, 2010).

BOX 5.2 The 'missing girls'

The strong cultural preference for sons rather than daughters in several Asian nations has deadly consequences for females. In combination, female foeticide (abortion) and infanticide and neglect of girl children have resulted in millions of 'missing girls'. On the assumption of a 'normal' sex ratio at birth and through childhood (i.e. around 105–106 boys for every 100 girls), China and India in 2010 are respectively missing over 17 million and 5 million girls under the age of 15. Sons are preferred as they will continue the family name, earn money and look after their parents in old age. Daughters are seen as a liability as they will ultimately be lost to another family. In China the 'One Child Policy' has accentuated pressure to have a boy. It is estimated that about 160 million girls, all told, are missing around the world.

Some gender-based inequalities in health originate in the different 'health risk environments' to which men and women are exposed. In both developing and developed countries men tend to dominate in physically demanding and high-risk work environments, such as mining, heavy manufacturing and construction, and thus carry the bulk of the burden of disease from those activities. Some female-dominated work environments also carry heightened health risks. For example, in Africa women account for about 70 per cent of agricultural workers, and with malaria endemic across the bulk of the continent they are especially vulnerable to attacks of the disease. The indoor home environment also poses a high health risk for many developing world women through air pollution from the use of biomass fuels (e.g. wood, dung, crop residues, charcoal) for household cooking and heating. Houses are frequently poorly ventilated and women (and their daughters) typically spend long hours inside exposed to dangerously high smoke levels and associated health risks. Men generally do not spend as much time indoors subjected to such conditions, but they are still exposed sufficiently to suffer substantial loss of life.

Gender inequalities are so deeply embedded in most societies that eliminating them and enabling all women and men to achieve their full health potential is unfortunately, but realistically, a long way off. At the end of this century there will almost certainly still be a significant global gender-based death and DALY toll. It is increasingly recognized that to overcome health problems caused by gender it is necessary to incorporate a gender perspective into all health policies and programmes – that is, *mainstreaming* gender (see Box 5.3). This involves both genders, not just adding a 'women's element' to policies and activities. Boys and men are central to reducing gender inequalities in health. Men must be involved as agents of change, in redefining and equalizing gender relationships and changing male attitudes and behaviour towards women. For example, the widespread acceptance of wife beating as justifiable (illustrated in Table 5.3) needs to be overturned. Likewise, it needs to be accepted by everyone that women have the right to insist on the use of condoms if they fear or know their partner is infected with HIV or some other sexually transmitted disease. Unless boys and girls and men and women are seen as of equal status, gender health inequalities will be perpetuated. Equally, mainstreaming involves addressing male health problems. For instance, the dangerous, risk-taking form of masculinity that exacts high death rates from road traffic accidents, suicide, homicide, illicit drug use and alcohol abuse in young men needs to be transformed into safer values and norms of being 'male'.

Mainstreaming should also recognize and address the health disparities associated with sexual orientation and gender identity. On top of 'standard' health challenges, lesbian, gay, bisexual and transgender (LGBT) people also experience heightened health risks and disadvantages related to their minority group. The most obvious examples for gay and bisexual men are their elevated HIV infection and prevalence rates. HIV prevalence among transgender women is also very high. Lesbian and bisexual women, meanwhile, are thought to get less routine healthcare (e.g. breast and cervical cancer screening) than other women. Difficulties in obtaining health insurance and finding healthcare professionals empathetic to LGBT people are common problems. Everyday societal opprobrium and discrimination are further obstacles to healthy living. Health data collection incorporating sexual orientation and gender identity is very limited, so the exact nature and extent of LGBT disparities are unclear. In June 2011 the United States Department of Health and Human Services announced it would begin to include sexual orientation and gender identity questions in the National Health Interview Survey (NHIS). Ideally, other countries will follow suit in their health data collections. Progress in this area, however, will likely be very slow in many countries. In 2011, there were seventy-six countries around the world in which homosexual acts were illegal, including five countries and parts of Nigeria and Somalia where such acts are punishable by death (Bruce-Jones and Itaborahy, 2011).

BOX 5.3 'Gender mainstreaming'

'Mainstreaming a gender perspective is the process of assessing the implications for women and men of any planned action, including legislation, policies or programmes, in all areas and at all levels. It is a strategy for making women's as well as men's concerns and experiences an integral dimension of the design, implementation, monitoring and evaluation of policies and programmes in all political, economic and societal spheres so that women and men benefit equally and inequality is not perpetuated. The ultimate goal is to achieve gender equality.'

(Source: United Nations General Assembly, 1997)

Ethnicity and race

In many countries large differences in health status and access to healthcare are found between ethnic and racial groups (Boxes 5.4 and 5.5). The term 'ethnicity' refers to population groups defined by shared social identity on such things as country of birth, cultural heritage, tribal affiliation, language and religion. 'Race', on the other hand, refers to inherited physical characteristics, such as skin colour, facial features, hair colour and texture. Historically, race was viewed as an indicator of distinct, genetically different population groups, but it is now recognized that there is more genetic variation within racial groups than between them. Accordingly, race is nowadays more seen and used as a socio-political construct than a biological one, although genomic research in the 1990s and 2000s has led to renewed debate on genetics and racial disparities in health (Frank, 2007; Fujimura *et al.*, 2008).

BOX 5.4 Ethnicity and health: the United Kingdom

'Black British people are 30% more likely than white people to describe their health as fair, poor or very poor.'

'Pakistani and Bangladeshi people, who generally have worse health than all other ethnic groups, are 50% more likely than white people to report fair, poor or very poor health.'

'Black African and Black Caribbean men have been found to be over-represented in mental health services and more likely to be held under a section of the Mental Health Act.'

'African-Caribbean people are also more likely to receive medication for mental health problems as the primary form of treatment . . . and less likely to receive psychotherapy.'

'[E]thnic minority people are more likely than white people to find physical access to their general practitioner (GP) difficult; have longer waiting times in the surgery; feel that the time spent with their GP was inadequate; be less satisfied; and less likely to be referred to secondary and tertiary care.'

(Source: Becares *et al.*, 2010, pp. 1, 1, 2, 2, 1)

BOX 5.5 Ethnic child mortality in eleven sub-Saharan African countries

'[T]his study has revealed large disparities in early child survival chances among ethnic groups in a wide range of African countries.'

'Descriptive statistics from households suggest a close correspondence of child mortality differentials with ethnic inequalities in household economic status, education of women, access to and use of health services, and degree of concentration in the largest city.'

'[M]ultivariate analysis shows that ethnic mortality differences are, in fact, closely linked to economic inequality in many countries.'

'[I]n the absence of policies to reduce economic disparities between ethnic groups, the targeted child health interventions are likely to have a limited impact on the inequalities or disadvantages for chances of survival in many countries.'

(Source: Brockerhoff and Hewett, 2000, pp. 36, 36, 36, 38)

With regards to ethnicity, routine national health data collection systems tend to focus on country of birth and cultural heritage/identification categorizations, while tribal affiliation, language and religion are more often canvassed in special-purpose health surveys. In the United States, health tabulations often report both race (American Indian or Alaska Native, Asian, Black or African American, Native Hawaiian or Other Pacific islander, White) and ethnicity (Hispanic or Latino, Not Hispanic or Latino) (see Figure 5.7).

Patterns of ethnic and racial health inequalities vary. Most frequently one or more minority ethnic/racial group(s) is/are particularly health disadvantaged. However, there are some cases where the majority ethnic/racial group rates most poorly. South Africa is probably the most marked such instance, with the white minority having a twenty-year life expectancy at birth advantage over the large black majority. Uzbekistan is another instance, with the 2002 DHS survey there finding that children born to women of Uzbek ethnicity had substantially higher infant and child mortality rates than children born to women of other ethnicities. Similarly, a 2000 MDG progress stocktake in Malaysia showed the Malay (Bumiputera) majority to have higher infant and child mortality than the Chinese and Indian communities. Malay maternal mortality is also higher.

While specific patterns vary from country to country, ethnic and racial health inequalities within all nations are 'social creations'. Biological susceptibility (see Box 5.6) may play a part in some cases, but overwhelmingly disparities can be linked to socio-economic disadvantage. This disadvantage usually intersects with discrimination, social and political powerlessness, poor housing and area environments, and healthcare deficiencies. Behavioural (e.g. smoking) and cultural (e.g. female status, language) factors also play a role. Address these issues, and inequalities will shrink. The causal interplay of factors is complex and far from fully understood, though. There are also occasional paradoxes: for example, the Hispanic mortality–social disadvantage paradox in the United States that was mentioned earlier in this chapter. Another case is the Bangladeshi community in England and Wales, which has one of the lowest infant mortality rates, despite high deprivation (Gray *et al.*, 2009). Adult Bangladeshis, however, fit the more usual deprivation pattern, reporting poorer health than the general population (Sproston and Mindell, 2006).

Life Expectancy at Birth (Years)

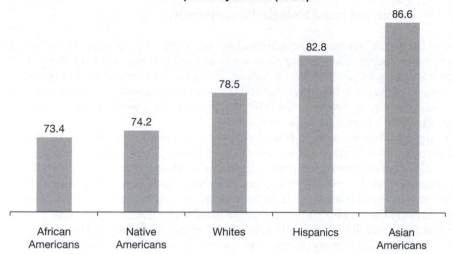

Infant Mortality Rate (per 1,000 live births)

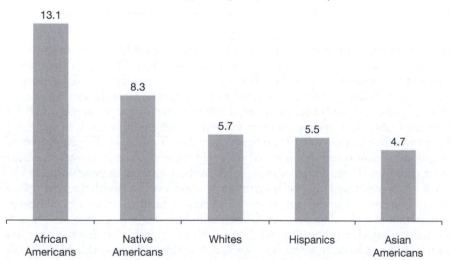

Figure 5.7 Life expectancy at birth (2007) and infant mortality rate (2004–06) in the United States, by race and ethnicity

Sources: Lewis and Burd-Sharps, 2010; NCHS, 2011.

BOX 5.6 Ethnic and racial biological susceptibility?

Ethnic and racial differences in morbidity and mortality raise the question of whether ethno-racial biological susceptibility plays any part. Genomic research over the past two decades has seen this question resurface. However, the far greater biological heterogeneity within than between racial and ethnic groups suggests that any intrinsic 'racial' or 'ethnic' population health effects are weak. Biological 'explanations', though, should be a legitimate topic for research.

Heart disease offers an example. It has long been suspected that South Asia carries an excess proportion of the global burden of heart disease. In turn, South Asians in the United Kingdom have higher rates of heart disease than the general population, and many researchers have thought biological differences could be involved. Research by a large international team across India and twenty-six other countries published in *Nature Genetics* (Dhandapany *et al.*, 2009) concluded that a common gene defect (a 25-bp deletion in MYBPC3) in South Asians is associated with chronic risk of heart failure. The 25-bp deletion was found to be a common variant in individuals from South Asia, present in Southeast Asia, but undetectable elsewhere.

Although biological factors may play a role, it is important not to lose sight of the primacy of the social determinants of health and effective social interventions to reduce inequities. Socio-economic status, not race or ethnicity, is the greater determinant of health.

One of the most unfortunate manifestations of ethnic/racial health disadvantage is the situation of indigenous peoples around the world (see Box 5.7). Generally, indigenous populations suffer considerably worse health than that of the overall national society of which they are part. When this topic is covered in the media and health texts, Australia, Canada, New Zealand and the United States are the usual contemporary examples cited. All four nations are highly developed, prosperous countries with enviable levels of aggregate health, but in which indigenes suffer large health gaps (see Table 5.4). The geography of disadvantaged indigenous health status in today's world, however, is by no means confined to those four countries. There are an estimated 370 million indigenous people worldwide, living in over 70 countries, and most have significantly lower levels of health than their non-indigenous counterparts. The problem of poor indigenous health is thus a global issue. European imperialism and colonialism set in motion indigenous demographic and health decline virtually everywhere they imposed themselves, but that health disadvantage has continued post-independence in many developing nations around the world. Also, not all indigenous marginalization and health disadvantage has its origins in European contacts and pressures. The aboriginal tribes of Taiwan, for example, lost much of their land and were gradually driven into the mountainous interior with the increase in Chinese settler numbers from the sixteenth century onwards. In turn, on mainland China itself, the growth and expansion of the Han Chinese majority has been to the disadvantage of many of the country's indigenous nationalities. The Ainu aborigines of Hokkaido, meanwhile, were persecuted and pushed northwards by ethnic Japanese settlement expansion over the centuries.

BOX 5.7 Who are indigenous peoples?

'An official definition of "indigenous" has not been adopted by the UN system due to the diversity of the world's indigenous peoples. Instead, a modern and inclusive understanding of 'indigenous' has been developed and includes peoples who:

- Identify themselves and are recognized and accepted by their community as indigenous.
- Demonstrate historical continuity with pre-colonial and/or pre-settler societies.
- Have strong links to territories and surrounding natural resources.
- Have distinct social, economic or political systems.
- Maintain distinct languages, cultures and beliefs.
- Form non-dominant groups of society.
- Resolve to maintain and reproduce their ancestral environments and systems as distinctive peoples and communities.'

(Source: WHO, 2007b, p. 1)

Table 5.4 The indigenous health gap in four developed nations, early 2000s

	Life expectancy at birth (years)		Infant mortality rate (per 1,000 live births)
	Males	Females	
Australia, 2005–07			
Aboriginal and Torres Strait Islander population	67.2	72.9	10.1
Total population	78.5	82.4	4.8
Canada, 2000–02			
Registered Indians	70.4*	75.5*	10–11
Total population	76.9	82.0	5.2
New Zealand, 2005–07			
Maori population	70.4	75.1	7.0
Total population	78.0	82.2	5.1
United States, 2004–06			
Native Americans and Alaska Natives	74.2 (Persons)#		6.8
Total population	78.3 (Persons)#		8.3

Notes: * 2001 figures; # 2006 figures.

Sources: Australian Bureau of Statistics, 2009; Statistics Canada, 2006; Smylie and Adomako, 2009; Statistics New Zealand, 2009; Lewis and Burd-Sharps, 2010; NCHS, 2011

All too often life for indigenous groups means social, cultural and economic marginalization, discrimination and powerlessness in the national societies in which they are embedded. Geographically, many are also on the margins, living in remote regions with limited access to modern healthcare services and education and employment opportunities. These conditions unsurprisingly frequently translate into multiple health disadvantages: high infant and child mortality (see Figure 5.8), poor maternal health, heavy morbidity and

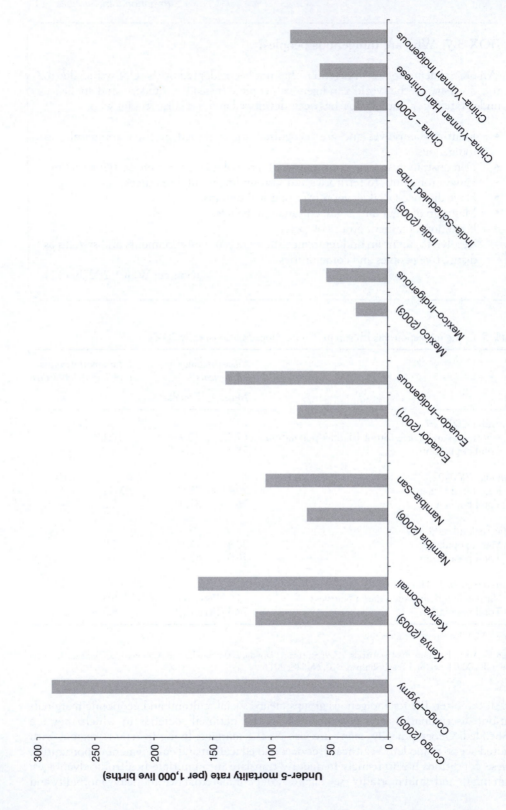

Figure 5.8 Indigenous and non-indigenous under-5 mortality rates in selected developing countries, early 2000s

Sources: Macdonald, 2010; Li *et al.*, 2008.

Table 5.5 Cause of death differences, indigenous and non-indigenous persons, Australia, 2009

	Indigenous persons	*Non-indigenous persons*
Median age of population (2006 Census)	20 years	37 years
Percentage of deaths due to:		
Ischaemic heart diseases	15.3	16.0
Diabetes	8.0	2.9
External causes	13.9	6.1
Suicide	4.0	1.5
Median age (years) at deaths due to:		
Cancer	62.7	75.3
Ischaemic heart diseases	58.1	84.2
Cerebrovascular disease	68.3	85.6
Diabetes	63.1	81.4
Respiratory diseases	65.3	82.7

Source: Australian Bureau of Statistics, 2011

shorter lives. Many developing world indigenous groups carry continuing 'old'-style disease burdens (e.g. tuberculosis, acute respiratory tract infections, diarrhoeal diseases) in combination with emerging 'modern' ones (e.g. diabetes, heart disease, mental disorders).

Indigenous populations in Australia, Canada, New Zealand and the United States have made the transition to 'modern' causes of death, but at disturbingly younger ages and higher rates than in the wider national populations to which they belong. Also, 'social pathology'-style deaths (e.g. motor vehicle accidents, suicide, violence) take an alarming toll. The indigenous life expectancy gaps in these developed countries are better than they used to be, but equity is still a long way off. Of the wealthy developed nations, Australia has by far the worst indigenous health record and the largest challenge ahead (Howitt *et al.*, 2005). Table 5.5 illustrates aspects of the very different mortality profiles of indigenous and non-indigenous Australians.

Geographic location

The other main type of health inequality found in most countries is geographical – that is, health and healthcare variations between different parts of countries (see Figure 5.9). These disparities are found at multiple levels: between macro sub-national divisions, smaller regions, towns and villages, right down to urban neighbourhoods. In addition, sizeable health differences commonly exist between aggregated 'types' of locations – for example, rural and urban areas, remoteness zones, etc. Some form of geographic classification is built into the routine health data collections of most countries, although the spatial detail varies from country to country. Virtually all developed nations now have both mortality and morbidity data collection, recording and dissemination down to a very fine scale, frequently to the unit record level. Developing countries in the main have more limited data collection and handling capabilities, but normally attempt to obtain at least broad regional information. Recognizing the importance and utility of geographic health data, most DHS health surveys produce regional statistics as regular output.

Geographical health inequalities come about in two broad ways – through *context* and *compositional* effects. 'Context' refers to features of the biophysical, social, economic and political environments within which people find themselves that influence their health: for example, weather and climate, exposure to hazards, the availability/unavailability of

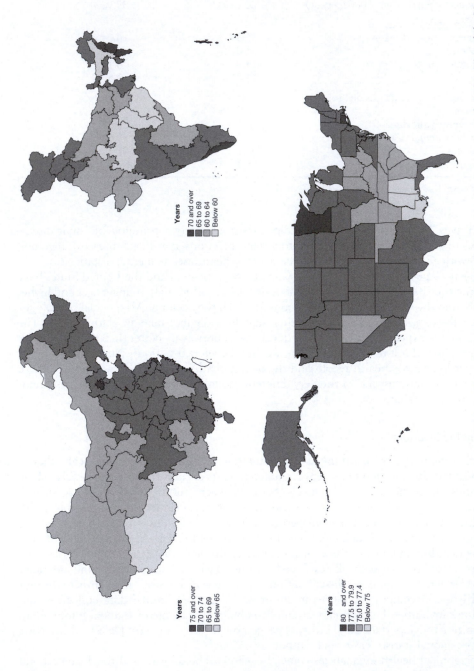

Years
■ 75 and over
■ 70 to 74
▨ 65 to 69
□ Below 65

Years
■ 70 and over
■ 65 to 69
▨ 60 to 64
□ Below 60

Years
■ 80 and over
■ 77.5 to 79.9
▨ 75.0 to 77.4
□ Below 75

Figure 5.9 Geographical inequalities in life expectancy at birth in China (provinces) 2000, India (states and union territories), 2001–06, and the United States (states), 2005

Note: The three countries are not drawn to exact geographic scale.
Sources: Heilig, 2004; Population Foundation of India and Population Reference Bureau, 2007; Burd-Sharps *et al.*, 2008

healthcare, the type of economy, the labour market, government policy, pollution levels, transport availability, and the like. 'Composition', on the other hand, refers to the individual characteristics of the people who live in a place: for instance, their age, sex, socio-economic status or ethnicity. Sometimes the factors are not as neatly classifiable as this. For example, being unemployed (and the health risks that involves) may be seen as an individual factor, but in reality the unemployment may be due to an area having a declining industrial base.

From the above, it will also have been seen that context as a determinant of health involves various scales: from the immediate living and working environment through to regional and national environments, and sometimes beyond. The disadvantaged health status of people in some regions may be due to policies and resourcing decisions by the national government. To reduce geographical disparities in health in a country, it is necessary to understand the respective roles (singular and joint) of composition and context in producing them.

Geographic disparities in health are often used as the basis for targeting health improvement interventions. Geographic targeting is attractive in the sense that 'needy' areas can be easily identified. Also, the geographic concentration of interventions simplifies programme implementation. However, not all people in need (i.e. in poor health or without sufficient healthcare services) will live in the targeted 'worst' areas and thus some may miss out on help by this approach. When focusing on health problems in targeted local areas, there is also the danger of overlooking that many such problems are generated at the broader state and national levels and need to be addressed at those levels. Local area-based health interventions can make a difference to health by improving such things as access to services, the provision of safe environments (e.g. roads, transport), the quality and quantity of housing stock, the availability of affordable, healthy food options and so on, but many of the forces producing health inequalities are rooted in broader societal and global processes.

Like socio-economic, sex/gender and ethnic/racial disparities in health, the magnitude of internal geographical health inequalities varies between countries. This is not surprising as those other disparities are the 'compositional' element of geographical ones. To some extent, geographical inequalities vary with stage of demographic and epidemiological transition. Countries with very high, early-transition mortality have limited regional mortality differences. There are always advantaged sections of such populations with lower mortality, but not enough to produce substantial geographical differentiation. Sierra Leone, and to a lesser extent Liberia, in Table 5.6 are examples of this. As mortality falls with progression further into the transition, some groups/areas benefit earlier and faster than others and a greater range and array of regional values emerge. The data for Nigeria and Kenya in Table 5.6 are illustrations. Further down the transition pathway to low mortality, geographical differences tend to narrow. For example, the three more demographically advanced nations shown in Table 5.7 – Japan, New Zealand and the United States – all have a narrower range and lower variability in regional life expectancy values than do the three developing world countries – China, India and the Philippines. The temporal data for China and the Philippines show narrowing is occurring, however. Interestingly, the fifteen-year period for New Zealand shows a small *widening* in regional health inequality. The differences in regional mortality range and variability shown between Georgia and Paraguay in Table 5.6, despite their reasonably similar total infant and under-5 mortality rates, show there is no absolute pattern, though.

Economic well-being is generally the main compositional factor behind geographical disparities. For the three countries shown in Figure 5.9 – China, India and the United States – for instance, the correlations of the displayed life expectancy levels with income measures are: China – real GDP per capita, PPP$, r = 0.75; India – per capita income, r = 0.59; United States – median household income, r = 0.62. The debate over income inequality (i.e. *relative*

Table 5.6 Regional variation in infant and under-5 mortality rates,* selected countries, early 2000s*

Countries	Infant mortality				Under-five mortality			
	Total rate	Highest regional rate	Lowest regional rate	Coefficient of variation (%) of regional rates	Total rate	Highest regional rate	Lowest regional rate	Coefficient of variation (%) of regional rates
Kenya, 2008–09	59.2	94.7	41.6	29.2	83.7	148.9	51.1	41.6
Georgia, 2005	29.0	47.5	8.8	41.8	32.7	57.2	10.6	41.1
Nigeria, 2008	86.8	109.5	58.9	18.2	171.0	217.5	89.1	29.7
Guatemala,– 2008	34.4	42.9	16.2	24.5	45.0	54.9	19.2	26.0
Cambodia, 2005	88.1	104.5	70.1	15.4	106.3	136.5	91.9	15.7
Liberia, 2009	100.9	120.3	79.4	14.9	157.8	187.5	124.5	14.7
Colombia, 2010	18.1	21.9	14.8	13.0	21.7	27.0	17.8	13.4
Paraguay, 2008	24.7	27.6	22.7	7.5	27.8	31.8	25.0	11.3
Sierra Leone, 2008	111.1	122.3	95.3	8.9	167.8	180.0	146.9	7.5

Notes: Countries are listed in descending order of under-5 mortality coefficient of variation; * rate per 1,000 live births; * data relate to the decade preceding the survey.

Source: Demographic and Health Surveys website

Table 5.7 Regional variation in life expectancy at birth (both sexes combined), selected countries, 1990s and early 2000s

Countries/regional units	Number of areal units	National life expectancy (years)	Highest regional life expectancy (years)	Lowest regional life expectancy (years)	Coefficient of variation (%) of regional values
China					
Provinces, 2000	32	68.0	78.1	64.4	4.4
Provinces, 1990	32	71.3	74.9	59.6	5.1
India					
States/union territories, 2001–06	35	63.6	74.7	58.2	6.7
Philippines					
Regions, 2005*	15	70.5	71.9	59.9	4.0
Regions, 1995*	15	67.5	69.5	54.9	5.2
Japan					
Prefectures, 2005*	47	82.4	83.2	80.5	0.6
New Zealand					
Regional council areas, 2005–07*	16	80.3	81.3	76.0	1.6
Regional council areas, 1990–92*	16	75.8	78.0	73.8	1.5
United States					
States, 2005	51	78.0	81.7	73.8	2.3

Note: * 'Both sexes' life expectancy figures are averages of published male and female figures.

Sources: Heilig, 2004; Population Foundation of India and Population Reference Bureau, 2007; National Statistical Coordination Board, 2005; Statistics Japan, *Prefecture Comparisons* website; Statistics New Zealand, 2009; Burd-Sharps *et al.*, 2008

versus *absolute* income) determining health outcomes (introduced in Chapter 4) also exists in relation to the sub-national scale. As for the international level, empirical research has produced mixed results. Certainly within some countries and at some scales, however, income inequality does clearly show up as a significant negative independent contributor to health levels. In the case of the US state life expectancy values of Figure 5.9, partial correlation analyses examining two income inequality measures – the Gini index and the ratio of the incomes of the top and bottom fifth of families – and controlling for household income revealed statistically significant income inequality contributions. Analyses of state infant mortality levels showed the same results. In both cases – life expectancy and infant mortality – the family income ratio variable had the slightly more powerful inequality effect. Absolute income, however, made the largest substantive contribution.

A virtually universal internal geographical health divide is between rural and urban areas. This reflects a mixture of contextual and compositional effects. Rural areas generally have fewer healthcare services and residents need to travel greater distances for care, especially specialist care. These disadvantages are in the main most pronounced in poor developing countries, but are also important in wealthy developed nations. People who live and work in rural areas also tend to have lower incomes and educational backgrounds and, accordingly, the health disadvantages that flow from those characteristics. Rural–urban under-5 mortality data collected in eighty-two recent DHS surveys show only five countries in which the rural rate was lower than the urban. On average, rural under-5 rates were 40 per cent higher than those in urban areas (WHO, 2011a).

While urban dwellers overall enjoy a health advantage, within cities there are usually further geographic divides. In general, children and adults in poor areas face worse health and shorter lives than residents of wealthier and better areas. In some cases, children in slums in large developing world cities have even higher morbidity and mortality than rural children (Montgomery, 2009; WHO/UN-HABITAT, 2010). Generally, the epidemiological transition is more advanced in the cities than in the rural areas of developing countries. City life brings exposure to 'modern' health risks – motor vehicle accidents, air pollution, new salt- and fat-rich diets, etc. Within individual cities, very different epidemiological profiles can be found side by side. Richer groups and locations tend to be characterized by modern disease profiles, while poorer groups and places often suffer more from old-style diseases. Table 5.8 presents the example of Cape Town, South Africa, highlighting the very different cause of death profiles of the poor Cape Flats district of Khayelitsha and the affluent South Peninsula area. Similar geographical variation in stage of epidemiological transition is found at the regional scale in middle-income developing countries (Stevens *et al.*, 2008).

Table 5.8 Leading causes of death, Cape Town and selected sub-districts of Cape Town, 2001

		Cape Town sub-districts			
Cape Town		*Khayelitsha (poor)*		*South Peninsula (affluent)*	
Cause of death	%	*Cause of death*	%	*Cause of death*	%
Homicide	10.5	Homicide	18.7	Ischaemic heart disease	12.8
Ischaemic heart disease	8.1	HIV/AIDS	15.0	Hypertensive heart disease	7.8
HIV/AIDS	7.4	Tuberculosis	14.9	Diabetes mellitus	6.9
Hypertensive heart disease	6.4	Lower respiratory infections	5.2	Homicide	5.7
Tuberculosis	5.9	Road traffic accidents	4.9	Stroke	5.2

Source: Groenewald *et al.*, 2003

Discussion topics

Find out the major health inequalities and inequities in your country.

• Do they show signs of narrowing or widening?
• What processes have led to these inequalities and inequities?
• Do global forces play any role in the existence of these inequalities and inequities?
• What policies and programmes would you advocate to reduce these inequalities and inequities?

6 Age and lifecourse transitions in health

Introduction: health and related changes over the lifecourse

As we saw in Chapters 4 and 5, health risks almost always differ over time and place; health variations are also often seen between different socio-economic and geographical locations. Moreover, as time evolves, different broad types of health disorders and health risks tend to affect people differently at different times of their lives, and these often underlie lifecourse patterns of change. In Chapter 4, we noted the broader patterns of changes in morbidity and mortality that have occurred over time and the major causes of death and DALYS in high-, middle- and low-income countries (Tables 4.6–4.9). In Chapter 7, we will look at some major contemporary health challenges that are likely to have major future impacts on patterns of health status and consequences for healthcare needs.

In this chapter, we look in more detail at patterns of health change as people and populations age. Many of today's risk factors identified by the WHO (see Table 4.10) raise the chances of people developing chronic conditions and diseases, such as heart disease, diabetes and cancers. Greater longevity is often associated with an increased risk of chronic physical and psychological health or degenerative mental conditions. From the preceding chapters, it is not only clear that aggregate changes are occurring in many aspects of global health but that these are affecting *different places, people and age groups differentially*, depending on how the various determinants in Figure 3.1 interact. Now, we examine how health changes and various types of health condition can affect different age groups across their lifespans, whether there are distinct patterns, and, as far as possible (as in Chapter 5), how they differ geographically, too.

In general, we see two patterns: lifecourse changes in health risks within countries; and those between countries at different stages of development and between social groups within them (see Table 4.10). These follow a fairly predictable epidemiological evolution from communicable, maternal, perinatal and nutritional as leading causes of deaths and DALYs among younger age groups (worldwide and especially influenced by countries' levels of income) towards non-communicable conditions in middle life and especially at older ages. The WHO's *Global Burden of Disease* website documents this for different countries and regions. Table 6.1 shows the example of burden of disease in DALYs for males at various ages in high-income and low-income countries.

Lifecourse and lifespan perspectives

At least two ways of looking at health-related changes over people's lives have emerged in recent decades: the lifecourse and the lifespan perspectives. These two terms are sometimes used interchangeably, though the disciplines from which they originated would not always agree this is appropriate. The lifecourse perspective tends to adopt a more sociological basis

Table 6.1 Burden of disease in DALYs among males (thousands), by age group and broad cause, 2004

		0–14	15–59	60+
World				
Total population (males, millions)	3,244	951	1,994	298
Total DALYs	796,133	283,314	403,131	109,688
Communicable, maternal, perinatal and nutritional conditions	294,075	209,259	75,063	9,753
Non-communicable conditions	378,693	47,526	235,848	95,318
Injuries	123,366	26,529	92,220	4,617
Low-income countries				
Total population (males, millions)	1,229	459	697	73
Total DALYs	418,206	210,789	172,662	34,754
Communicable, maternal, perinatal and nutritional conditions	227,259	171,013	50,652	5,595
Non-communicable conditions	137,727	24,654	85,417	27,655
Injuries	53,220	15,122	36,593	1,504
High-income countries				
Total population (males, millions)	482	92	308	83
Total DALYs	64,189	5,277	37,789	21,124
Communicable, maternal, perinatal and nutritional conditions	3,482	1,423	1,288	770
Non-communicable conditions	52,701	3,109	29,932	19,659
Injuries	8,007	744	6,568	694

Source: Adapted from WHO, 2008b, Table A6

and has become a leading theoretical orientation for the study of patterns of people's lives as they unfold over time. The perspective has potential to help understanding of behavioural aspects underpinning global health and, therefore, how it might change in the future. It encompasses at least three kinds of outcome: individual, collective and socio-cultural. Lifespan development is more based in psychology and psycho-social development, and attempts to describe and explain age-related changes (outcomes) in individual people, and examines multiple aspects of the individual (Baltes *et al.*, 1999; Berger, 2007, 2012).

As the WHO (2007a, p. 13) notes, 'a life course approach explicitly recognizes the importance of time and timing in understanding causal links between exposures and outcomes within an individual life course, across generations, and in population-level diseases trends'. A lifecourse perspective directs attention to how social and other determinants of health operate at every level of development – early childhood, childhood, adolescence and adulthood – and can immediately influence health and also provide the basis for how health or illness develop later in life. The WHO, in the naming of its Department of Ageing and Lifecourse, explicitly recognizes the importance of health developing over all stages of one's life.

The lifecourse perspective can help us see how processes operating across the lifecourse of one cohort may be related to earlier and subsequent cohorts and may be manifested in disease trends over time at the population as well as individual level. It can give a useful multi-disciplinary perspective for public health in the epidemiology of a number of chronic diseases (including coronary heart disease, type 2 diabetes, chronic obstructive pulmonary disease and breast cancer), providing a framework to understand time, exposure and outcomes at both individual and population levels (Lynch and Smith, 2005; Osler, 2006). Factors such as time lags between exposure, the start of a disease and clinical recognition ('latency period') suggest that exposures early in life are often involved in starting disease processes long before the condition can be clinically detected. However, even if we recognize and acknowledge any early life influences on chronic diseases in particular, this does not mean interventions to improve health or change behaviour in later life are of no use.

The WHO cites two main mechanisms. The *critical periods* model occurs when a certain exposure, acting during a specific period, has lasting or lifelong effects (on the structure or function of organs, tissues and body systems) that are not substantially modified by later experiences. This implies biological programming, or a latency model, the basis of hypotheses on the foetal origins of adult diseases. The *accumulation of risk* model suggests that factors that increase disease risk – or, conversely, promote good health – may accumulate gradually over the lifecourse. There may be developmental periods when their effects have greater impact on later health than those operating at other times. This complements the idea of cumulative damage to biological systems as the intensity, number and/or duration of exposures increase.

The lifecourse and lifespan perspectives have similarities in that they recognize that people's experiences are lifelong, contextual and dynamic. Health is influenced by experiences which may include micro and macro features, gains and losses, risks and resiliencies. As noted in Chapter 3, some will be within and others beyond an individual's control. These two perspectives have increasingly been used explicitly and implicitly in research on health and health behaviour across people's lives in public health, medicine, sociology and education. To some extent, they help bridge disciplinary boundaries between the health and social and behavioural sciences. However, confusingly to the student of global health, these two perspectives have not always interacted effectively. Key aspects of the relations between lifespan/lifecourses and context remain largely undeveloped, partly because of their disciplinary origins. Nevertheless, as Dannefer and Daub (2009) note, particularly with respect to ageing, while both perspectives deal with somewhat disparate outcomes, they tend to share common explanatory strategies. An important aspect is recognition of risk.

Risk over time

We know that certain diseases are becoming more prevalent, some are emerging at ever younger ages, and others are manifesting themselves widely in older populations. An important feature is age, length and exposure to risk factors, many of which are now being seen at earlier ages. Epidemiologists and medical scientists note that, in terms of health changes, many factors in early life and at intermediate ages will affect individual health and, ultimately, the population's health. Obvious factors have long been recognized, such as people's occupations and their duration, which affect exposures to various substances and forms of occupational danger. Other factors are social behaviours, especially consumption patterns. These have led to sometimes very marked socio-economic and occupational differences in health status and health life expectancy, as noted in Chapter 2. Today, even earlier events in life are being recognized as significant, such as early childhood diets and environmental exposures, including *in-utero* gestational exposures (such as toxins or radiation) and mothers' behaviour (dietary, smoking, exercise, etc.) and even pre-conceptional features that may have predisposed to genetic damage. These factors may affect not only childhood and adolescent health but long-term adult health. Potential influences are complex, manifold and often highly interrelated. As discussed below, one example being considered is the link between very young feeding habits, childhood obesity and the early onset of degenerative diseases such as diabetes and heart disease previously considered mainly conditions of middle and old age.

Risk transition

'Health risk' is defined by the WHO (2009a, p. v) as 'a factor that raises the probability of adverse health outcomes'. Adverse outcomes could include subsequently developing any given disease or health condition – physical, mental or emotional. Risk transition relates to the changing sources and levels of risk over time, for individuals, groups and places, so it is very relevant to age and lifecourse transitions in health. The WHO (2009a) sees, over time, major risks to health shifting. This shift would tend to be from 'traditional' risks (such as inadequate nutrition or exposure to infections via unsafe water and sanitation, often associated with poverty and affecting low-income populations) to modern risks with a greater lifestyle component (such as overweight and obesity, inactivity, or exposure to carcinogenic substances), often associated with chronic and non-communicable diseases. There are also varying health risk environments to which people are differentially exposed, as noted in Chapter 5.

Risks often take different trajectories in different countries, depending on the particular risk and the context in which it is set. To an extent, this mirrors epidemiological transition, insofar as, when a country develops, with social, environmental and healthcare changes, the types of diseases that affect a population almost always shift from primarily infectious to primarily non-communicable conditions. These conditions also tend to have different incidence and prevalence rates within different age groups, though their expression may be at earlier or later ages, depending on the country, region and/or social group in question. The WHO (2009a, p. 2) notes that this risk shift is caused by various factors:

*   improvements in medical care (so children no longer die as frequently from easily curable or preventable conditions, such as diarrhoea);
*   the ageing of the population (as non-communicable diseases tend to affect older adults more);
*   public health interventions, such as vaccinations; and
*   the provision of clean water and sanitation (both reduce the incidence of many infectious diseases).

This general pattern can be observed across many countries, with wealthy countries usually further advanced along the road of epidemiological transition (see Chapters 1, 3 and 4). In many ways, the second point above – the gradual ageing of populations, often growing healthier with greater longevity – is the major expression of risk transition. This suggests it is important to consider changes in health by place as much as by stage of life, as there is considerable regional variation in demographic ageing.

Age and life changes in health

In the context of the global trend of population ageing, ideas on the effects of *age stratification* have emerged, with respect to health as much as to other human areas (Bond *et al.*, 2007). Age stratification recognizes the influence of social factors on individual ageing and the stratification of age in society. In health terms, it also helps us recognize that health risks tend to affect different age groups with varying degrees of severity.

Members of different age cohorts comprise 'age strata', age bands (such as 0–5 years, 6–10, 65-plus, etc., or children, young adults, middle aged, older adults, etc.) whose members will potentially exhibit health differences according to both their age and their historical experiences. This has similarities to the established concept of the life cycle, another term used within developmental psychology and related fields, and sometimes, incorrectly, used interchangeably with the terms lifespan and lifecourse. The life cycle is usually thought of as sequential chronological eras, such as infancy (conception to, say, age 5), pre-adulthood (age 6–22), early adult transition (age 17–22), etc., until late adulthood (age 60–death). Sometimes the life cycle is divided into only three broad periods, such as evolescence (up to young adulthood), senescence (middle and later adulthood) and senility (involving the decline of the individual in old age).

This form of the life cycle may be over-simple and over-dependent on age categories and the implication that people within them are somehow uniform. Nevertheless, the life cycle does provide a *framework* for looking at health changes in different age groups over time. The WHO's approach of looking at disease and health changes, risk and evolution through the life cycle is practical. Jenkins (2003) outlines health improvements and risks through the life cycle in four main age groups:

- pregnancy, infants and children up to 14 years;
- adolescents and young adults: 15–24 years;
- the 'prime of life': ages 25–64 years; and
- the older years: 65–100.

While recognizing its simplistic, age-based categorization and the possibility of exaggerating the uniformity within and importance of age groupings, this approach has utility (Phillipson and Baars, 2007). First, we see in the lifecourse that people age from birth to death, hopefully reducing a predilection to focus only on, say, 'the elderly'. Second, lifelong ageing involves social, psychological and biological processes. Third, the *experience* of ageing, especially in health and psycho-social terms, is often affected by cohort–historical factors, especially in particular geographical situations.

This geographical feature is very important for global health patterns, as was highlighted in Figure 3.1. Local environmental experiences and risk exposures will change considerably over time in specific places, so the health status and causes of disease of age cohorts born in previous eras are likely to be very different from those of the same age cohort born in later eras, even though living in the same locations. This seems to happen even over quite short time scales. Even more so when we attempt to compare the health of similar age groups over time, but living in different places, variability of risk and exposures, as well as services, makes comparison even more difficult or impossible. Therefore, direct extrapolation of health status influences from past generations to current or future ones is of very questionable value. Health is increasingly likely to be an evolutionary feature of succeeding cohorts, and population movements and change make this issue ever more complex. Health is likely to be an evolutionary feature of succeeding cohorts. Therefore, from a global health perspective, the same chronological cohorts (say, today's 70–75-year-olds) but who were born and have lived their lives in different countries or neighbourhoods will be unlikely to have identical health statuses (see Chapter 5). Likewise, by 2030, the 70–75-year-old cohort will probably have very different health profiles and needs to those of this age group today, even in the same locations.

The *lifecourse perspective* can also be used to examine racial and ethnic disparities in birth outcomes (Lu and Halfon, 2003) and attempts to understand and suggest how to address longstanding social differences in health across populations. The perspective sees, for example, that birth outcomes are not just the end-product of nine months of pregnancy but reflect the entire lifecourse of the mother leading up to conception, and to some extent that of the father, and the mother's behaviour during the pregnancy itself. Disparities in birth outcomes, within this perspective, reflect both differential exposures during pregnancy and differential developmental experiences of the mother (and perhaps the father) across their lifespans. This perspective is entering many areas of health research and policy, although it is currently prominent particularly in mother and child health (MCH).

A lifecourse perspective, looking at health changes and consequences through the life-cycle framework, therefore has considerable implications for how health professionals and others develop ways to improve individual and public health. It also has potentially very wide implications for addressing geographical, social and ethnic disparities, and disparities across income groups, communities, states and nations. In other words, a global health approach is possible and allows for many local variants. The lifecourse perspective may also have policy relevance and help identify certain critical periods for intervention. It may be yet more important in emphasizing the *cumulative* impacts of environmental and behavioural factors on health as these develop over time (Fine *et al.*, 2009). A lifecourse perspective also enables a view to be taken by gender, social class and geographical location, where data are available. The WHO shows there are distinct patterns of causes of death and disease for women at different ages (Boxes 6.1–6.3)

Health changes and transitions over life: some examples

The younger years: mother and child health (MCH)

Here we focus on the main causes of childhood ill-health and mortality in different regions. Healthy pregnancy and safe delivery are essential foundations for healthy life, but both vary greatly internationally and even locally. Poor nutrition, infections and toxins are the three most frequent causes of infant morbidity and mortality. They are also the three most pre-ventable. We also note that children worldwide – both rich and poor – are becoming heavier and increasing their risk of developing early various non-communicable or degenerative conditions, such as diabetes and even heart disease.

Childhood health risks and transitions

There is naturally enormous interest in whether infants' and children's health is improving in specific locations or groups and internationally (recall Figure 3.1 when thinking about spatial scale and influences). In health terms, 'childhood' generally refers to those aged under one and under 5, and school-age children, usually aged between 6 and 18, so it covers a wide range of human developmental stages, with the higher ages overlapping with young adulthood. The picture is varied almost everywhere but, in general, over the past few decades, most children have been becoming healthier and less subject to infectious con-ditions and neonatal or perinatal deaths, although these remain a huge burden in specific countries (see Figures 6.1 and 6.2; Black *et al.*, 2008, 2010; United Nations Inter-agency Group for Child Mortality Estimation, 2011). While all hope that such improvements continue in the future, in some places, specific problematic circumstances have turned back the clock, sometimes temporarily. War, natural disasters, related disease outbreaks and famine have led to much loss of life and excess morbidity. Children are often resilient but, along with older people, the most vulnerable in emergencies.

Broad patterns can be seen. In nations with higher rates of early childhood deaths, the main causes of mortality are infectious and parasitic diseases; for nations with lower childhood mortality, external causes (accidents, neglectful or intentional trauma) are commonest, with congenital anomalies and infectious and parasitic conditions usually second. Environmental risks appear to be becoming more important almost everywhere, especially accidents and lifestyle factors (such as nutrition, education, parental attention and environmental safety).

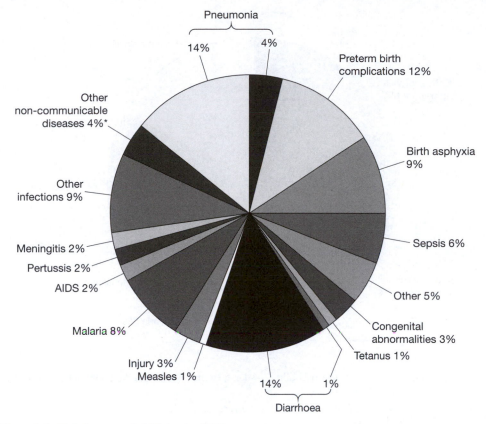

Figure 6.1 Global causes of child deaths, 2008

Notes: * Includes data for congenital abnormalities; data are separated into deaths of neonates aged 0–27 days and children aged 1–59 months; causes that led to less than 1 per cent of deaths are not presented.
Source: Black *et al.*, 2010. Reprinted from *The Lancet*, 375 Black, R.E. *et al.*, for the Child Health Epidemiology Reference Group of WHO and UNICEF (2010). "Global, regional, and national causes of child mortality in 2008: a systematic analysis", pp. 1969–1987. Copyright (2010) with permission from Elsevier.

In many countries, the broader social and economic environment is paramount and, in this, MDG 1 (eradicate extreme poverty and hunger) and MDG 4 (reduce child mortality) should support each other (see Box 7.2). Globally, in 2010, the four main killers of children under five were pneumonia, diarrhoeal disease, pre-term birth complications and birth asphyxia (see Figures 6.1 and 6.2). The environment is the setting for malnutrition among both mothers and children (underweight, slowed linear growth, or with vitamin and mineral/micronutrient deficiencies). Undernutrition was a factor in more than one-third of the deaths and the underlying cause of 3.5 million deaths and 35 per cent of the disease burden in children under 5 (Black *et al.*, 2008; United Nations Inter-agency Group for Child Mortality Estimation, 2011). However, as under/malnutrition does not usually play the most direct role, it does not usually attract the attention or receive the resources allocated to specific disease programmes. Malnutrition has therefore been targeted by the Bill and Melinda Gates Foundation, among others, to help raise its visibility and enhance initiatives such as the Scaling Up Nutrition (SUN) global framework for action, which is endorsed by more than 100 donor, non-profit and research organizations (Population Reference Bureau, 2010).

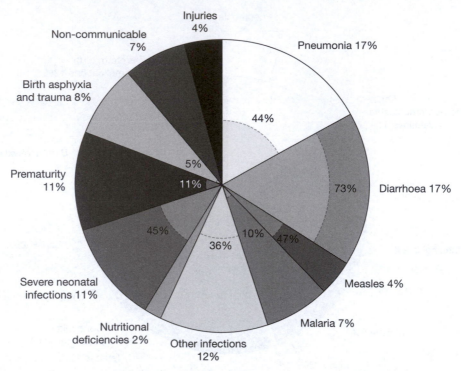

Figure 6.2 Major causes of death in children under 5 (with disease specific contribution of under-nutrition), 2004

Note: Dotted line = contribution of undernutrition to each cause of death.
Source: WHO, 2009a, Fig. 8, p. 14

Children aged 1–4 tend to experience more injuries than those under 1. They are more mobile, curious, less restrained and often less easy to monitor than babies. They explore, get into water and into road traffic, and they know less about local and household dangers than older children. Boys, in particular, are at risk and experience 150–250 per cent the rate of injuries of girls at all childhood ages (Jenkins, 2003). Globally, the WHO (2009b) notes that girls under 5 years are more likely to be overweight than boys. This, with obesity, is a risk factor for cardiovascular disease, diabetes, musculoskeletal disorders and some cancers later in life. Girls are about three times more likely than boys to suffer sexual violence and any form of sexual abuse (see also Chapter 10).

For slightly older children, death rates for those aged 5 to 14 are generally 50–80 per cent lower than among those aged between 1 and 4 in any country. Mid-to-early teen children not only gain experience and some awareness of dangers but have greater biological immunity and physiological reserves. However, this 'benign health situation' begins to deteriorate with the onset of puberty (Jenkins, 2003). We shall see below that mortality rates, especially for adolescent and young adult males, start to rise, with trauma becoming the leading cause of death. Moreover, many behaviours established in people's teens, such as smoking, will heavily influence health in later years, as discussed later.

In spite of global improvements, in some areas, especially after natural and human-induced disasters, child mortality and ill-health spike. In more detail than given above, a study of the distribution of causes of death under age 5 for 191 countries showed that, of the almost 9 million estimated worldwide deaths in 2008, almost half (49 per cent, or 4.294

million) occurred in just five countries: India, Nigeria, the Democratic Republic of the Congo, Pakistan, and China (Black *et al.*, 2010). Infectious diseases caused over two-thirds (68 per cent, 5.970 million). The largest percentages were due to pneumonia (18 per cent), diarrhoea (15 per cent) and malaria (8 per cent). About 41 per cent (3.575 million) of deaths occurred in neonates (aged 0–27 days), with the most important single causes being pre-term birth complications (12 per cent), birth asphyxia (9 per cent), sepsis (6 per cent) and pneumonia (4 per cent) (see Figures 6.2 and 7.1; Figure 6.2 shows the contribution of undernutrition). This analysis repays careful reading as it illustrates the use of various models to estimate mortality. It also highlights the importance of access to good health services, especially midwifery, and healthy environmental conditions for newborn children.

Variations in child health by place and cause

There are many variables concerning child health, though the focus has, understandably, tended to be on mortality. Of the MDGs listed in Boxes 7.1 and 7.2, the fourth MDG target of reduction in under-5 mortality by two-thirds between 1990 and 2015 implies that this would have to decline by 4.4 per cent every year over the twenty-five-year period. Actual achievements have often been below that target, though the picture is varied and some very good gains were made by 2010, with child deaths falling from 8.1 million in 2009 to 7.6 million in 2010 (see Figure 6.3). Overall, however, the average reduction in under-5 mortality was only 2.2 per cent globally, so, to have any chance of reaching the target, improvement will have to accelerate considerably. The United Nations Inter-agency Group for Child Mortality Estimation (2011) note that rate of decline has accelerated, from 1.9 per cent annually between 1990 and 2000 to 2.5 per cent annually over 2000–2010, but this is still insufficient to reach MDG 4's target, particularly in the regions noted below.

Even the moderate global improvements in under-5 mortality rates hide considerable regional and local disparities (Figure 6.3 shows distribution by MDG regions). Table 6.2 indicates that several regions (East and South-east Asia, China, Latin America and the Caribbean, North Africa) had either achieved or almost achieved the requisite 4 per cent annual target by 2010 and were considered to be on track for achieving the MDG 4 for reduction in child mortality. However, the under-5 mortality rate in sub-Saharan Africa has declined by just 1.8 per cent annually, on average, since 1990. The Countdown Group, looking at progress of sixty-eight countries towards health-related goals, found that, in 2010, the vast majority of countries rated as making no progress towards MDG 4 were in sub-Saharan Africa and South Asia (Requejo, 2010; United Nations Inter-agency Group for Child Mortality Estimation, 2007, 2010, 2011). In recent years, the picture for under-5 mortality has become quite varied sub-regionally, actually increasing in a very few countries, though between 2000 and 2010, six of the best-performing countries were in sub-Saharan Africa. Regionally, nevertheless, sub-Saharan Africa and South Asia combined still account for many global under-5 deaths each year. As the United Nations Inter-agency Group for Child Mortality Estimation (2011) notes, global child mortality is generally falling and considerable progress has been made towards MDG 4. However, as noted above, just under half of under-5 deaths occurred in only five countries, with India (22 per cent) and Nigeria (11 per cent) together accounting for one-third. Moreover, almost 30 per cent of neonatal deaths occurred in India. By contrast, some countries, such as Malawi and (since 2000) Botswana, have made great improvements and are on track for the targets (Requejo, 2010). However, unless mortality in many countries is significantly reduced, the global MDG targets will not be met (United Nations Inter-agency Group for Child Mortality Estimation, 2007, 2010, 2011).

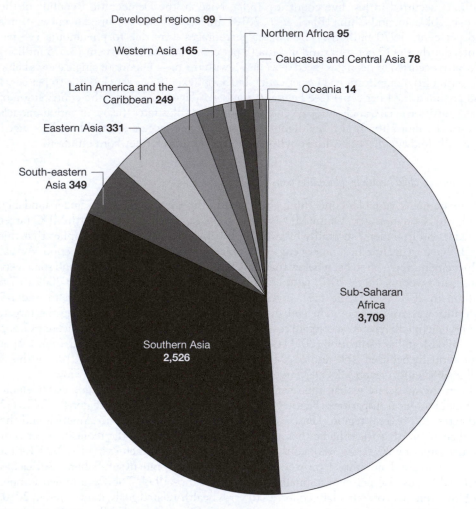

Developed regions **99**

Northern Africa **95**

Western Asia **165**

Caucasus and Central Asia **78**

Latin America and the
Caribbean **249**

Oceania **14**

Eastern Asia **331**

South-eastern
Asia **349**

Sub-Saharan
Africa
3,709

Southern Asia
2,526

Figure 6.3 Number of under-5 deaths, by Millennium Development Goal region, 2010 (thousands):
7.6 million children died aged under 5 in 2010

Source: United Nations Inter-agency Group for Child Mortality Estimation, 2011, Fig. 3, p. 7

Changes in life expectancy at birth (ELB)

Looking forward over the lifespan, in many countries, life expectancy at birth (ELB, as seen in Chapters 2 and 4) has been steadily increasing over recent decades. In some parts of the world, such as the Asia–Pacific, this has been spectacular in some countries, but not in all (see Figure 6.4). While ELB is a somewhat theoretical figure, based on extrapolations assuming current health and social circumstances, the gradual increases in many middle-income countries globally are nevertheless impressive; in many richer countries, the increase in ELB has slowed somewhat (see Chapter 7). In most of the Asia-Pacific, as in almost all rich countries, the expectation is that children born today will live to their high-seventies and even into their mid-eighties. However, in some places, gains have not been so great. ELB in the less developed country group averages 65 years, and in the least developed

Table 6.2 Levels and trends in the under-5 mortality rate, 1990–2010 (deaths per 1,000 live births)

Region	1990	2000	2009	Decline, 1990–2009 (%)	Average annual rate of reduction, 1990–2009 (%)	Progress towards Millennium Development Goal 4 2009
Developing regions	99	84	66	33	2.1	Insufficient progress
Northern Africa	80	46	26	68	5.9	On track
Sub-Saharan Africa	180	160	129	28	1.8	Insufficient progress
Latin America and the Caribbean	52	33	23	56	4.3	On track
Eastern Asia	45	36	19	58	4.5	On track
Eastern Asia Excluding China	28	29	17	39	2.6	On track
Southern Asia	122	95	69	43	3.0	Insufficient progress
Southern Asia Excluding India	131	101	78	40	2.7	Insufficient progress
South-eastern Asia	73	48	36	51	3.7	On track
Western Asia	66	44	31	53	4.0	On track
Oceania	76	65	59	22	1.3	Insufficient progress
Countries of the Commonwealth of Independent States	46	39	23	50	3.6	On track
In Europe	26	23	13	50	3.6	On track
In Asia	78	62	37	53	3.9	On track
Developed regions	12	8	6	50	3.6	On track
Transition countries of South-eastern Europe	31	20	11	65	5.5	On track
World	89	77	60	33	2.1	Insufficient progress

Note: 'On track' under-5 mortality is fewer than 40 deaths per 1,000 live births (2010) or the average annual rate of reduction is at least 4 per cent (1990–2010).

Source: Based on data in United Nations Inter-agency Group for Child Mortality Estimation, 2007, 2011

countries only 56 years. In Africa as a whole, it is 55 years, but only 51 years in sub-Saharan Africa. Gender differences also persist almost everywhere, with females living from one to five (or more) years longer than males. There are almost no exceptions (aside from Swaziland) to the 'rule' that females have longer life expectancy at birth than males.

A retreat of childhood infectious diseases?

Which conditions still cause child mortality (and morbidity)? Children worldwide, and especially in developing and transitional-economy countries, have been at risk from many causes of ill-health and death, especially from infectious diseases, pre-term birth complications, perinatal and neonatal events and, of course, accidents. Have things been changing over recent years? As we saw above, there are still far too many deaths of children under five, but there have been success stories, such as reduced deaths from the infectious childhood disease measles. Alliances such as the multi-partner and sector organization GAVI (formerly the Global Alliance for Vaccines and Immunization) stress the need for momentum in immunization and focus on the poorer countries. In June 2011, a number of major

Expectation of Life at Birth – a longevity boom

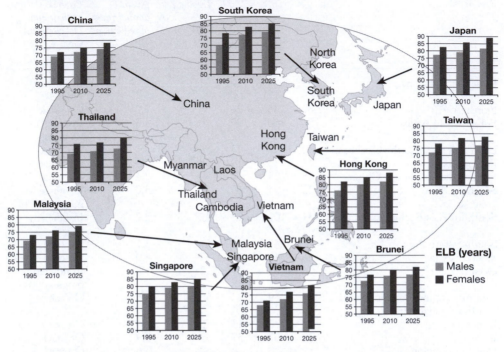

But not everywhere in the Asia–Pacific

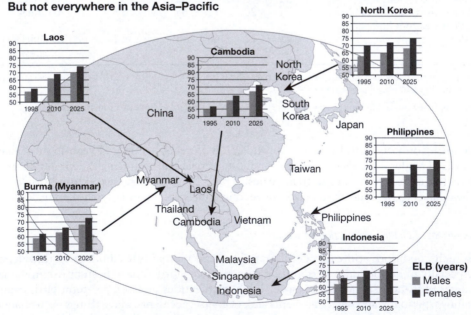

Figure 6.4   Life expectancy at birth: examples of differential increases in selected Asia-Pacific countries, 1995–2025

Source: Data from UNDESA-PD (2011) and others

pharmaceutical multinationals announced they would provide GAVI countries with certain essential vaccines (such as against rotavirus) that donors could purchase at 5 per cent of the cost in richer countries. This is an important example of a move towards multiple-tier pricing in which the poorest countries do not have to pay for the research and development elements of some drugs.

Experts in public health tend to attribute the decline in childhood deaths and generally improving child health in many places, even if variable, to the interplay of numerous key health and social care interventions. These include immunizations, such as measles vaccinations and combined vaccines, malaria prevention strategies (e.g. insecticide-treated bed nets) and vitamin A supplementation. Social improvements, including maternal education, nutrition, access to clean water and better communication, are also essential underlying changes. While the focus tends to be on the poorest countries and groups within them, as childhood ailments also affect rich countries, where the demand for information and safety is huge, these children must also not be overlooked.

Measles

Measles has historically been a major cause of childhood deaths and remains among the world's most contagious diseases and one of the leading causes of death among children, especially in poor countries. One of the indicators for achievement of MDG 4 is the proportion of 1-year-old children immunized against measles.

Even when it does not kill, measles can leave many impairments, such as deafness, partial deafness, blindness and even brain damage. Sometimes healthy and well-nourished children without immunity are at risk, but the vast majority of measles deaths occur in developing countries, especially where immunity rates are low. The development of the measles vaccine and subsequent delivery campaigns (often delivered as MMR, measles–mumps–rubella in developed countries and previously via the EPI in poorer countries) have had dramatic effects over the past thirty-plus years. An Expanded Programme on Immunization (EPI) was introduced by the WHO in 1974 and was pushed strongly through the 1980s and 1990s, including a Universal Child Immunization Programme (Phillips, 1990). The EPI focused especially on diphtheria, pertussis (whooping cough), tetanus, measles, poliomyelitis and tuberculosis. Millions of child deaths have undoubtedly been averted and, for measles alone, an estimated 4.3 million deaths were prevented between 2000 and 2008. GAVI has stressed the use of the pentavalent vaccine for coverage of new and under-vaccinated childhood diseases (diphtheria, tetanus, pertussis, Hib and hepatitis B), illustrating the range of approaches and combinations possible.

Between 2000 and 2008, nearly 700 million children were vaccinated through large-scale immunization campaigns and increased routine immunization coverage (UN Foundation, 2009). In December 2009, the Measles Initiative noted that measles deaths worldwide had fallen from an estimated 733,000 in 2000 to 164,000 in 2008, an impressive decline of 78 per cent. All regions, with the exception of one, achieved the UN goal of reducing measles mortality by 90 per cent from 2000 to 2010, two years ahead of the target date. Only South-east Asia, which includes the very populous South Asian countries, missed out. It had a 46 per cent decline, mainly attributable to India, where UNICEF estimated that three out of four children who died from measles in 2008 were located. The Indian government proposes vigorous campaigns to improve this situation.

Success against specific infectious diseases can, however, mean they fall off the radar. They can then lose crucial funding or the impetus to continue programmes, and agencies therefore fear complacency. This, with lack of sustained funding and follow-up and poor surveillance, can easily allow the resurgence of very infectious diseases, such as measles. Follow-up campaigns every two to four years, with healthcare systems aiming to provide two doses of measles vaccine for all children, are seen as key. Disease surveillance and treatment facilities are also crucial, to detect and control outbreaks as soon as possible. The WHO's Director-General (2012a, p. 1) notes that measles is 'a highly contagious disease that can quickly take advantage of any lapse in effort'. In this respect, maintaining and increasing funding is essential, as the Measles Initiative fears a funding gap could allow a resurgence of measles deaths. Decreased political and financial commitment, instability and inefficient systems could mean as many as 1.7 million measles-related deaths between 2010 and 2013, with more than half a million deaths in 2013 alone, compared to 164,000 in 2008. Indeed, the WHO reported resurgences of measles cases in thirty African countries in 2009–2010, and even in rich countries, such as Britain, following a sharp drop in immunization there in the late 1990s, with a tenfold increase over the decade to 1,000 cases annually. Outbreaks in Europe and Africa in 2010 led to more than 60,000 cases globally over 2009 (CDC, 2012). These outbreaks have been linked to low vaccination coverage, perhaps due to poor access to health services, but also sometimes because of religious or philosophical opposition to vaccination by some parents. Some blame a methodologically flawed paper that linked autism to the combined measles–mumps–rubella vaccine may well have dissuaded many parents from vaccinating their children. Hence, the need remains for combined, sustained efforts, such as the Measles Initiative (involving the American Red Cross, CDC, UNICEF, UN and WHO), for fundraising and promotion, especially targeting sub-Saharan Africa.

Childhood and maternal mortality

Maternal and child health programmes and services have been major features of many local and international health efforts over many decades. Their impacts go far beyond the actual perinatal and infant period, although MCH has tended to use a relatively narrow time frame for intervention and for assessing outcomes (Fine *et al.*, 2009). For example, efforts to improve birth outcomes typically tend to address only the nine-month period of a woman's pregnancy and the more immediate medical, behavioural and, to some extent, individual social conditions surrounding conception and birth. Of course, these are very important, but longer-term social, economic or environmental factors may be even more influential – as recognized previously, for example, in terms of infant mortality, where a major factor is mother's education (see Figure 5.4). (We return to the MDG and other goals on maternal and child health in Chapter 7.)

Adopting a lifecourse or lifespan perspective can provide a broader way of looking at mother and child health, integrated over a lifespan rather than as disconnected or discrete stages, such as infancy, latency, adolescence, childbearing years and old age. This recognizes that a complex interplay of biological, behavioural, psychological, socio-economic and environmental factors contributes to health outcomes across the course of a person's life. It also builds on recent social science and public health literature and the WHO's programme on social determinants of health, which support the lifecourse proposition that each life stage influences the next, and that social, economic and neighbourhood environments acting across the lifecourse have a profound impact on individual and community health (Marmot and Wilkinson, 2006; WHO, 2007a, 2008c). This has huge implications for the types of services planned, when and how. It also highlights the importance of longer-term impacts, such as environmental factors and community and individual behaviours, on health. In many ways, it will enhance, say, the role of education as well as curative health services.

Childhood obesity

While measles is an example of a targetable infectious disease with a specific intervention (immunization), several chronic and potentially serious problems associated in part with lifestyles and poverty have emerged recently. One in particular – obesity – is almost globally appearing ever earlier in the lifecourse. The WHO (2010b) identifies childhood obesity as one of the most serious public health challenges of the twenty-first century, and it is increasingly recognized as a lifecourse risk factor for mortality and a range of chronic diseases in adult life. Its incidence and prevalence are increasing and global – seen in developing and richer countries alike. Many countries and areas have become particularly concerned about the 'epidemic' of childhood obesity, which will be curbed only through sustained political commitment and collaboration of societies, families and individuals.

Obesity is generally viewed as a condition where weight gain has reached the point that it poses a serious threat to health. A common measure is a person's body mass index (BMI), determined by weight and height. BMI cut-off points have been agreed for obese and overweight adults. For children, BMI is more complex, as a child's BMI varies with age, so differing cut-off points have to be used to define overweight and obese children depending on age. We look further at the causes and consequences of obesity in children and adults in Chapter 7.

International trends in childhood obesity: global, England, USA and China

There is worldwide concern over children's increasing weight, and, while some find childhood obesity more alarming because of its future health implications, adults are also frequently affected (see Chapter 7). In 2010, the WHO estimated 43 million children under the age of 5 were overweight throughout the world, though more than 75 per cent of overweight and obese children were in low- and middle-income countries. Overweight and obesity are included within non-communicable disease prevention advocacy (WHO, 2010b). Globally, it has been estimated that 170 million children aged under eighteen are overweight or obese. This includes more than 25 per cent of all children in some countries, and it is more than double the figure at the start of the 'epidemic' in the early 1970s. Children in both rich and poorer countries are affected (Swinburn *et al.*, 2011; see Figure 6.5).

In some countries, such as England, childhood obesity has been emerging over some decades but has increased recently: its prevalence doubled between 1984 and 1994 among 4–12-year-olds – from 0.6 to 1.7 per cent in boys and from 1.3 to 2.6 per cent in girls. By 2001, some 8.5 per cent of 6-year-olds and 15 per cent of 15-year-olds were defined as obese. Similar rises in the prevalence of obesity have also been reported in children in Scotland and in many other developed countries. In many developing countries, especially rapidly modernizing ones such as China, concern has arisen since the 1990s, since when rates have been increasing much more quickly.

Studies in the USA have found childhood obesity to affect as many as one in five children, varying by ethnic groups, and almost one-third of children aged over 2 are already overweight or obese (Wojcicki and Heyman, 2010; McCormick *et al.*, 2010). While some children are somewhat overweight, others are excessively so. Southern California is considered to have only a moderate obesity problem in the USA, but more than 6 per cent of 710,000 children aged 2–19 studied were *far* too heavy, with potentially some 45,000 children affected in this area of the state alone (Koebnick *et al.*, 2010). Extreme obesity was also noted in 7.3 per cent of boys and 5.5 per cent of girls, with prevalence peaking at 10 years among boys and 12 years among girls, with a second peak at 18 years. Extreme obesity varied in ethnic/racial and age groups, with the highest prevalence in Hispanic boys (up to

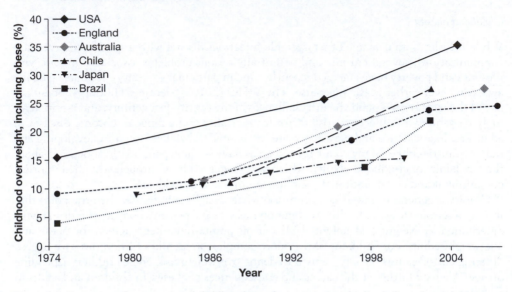

Figure 6.5 Estimates of percentage of childhood population overweight (including obese) in a
        selection of countries (from c. 1974)

Source: Swinburn *et al.*, 2011. Reprinted from *The Lancet*, 278, Swinburn, B.A. *et al.*, "The global obesity
pandemic: shaped by global drivers and local environments", pp. 804-814. Copyright (2011) with permission from
Elsevier.

11.2 per cent) and African-American girls (up to 11.9 per cent). The percentage of extreme
obesity was lowest in Asian-Pacific islanders and non-Hispanic white children. This may be
one of the first studies to provide a snapshot of the prevalence of *extreme* obesity in a
contemporary cohort of children aged 2–19 years from a large racially and ethnically diverse
population using the 2009 US Centers for Disease Control and Prevention 'extreme obesity'
definition.

Rapidly industrializing countries (or sub-regions), especially in Asia and Latin America,
are also noting increased childhood weight. In China, the phenomenon of one-child families
has compounded this, to some extent, with single children, especially boys ('little emperors'),
accorded all the food and treats they demand, and with academic achievement often placed
ahead of physical activities. By 2002, of the 155 million overweight or obese children worldwide, 12 million lived in China. This has happened relatively quickly, associated with the
country's rapid modernization and economic boom. In the 1980s, prevalence of childhood
overweight was only around 5 per cent and obesity 2 per cent. However, research in 2008 in
the major city of Guangzhou, southern China, involving 1,800 schoolchildren aged 7–14
years, found more than 11 per cent were overweight and over 7 per cent obese. Many displayed a cluster of cardiovascular disease risk factors, including insulin resistance, impaired
glucose, elevated blood pressure and triglycerides and cholesterol problems (Liu *et al.*, 2010).

Causes of obesity among children

Obesity can occur when an individual takes in more energy than they expend, although
some people appear genetically more susceptible than others. Many feel the rise in obesity
has been too rapid to be attributed solely to genetic factors and that it principally reflects
changes in eating patterns (amounts and types of food) and reduced levels of physical

activity. Wojcicki and Heyman (2010) note that other factors associated with an increased risk of becoming overweight for infants and young children include:

- mother's excessive weight gain or smoking during pregnancy;
- shorter than recommended breastfeeding; and
- lack of sleep during infancy.

These behavioural or lifestyle factors may somehow programme long-term regulation of energy balance, with subsequent effects on ability to regulate body weight. For example, long-term benefits of breastfeeding appear to include reduced risk of obesity in adulthood, with a consequent lower risk of type 2 diabetes, lower blood pressure and total cholesterol levels. Energy intake, often thought the key dietary factor in obesity, may be only one in a sequence of risk factors. Indeed, in the UK, for example, average energy intakes appear to have *declined* since the early 1970s, but other factors, such as sources and timing of food intake, may have changed and influenced obesity. For example, increased consumption of alcoholic drinks, confectionery and food and drink outside the home and regular mealtimes occurred over this period. Some studies implicate reduced physical activity and emergence of more 'sedentary' lifestyles. In many countries, and especially in some groups, research and anecdotal evidence do indicate decline in engagement in physical sport, team games and outside activities by young people, with clear increases in sedentary pastimes, notably television, computer gaming, internet surfing and school work on computers.

Consequences of obesity in children and young adults

As we seem to be able to detect the causes, why is the increase in childhood and youth obesity now a major cause of concern? It may often affect a child's behaviour and development and, moreover, obese youngsters may be at greater risk of a number of 'adult' chronic conditions, appearing at much younger ages than otherwise expected. The southern California study raised the alarm as extreme obesity is increasingly seen at relatively young ages. The shift towards more extreme body weights is predicted to cause an enormous burden of adverse health outcomes once these children and adolescents grow older (McCormick *et al.*, 2010). In the California study, Koebnick *et al.* (2010) and Kaiser Permanente (2010) note that extremely overweight children may continue to be extremely obese as adults, so the many health problems associated with obesity will lie in their futures. They state frankly that, without major lifestyle changes, such children face lifespans ten to twenty years shorter, and will be likely to develop health problems in their twenties that are more often found in 40–60-year-olds. Extremely obese children have higher risk of developing heart disease, type 2 diabetes, fatty liver disease and joint problems, among many others.

'Our focus and concern is all about health and not about appearance. Children who are morbidly obese can do anything they want – they can be judges, lawyers, doctors – but the one thing they cannot be is healthy' (Amy Porter, in Kaiser Permanente, 2010, p. 1).

Obesity not only increases mortality but, as seen above, it is an important risk factor for many chronic conditions, principally in adult life. Moreover, it raises the risk of chronic conditions appearing at ever-younger adult ages. Overweight adolescents have a 70 per cent chance of becoming overweight or obese adults. During childhood, problems that can be associated with youth obesity include:

- social and psychological consequences: stigmatization, discrimination, bullying and prejudice, low self-esteem, self-image and depression (in children and adults);
- reduced physical activities which itself can increase social isolation;

- type 2 diabetes, previously considered a disease of adulthood, but increasingly seen in obese schoolchildren;
- coronary heart disease (the most common cause of premature death among obese people);
- osteoarthritis and back pain; and
- cancers: there are few clear links between cancer and obesity, but there is evidence of both dietary and overweight links in some, such as colon cancer (obesity increases the risk by nearly three times).

Strategies on obesity

These possible consequences and the risk factors suggest strategies may need to go beyond targeting just young heavy eaters themselves. It has been suggested that interventions should specifically involve pregnant women, infants and pre-schoolers, for example, to reduce excessive weight gain in pregnancy, to increase duration of breastfeeding and to increase sleep during infancy. Existing health campaigns already often try to reduce smoking rates, especially among women who wish to become pregnant and mothers of young children. Policies increasingly attempt to incorporate families and communities, involving the education of parents and would-be parents. They include public education, school healthy-eating and exercise campaigns, and labelling of food. Campaigns are appearing everywhere, such as the high-profile US national 'Let's move' campaign launched in February 2010 by the President's wife, Michelle Obama. This is an example of a multifactor campaign that aims to prevent childhood obesity from pregnancy and infancy, and tries to change national attitudes to eating habits, physical exercise and knowledge of foods (Wojcicki and Heyman, 2010). In most developed countries (and, increasingly, in many transitional, middle-income economy and developing countries), childhood obesity campaigns at various social and geographical levels are also being implemented.

Diabetes in children and adolescents

Apparently closely associated with widespread increases in childhood obesity, diabetes is also becoming a global issue. Diabetes, discussed further in Chapter 7, was previously thought of mainly as a condition of adulthood or of older people. Today, it is becoming one of the most common chronic diseases of childhood, and worldwide estimates suggest that 490,000 children are living with type 1 diabetes. Diabetes can affect children at any age and 78,000 children under 15 annually develop type 1 diabetes, the causes of which remain unknown. Type 1 diabetes is growing globally at an estimated 3 per cent annually in children and adolescents, and at an alarming 5 per cent among children aged 5 years and under (International Diabetes Federation, 2003, 2009, 2011). There are considerable regional variations in type 1, and of the approximately 490,000 cases in 2011, 23 per cent were in South-east Asia and 24 per cent in Europe, but only about 6 per cent in the Western Pacific region, in spite of its large child population, and few in sub-Saharan Africa, where data are very sparse (International Diabetes Federation, 2011). Perhaps due to a paucity of research and data in poorer countries, all of the 'top ten' countries for new cases of type 1 diabetes are developed, where data are most complete. Top of the list are Finland, Sweden, Norway, the UK and the USA (Soltesz *et al.*, 2009).

Of equal or greater concern is the emergence of type 2 diabetes among children globally, whereas once this was almost exclusively an adult disease of the 40-plus age group. The CDC (2011a) suggest that epidemics of obesity and low levels of physical activity among young people, and possibly exposure to diabetes *in utero*, may be major underlying factors in the increase in type 2 diabetes in childhood and adolescence. It is already a considerable and growing problem among children and adolescents in the USA, several European and other countries. Type 2 diabetes in children, rare thirty years ago, now accounts for over 40 per cent of new-onset cases in children in the USA, and 10 per cent in Asia. Looking at change over time, Japan and Taiwan found type 2 is now more common among children or school-children than type 1 and, at diagnosis, it was not unusual for young people to be displaying multiple risk factors for heart disease (Kaufman, 2007).

Despite treatment, many children with diabetes develop complications about twelve years after diagnosis, although early diagnosis, appropriate care, access to medication, education and support can enable children with diabetes to live full and healthy lives. Unlike type 1, type 2 diabetes has known risk factors, discussed more in Chapter 7, so avoiding the avoid-able ones is crucial. The public health campaigns related to obesity noted above will become increasingly important. As Kaufman (2007, p. 35) notes, it is now 'widely recognized that the current tide of type 2 diabetes in young people can be turned back through the develop-ment and implementation of anti-obesity initiatives and diabetes prevention strategies for children'. This will require the concerted collaboration of many sectors, involving health-care, governments, schools, business, communities, families and individuals globally.

Middle-age (and earlier) health transitions

The middle years cover a wide range of health-status potential changes occurring from young adulthood to middle age (see Boxes 6.1 and 6.2). By age 15, mortality rates are generally starting to climb, which continues for the rest of the adult life cycle. Lifetime's lowest age of mortality is between 5 and 14 and thereafter death rates rise by 50 to 100 per cent for ages 15 to 24 (Jenkins, 2003). Teenage years, in particular, are increasingly seen as crucial for future health. It is estimated that two-thirds of premature deaths in adults are traceable to behaviour that started during teenage years, especially (notably in lower-income countries) smoking, but also other risky activities (Hammond, 2011).

Leading causes of morbidity and disability have a mixed pattern in the adolescent/young-adult age group, 15–24; for females aged 10–19, examples are given in Box 6.1. At this stage,

---

BOX 6.1 Adolescent girls (10–19 years): major causes of death and ill-health

- *Unintentional injuries*: road traffic accidents are the leading cause of death among adolescent girls (10–19 years) in high- and middle-income countries.
- *Mental health*: suicide and mental health disorders become significant in ill-health and death in all regions.
- *HIV/AIDS*: HIV infection is high in countries that have generalized HIV epi-demics. Adolescent girls are at risk of unsafe, often unwanted, forced sexual activity. Risk of HIV/AIDS, other sexually transmitted infections, unwanted pregnancy and unsafe abortion.
- *Adolescent pregnancy*: pregnancy-related complications are a leading cause of death among girls aged 15–19 years in developing countries, with unsafe abortion a major factor.
- *Substance use*: 'adolescent girls are increasingly using tobacco and alcohol'. There is some evidence of tobacco advertising targeting young girls and women.

(Source: WHO, 2009b, pp. 1–2)

BOX 6.2 Reproductive age (15–44 years) and adult women (20–59 years): major causes of death and ill-health

- *HIV/AIDS*: this becomes a leading cause of death and disease worldwide, with unsafe sex 'the main risk factor in developing countries.'
- *Maternal health*: 99 per cent of the half a million maternal deaths occur in developing countries.
- *Tuberculosis*: often linked to HIV infection, this is the third leading cause of death among women of reproductive age in low-income countries and worldwide. 'It ranks fifth worldwide among women aged 20–59 years.'
- *Injuries and violence*: injuries from road traffic accidents are in the top ten causes of death of adult women (20–59 years) globally. Women are at greater risk of fire-related deaths/injury. Violence against women is widespread globally. Most is perpetrated by an intimate male partner but it is also often a tactic of war.
- *Cervical cancer*: the second most common type of cancer among women, mainly linked to infection with human papillomavirus (HPV). 'Almost 80 per cent of cases and a higher proportion of deaths from cervical cancer are in low-income countries' (due to lack of access to screening and treatment).
- *Depression and suicide*: women are more susceptible to depression and anxiety than men. 'Suicide is the seventh top cause of death globally for women aged 20–59 years.'
- *Chronic obstructive pulmonary disease (COPD)*: tobacco use and burning solid fuels for indoor heating/cooking are primary risk factors for COPD.

(Source: Based on WHO, 2009b, pp. 2–3)

---

rates of fatal biological diseases (cancers, heart and blood vessel pathology) begin to increase. However, trauma and injury, especially motor-vehicle related, become the main causes of death. Homicides and suicides kill many young males, especially in certain regions (such as the Americas and some Middle Eastern countries). Suicide starts to appear as a major cause of death around age 15, although geographical variations are considerable. For example, Hispanic countries have relatively low rates for attempted and actual suicides, while China has high rates among young women (and among older people). In the 15–24 age group, risk behaviours start to emerge seriously (Jenkins, 2003; WHO, 2009b).

Tobacco use, misuse of alcohol and related activities involving unsafe sex, motor-vehicle and pedestrian injuries, drownings, assaults, suicides and chemical dependencies appear in this age group. Unsafe sexual behaviours risk unwanted pregnancies, and any one of twenty or more other sexually transmitted diseases (STDs) as well as HIV/AIDS. Lack of regular exercise, unhealthy eating habits and psychologically driven eating disorders may emerge among young males and females. Broader psychological and psychiatric concerns also often manifest themselves and the psycho-social foundations of many health problems emerge: hormonal changes, competitiveness and a sense of invulnerability may all lead to impulsive risk taking (Jenkins, 2003).

The middle-adult years, 25–64, are the main economically active ages (varyingly interpreted) – years when many people settle down, build households and raise families. It is a very heterogeneous stage. For example, by age 50, the older period, many people are beyond parenting and indeed may be caring for older relatives, but many are still looking after children at the same time. Health-related influences change considerably and many lifestyle-related diseases may emerge. These include work-related stress, overweight, obesity and diabetes, with concomitant cardiovascular and other physiological deterioration and risk factors (discussed in more detail in Chapter 7). Between 25 and 64, the full range of risk factors and health problems emerges. There is considerable differentiation between and within countries, between social groups and occupations, and among individuals.

Health transitions in the later years: older persons and the oldest old

Impacts of global ageing

Worldwide – in most countries – the major feature of lifecourse transitions has been the lengthening of life expectancy and demographic ageing. (However, as noted in Chapter 4, there are some exceptions.) Considerable changes in health patterns have been associated with demographic ageing (see, for example, Box 6.3). It is difficult to predict the ultimate demographic patterns in any given country or locality, as these will be heavily affected by reproductive behaviour, life expectancy and migration patterns. Nevertheless, generally increasing numbers and percentages of older people, with an almost universal female preponderance, are major features almost everywhere (UNDESA, 2008; NIA, 2007; Dannefer and Phillipson, 2010). The social and health ramifications of demographic ageing are manifold (Kinsella and Phillips, 2005; Kinsella and He, 2009). In many countries, the bulk of deaths are being pushed into the age group 65 and over, which has enormous implications for healthcare provision, societies, families and carers.

BOX 6.3 Older women (60-plus years): major causes of death and ill-health

Women form the growing majority of older people (in 2011, almost 55 per cent of people aged 60 and over were women, reaching 60 per cent at 75 and over). 'Chronic conditions, mainly cardiovascular disease and COPD, account for 45 per cent of deaths in women aged 60 and over worldwide'; 15 per cent of deaths are caused by cancers, mainly of the breast, lung and colon.

- *Lifecourse accumulation of health risks:* many women's health problems in older age stem from risk factors of their adolescence and adulthood (smoking, sedentary lifestyles, unhealthy diets). Debilitating problems include poor vision, hearing loss, arthritis, depression and dementia.
- *Cardiovascular disease: heart attacks/ischaemic heart disease and strokes:* often thought a 'male' problem, cardiovascular disease is the main killer globally of older women. Women tend to develop heart disease later in life than men.
- *Breast, lung and colon cancer:* these cancers are among the 'top ten' causes of death of older women globally. Breast cancer incidence is much higher in high-income countries than low- and middle-income countries, though mortality is similar. Incidence and mortality for lung and colon cancer are currently higher in high-income countries; 71 per cent of lung cancer deaths globally are linked to tobacco use.

(Sources: WHO, 2009b, p. 3 and US Census Bureau, *International Database* website)

There are many actual and potential health changes in later years, but several specific features are important, especially among the oldest old:

- There are often multiple causes of morbidity and death in old age. Among older adults, several potentially fatal disease processes may be present and may jointly contribute to death. For example, many older men may have slowly developing prostate cancer, live with it and die from a cause such as heart disease or stroke.
- In developed countries and those with organized reporting systems, a certifying physician usually determines which conditions 'caused' death (see Chapter 2), but this may sometimes be an arbitrary decision. On average, three causes are listed on death certificates of older deaths. However, in many countries, especially the poorer ones, deaths may be only verbally reported or not at all, so there is little reliable information on actual causes of death of older people.
- Heart disease and cancer, the leading underlying causes of death, are also the most prevalent when all causes on the death certificate are considered, so these data may not be helpful for refined analyses of mortality trends.
- According to US studies, one in every three people aged 65 and older suffers a fall each year. This problem can be hidden, as many older people do not talk to healthcare providers about their falls. However, among this age group, falls are the leading cause of injury death and the most common cause of non-fatal injuries and hospital admissions for trauma. Falls can cause moderate to severe injuries, including hip fractures and head traumas. Importantly, they increase the risk of early death (82 per cent of fall deaths were among people aged 65 and over). Falls are seen as a public health problem that is largely preventable, but death rates from falls among older men and women have risen sharply over recent years. The direct and indirect medical costs of falls are considerable. Falls may mean older people are unable to live independently, they lead to high rates of hospitalization and can lead to a fear of falling. Moreover, the chances of falling and of being seriously injured from the fall increase with age. The rate of fall injuries for those aged 85 and over in 2009 was almost four times that for people aged 65–74 (CDC, 2011b).
- Perhaps most significant for the future, psycho-social conditions and especially cognitive impairment from dementias increase greatly as people and populations age. As we shall see subsequently (Chapters 7, 8 and 11), dementias will pose an ever more significant challenge for the poorer countries, as well as the already-aged countries. The prevalence of dementias nearly doubles every five years after age 65, and at 85-plus close to a quarter of people can have some degree of dementia (see Chapters 7 and 11).
- Importantly, not all older persons are ill or even in need of assistance. There is considerable debate about longer life and whether health is improving or deteriorating and whether morbidity is compressing into a short period before death (see below and Chapter 11).

The 'speed' of population ageing

The recent apparent rapidity of demographic ageing of populations has become a global feature (see also Chapter 11). Over the last three or four decades, this phenomenon has been seen strongly in many, if not all, former developing and transitional countries.

Most developed countries, especially those in Western and Northern Europe and North America, were effectively 'aged' by the 1970s. They had typically taken between fifty and a hundred years for the percentage of older people (arbitrarily, those aged over 65) in their populations to increase from 7 to 14 per cent. By contrast, many erstwhile developing countries have taken only between twenty and thirty years for this to occur, mainly since 1970 (Kinsella and Phillips, 2005; NIA, 2007; Victor, 2010). This has included huge-population countries such as China, Brazil and many others. This clearly shifts the balance of many such population pyramids upwards, towards the older age groups. Similarly, several countries now have 18–20 per cent of their populations aged over 65 (Italy, Germany, Sweden) and numerous have between 15 and 20 per cent, including almost all countries in Europe. Many are seemingly in almost a 'steady state' in terms of this age group. The demographically oldest country (Japan) had 23 per cent aged over 65 in 2011.

By contrast, although numbers of older people are increasing in most poorer countries, many still have relatively small percentages aged over 65, due partly to the sustained high birth rates which dilute the percentages of older people and partly to somewhat lower life expectancies. Countries in this category include many in Western Asia and almost all of sub-Saharan Africa. Almost all the countries in the less and least developed groups have between 3 and 5 per cent of their populations aged over 65. However, this is likely to change substantially over the next two to three decades, when demographic ageing accelerates in these nations. This existing and predicted 'compression of ageing' means local and national institutions will have to adapt quickly to their new population structures.

Life expectancy at 60 or over 65

The somewhat theoretical figure of expectation of life at birth (ELB) (see Chapters 2, 4 and 11) is generally increasing worldwide, although there have been some notable reversals. The regional patterns and some specific examples are considered later (in Figures 11.1 and 11.2). More important in terms of regional health patterns in old age is perhaps life expectancy at 60 or over 65 (see Table 6.3). This has often been increasing, given the growth in many countries of what is sometimes called the 'oldest old' – people aged over 80 or 85 years.

Survival curves moving out over the last century

Following the detailed discussion of changes in life expectancy in Chapter 4, one question that has persistently intrigued humanity becomes more poignant: how long can human beings be expected to live? As well as being a historical and philosophical dilemma, this question has technical demographic aspects seen in the debate on limits to human life expectancy. Survival curves are 'moving out' but vary internationally (see Figures 4.1 and 4.5). As Bongaarts (2006) notes, since 1800, life expectancy at birth has more or less doubled from around 40 to nearly 80 years. However, many demographers and biologists disagree about what lies ahead. 'Pessimists' believe limits to life expectancy are now being approached, at around 85 years. The 'optimists' tend to foresee continued rapid improvements with almost no finite limits. Biologists also sometimes suggest that 'mortality after the reproductive ages' lies 'beyond the reach of Darwinian forces of natural selection'. A biologically determined age pattern of *senescent* mortality is said to exist, 'which rises steeply with age after about 30 in humans'. Bongaarts (2006, p. 623) suggests that a 'steady upward trend in senescent life expectancy in recent decades' supports the more optimistic view, and that there is no evidence that humanity is approaching limits to longevity. He presents calculations suggesting that life expectancy is likely to increase by an average of about 7.5 years over the next fifty years, plus any (likely to be minor) effects of further declines in juvenile, background and smoking mortality. There seems little or no reason to believe that 'advances in biotechnology, preventive and curative medicine will be less effective in reducing senescent mortality in the future than in the past' (p. 623). Indeed, Bongaarts suggests that an *acceleration* of improvements cannot be ruled out. This school of thought implies an

Table 6.3 Life expectancy (years) at age 65, 1960–2009

	Males	Females
Japan		
1960	11.6	14.1
1970	12.5	15.3
1990	16.2	20.0
2009	18.9	24.0
United Kingdom		
1960	11.9	15.1
1970	12.0	16.0
1990	14.0	17.9
2009	18.1	20.8
Australia		
1960	12.5	15.6
1970	11.9	15.6
1990	15.2	19.0
2009	18.7	21.8
Spain		
1960	13.1	15.3
1970	13.3	16.0
1990	15.5	19.3
2009	18.3	22.4
South Korea		
1960	–	–
1970	10.2	14.6
1990	12.4	16.3
2009	17.1	21.5

Source: OECD website

ever-ageing global population, but what will be the concomitant health and social care consequences of that?

As more people survive longer in most countries, their health and functioning in old age become ever more important. However, the WHO (2011c) notes that higher disability rates among older people reflect the accumulation of health risks of disease, injury and chronic illness over the lifespan. Rates vary according to development status, with disability prevalence among people aged over 45 in low-income countries being higher than in high-income countries, and also higher among women than men. In most places, older people are disproportionately represented among disabled populations. For example, while older persons comprise 10.7 per cent of Australia's population, they are 35.2 per cent of people with disabilities. Similarly, people aged over 65 comprise 6.6 per cent of Sri Lanka's population but 22 per cent of people with disabilities. Given the growth of the 'oldest old' mentioned above, it is important to recognize that rates of disability are generally much higher in the 80–89 year group – the fastest-growing age cohort worldwide – which is projected to comprise one-fifth of the world's population aged over 60 by 2050.

Canadian research indicates that five types of chronic conditions contributed the main causes of activities of daily living (ADL) and instrumental ADL (IADL) disability among people aged over 65: foot problems; arthritis; cognitive impairment; heart problems; and vision (Griffith *et al.*, 2010). Other important problems include hearing impairment, chronic obstructive pulmonary disease (COPD) (probably more common in older people than is often recognized), and falls and hip fractures. Similar conditions feature in the 'top ten' associated with functional limitation or disability among older people (65 and over) in the USA:

1 Arthritis/rheumatism: 30.0 per cent
2 Heart problems: 23.2 per cent
3 Hypertension: 13.7 per cent
4 Back/neck problems: 12.6 per cent
5 Diabetes: 12.1 per cent
6 Vision problems: 11.8 per cent
7 Lung/breathing problems 11.1 per cent
8 Fractures/bone/joint injury: 10.7 per cent
9 Stroke: 9.2 per cent
10 Hearing problems: 7.0 per cent.

(Based on Freedman *et al.*, 2004 and Lafortune *et al.* 2007; the numbers add up to more than 100 per cent because of co-morbidities)

Compression of morbidity?

An important question in the discussion of life expectancy and disability-free life is, as the WHO maxim suggests, whether 'life is being added to years' as well as 'years being added to life'. Life expectancy may generally be increasing but are people living healthier lives as well as longer years, or are they suffering poor health for longer (NIA, 2007)? The quality of the added life years is crucial, both socially and economically.

The debate effectively revolves around a question posed by Lois Verbrugge in 1984: is there 'longer life but worsening health'? (See also Chapter 4.) Will longer life be accompanied by worsening (chronic) health or morbidity or might serious illness be pushed into the final few months or years of life in a compression of morbidity? Christensen *et al.* (2009) similarly ask whether increases in life expectancy are accompanied by a concurrent postponement of functional limitations and disability. They feel this is still an open question, although research suggests that ageing processes are modifiable and that people are living longer without severe disability.

The compression of morbidity concept was suggested by Fries in 1980, but evidence is still mixed. As we saw in Chapter 4 with regard even to death rates, data are often too scanty. When it comes to morbidity, things are even more difficult to resolve and the crucial question – will people be healthier and more active as well as longer lived? – remains very awkward. This will have overwhelming importance to older people and their families in terms of well-being, but it will also have huge implications for the costs and needs for long-term care and support.

International comparisons

In recent years, a number of researchers have identified potential compressions of morbidity, under which ill-health, disability and dependency are pushed further back into a shorter period towards the end of a person's life. While evidence is mixed, Kinsella and He (2009) note that research has attempted to take account not only of mortality but of variations in morbidity to determine 'health expectancy'. This could be years of good health or years free from specific diseases, healthy life expectancy (see Chapter 2). Unfortunately, strict comparisons of the various estimates of healthy life expectancy among nations are often impossible due to differences in ways these are calculated and varying definitions of such things as impairment, disability and handicap. Nevertheless, comparative studies have been conducted. One using late twentieth-century data in nine developed countries plus Taiwan suggested disability was in general declining in older age (Waidmann and Manton, 1998). On the whole, it appears that there is a general decline in levels of disability among succeeding cohorts of older people, especially in the richer countries and parts of East Asia. However, improvements may be confined to people in certain geographical areas and maybe only to those in certain social groups.

Further evidence for a mixed picture of disability change is seen in a study of twelve OECD countries for people aged over 65. The data give clear evidence of annual decline in severe disability in only five of the twelve countries studied: Denmark, Finland, Italy, the Netherlands and the United States (Lafortune *et al.*, 2007). In these, the average decline over the period was around 1–2 per cent per annum. However, the reduction could be due to a decline in less severe levels of disability in some countries: that is, only a reduction in functional limitations. Three countries (Belgium, Japan and Sweden) actually showed an *increasing* annual rate of severe disability of around 2.5–3.5 per cent among people aged over 65 during the previous five to ten years. Two countries (Australia and Canada) reported relatively stable rates. Because data from different surveys in France and the United Kingdom showed different trends in ADL disability rates, it was impossible to state definitively the direction of their trends.

National changes in disability-free life expectancy

In terms of national studies, considerable research has been conducted in the USA, using national and other data sets, focusing principally on older groups. Some studies indicate decline in disability, others do not. Manton *et al.* (2006) noted good news in an increase in non-disabled people in the USA aged over 65 from 73.5 per cent in 1982 to 81 per cent in 2004–05. Data from a number of other US studies over varying periods also indicate declines in disability rates and/or percentages of older people reporting disability. However, the results are by no means clear. Seeman *et al.* (2010), for example, noted that, between 1988–94 and 1999–2004, except for functional limitations, there were significant increases in other types of disability among 60–69-year-olds, regardless of socio-economic variables, health status, behaviours and weight. However, they found no particular trends among people aged 70–79, and among the oldest group (over 80), trends indicated lower prevalence of functional limitations among the recent cohorts. They note studies indicate that, while the older groups may be experiencing somewhat less disability, the younger old groups, including the oldest baby boomers, 'may be experiencing worse health status and more disability than their earlier counterparts' (p. 100). This has worrying implications for long-term healthcare needs and costs.

There are ethnic and social differences, even in developed economies, and Seeman *et al.* (2010) suggest that the changing composition of the upcoming older groups in the USA will be important. For example, greater increases in disability occurred among non-whites and persons who were obese or overweight, two of the fastest-growing sub-groups of the USA's upcoming-old population. These are also very important, large groups of future older people in many other countries. Looking across countries, comparing the USA and England, studies suggest that middle-aged white, non-Hispanic, middle-aged Americans are not as healthy as their English peers. Indeed, among three socio-economic groups, the healthiest Americans (those with highest education and income levels) had rates of heart disease and diabetes comparable to the least healthy group in England (those with lowest education and income levels) (Banks *et al.*, 2006; Kinsella and He, 2009).

Among factors promoting declines in disability, changes in the prevalence of heart and circulatory conditions and visual limitations have played major roles (Kinsella and He, 2009). However, factors such as increases in obesity may have an escalating longer-term counter-effect, and limit healthy life expectancy, especially if obese young–middle-aged people develop disabilities earlier. Some factors can help reduce disability, or its impacts, such as a greater use of assistive technology, increasing education levels and declines in poverty. In some countries, and among some groups, declines in smoking have also been important in reducing later-life morbidity and premature mortality, although there are huge global and social variations.

To judge how any people or groups are affected we need more refined analyses of types of disability, its onset, people's environments and many other factors. In the USA, for example, it seems that less severe disability has declined since the 1980s, and more severe disability has declined since the 1990s (Crimmins *et al.*, 2009, p. 627). Crimmins *et al.*'s detailed study considered changes in life expectancy free of disability, using longitudinal data from 1984–2000. 'At age 70, disability-free life expectancy increased over a 10-year period by 0.6 of a year in the later cohort . . . the same as the increase in total life expectancy.' However, average length of expected life with ADL and IADL disability did not change. Changes in disability-free life expectancy seemed to stem from decreases in disability incidence and increases in *recovery* from disability across the two cohorts. After age 80, age-specific mortality among ADL disabled persons declined significantly in the later cohort but did not change significantly for IADL disabled and the non-disabled people. People with ADL disability at age 70 showed 'substantial increases in both total life expectancy and disability-free life expectancy'. These complex findings indicate the importance of efforts both to prevent and delay onset of disability and to promote recovery from disability for increasing life expectancy without disability. Therefore, development of both treatment and rehabilitative services for people who have suffered disability is crucial. However, greater survival can work in several ways. Reductions in incidence and increases in recovery may help decrease population prevalence of disability, but declining mortality among the disabled groups can perhaps be a factor underlying increasing the *prevalence* of disability.

There may be other reasons why some studies have found an apparent decrease in the onset of disability (Crimmins *et al.*, 2009). Some diseases may have become less disabling over time, perhaps because of earlier diagnosis and/or better treatment and disease management. Recent cohorts of older people may also have reached any given older age in better condition and therefore with less chance of ADL/IADL problems. Once can speculate that factors such as lifetime advantages of better education, less physically demanding jobs, better nutrition and healthcare might all play a part, though this is rather difficult to quantify. Environmental factors could also be important as permissive factors. An age-friendly environment should make life much easier, allowing people with lower-level ADL problems to manage for longer. More appropriate or less challenging housing, along with assistive technology or social support, or alternatives to traditional housing, will also very likely enhance person–environmental fit. Its availability might benefit many older people in more recent cohorts and might mitigate the impacts of any declining ADLs. It is clear that more country-specific and cross-national studies are needed. Given the international increases in the oldest-old cohorts, who have the likelihood of greater disability, this topic has huge implications for integrated health, social and welfare.

What do the data mean?

Attempting national and international comparisons soon shows that many factors could affect findings and influence data on disability. These include better and earlier diagnosis, especially in richer countries; greater awareness of conditions (such as dementias); better reporting; better treatments and longer survivorship with chronic conditions; and rising expectations of good health (Kinsella and He, 2009). More pessimistic policy implications can be drawn from the OECD and some US studies. It might therefore be unwise for policy-makers to rely on future reductions in the prevalence of severe disability among elderly people wholly to offset the likely rising demand for long-term care coming from population ageing (Lafortune *et al.*, 2007). Indeed, while disability prevalence rates may have declined in some countries, and may decline further, population ageing and greater longevity of individuals may be expected to lead to increasing numbers of people at older ages with severe disabilities and hence need of long-term care. We return to these effects of global health changes and policy in Part III.

Dementias

Undoubtedly, one of the major global challenges of demographic ageing is the increase in number of people with psycho-social problems and especially degenerative mental and physical conditions, such as dementias. For example, data in an ageing Asian society, such as Hong Kong, indicate that, at age 60, people with dementia have on average seven years less life expectancy than the general population, although males with dementia might still expect to live another sixteen years (Yu *et al.*, 2010). We introduce this here to acknowledge the emerging pre-eminence of these lifecourse conditions, with more detailed consideration given in Chapters 7 and 11, especially as dementias are likely to become an ever-increasing future challenge.

Discussion topics

1   What differences do you see in the main threats to childhood health between high-income and middle- and low-income countries?
2   How far do you feel that population ageing is a great benefit to humanity or something that brings insurmountable health and welfare challenges?
3   How might the poorer countries develop strategies to cope with great predicted increases in 'lifestyle' conditions, such as obesity, and NCDs, such as diabetes, cancers and dementias?

7 Major contemporary challenges in global health

Risk factors and contemporary disease control priorities

In terms of burden of disease measured by DALYs (defined in Chapters 2 and 4), the leading global risks for burden of disease are underweight (6 per cent of global DALYs); unsafe sex (5 per cent); alcohol use (5 per cent); and unsafe water, sanitation and hygiene (4 per cent). The distribution of these risk factors tends to underlie the differing regional patterns of major causes of death and DALYs seen in Table 4.9. Three of these risks particularly affect populations in low-income countries, especially in the regions of South-east Asia and sub-Saharan Africa. The fourth risk (alcohol use) has a somewhat different geographic and sex pattern, with its burden highest for men in Africa, in middle-income countries in the Americas and in some high-income countries (Jamison *et al.*, 2006; WHO, 2009a).

Box 7.1 summarizes the WHO's overall global burden of disease findings. It is important to note at the outset, however, that these tend to reflect a focus on acute and infectious diseases, especially in low-income countries. But as we discuss below, non-communicable diseases (NCDs) are rapidly becoming a major burden in these as well as in richer countries.

In terms of global patterns of health risk, for mortality, the WHO's *Global Health Risks* (2009a, p. 9) notes that more than one-third of the world's deaths can be attributed to a small number of risk factors. It notes twenty-four risk factors in the report, which are responsible for 44 per cent of global deaths and 34 per cent of DALYs; the ten leading risk factors account for 33 per cent of deaths. In terms of developing effective strategies for improving global health, knowledge of the role of these risk factors and how they can be modified is crucial. As noted in Chapters 4 and 6, the five leading global risks for mortality in the world are identified as:

- high blood pressure (13%);
- tobacco use (9%);
- high blood glucose (6%);
- physical inactivity (6%); and
- overweight and obesity (5%).

These five factors are responsible for raising the risk of many chronic NCDs, such as heart disease and some cancers (a very varied disease group), and they can also lead to acute episodes, such as heart attacks. They affect countries at all levels of incomes and development, although with varying impacts, as we saw in Table 4.10. The WHO (2009a, p. 5) selected its risk factors according to whether they filled specific criteria, with:

- a potential for a global impact;
- a high likelihood that the risk causes each associated disease;

BOX 7.1 The global burden of disease (GBD) and injuries

The GBD 2004 update is a comprehensive assessment of the causes of loss of health in the different world regions. It assesses the comparative importance of diseases and injuries in causing premature death, loss of health and disability in different populations (by age, sex and for a range of country groupings). Estimates are given for 135 disease and injury cause categories. Findings include:

- Worldwide, Africa accounts for nine out of every ten child deaths from both malaria and AIDS, and half the global child deaths due to diarrhoeal disease and pneumonia.
- In low-income countries, pneumonia is the leading cause of death, followed by heart disease, diarrhoea, HIV/AIDS and stroke. In developed or high-income countries, heart disease is first, followed by stroke, lung cancer, pneumonia and asthma or bronchitis.
- Men aged 15–60 years have much higher risks of dying than women in this age category in every world region, mainly because of injuries, including violence and conflict, and higher levels of heart disease. Differences are most pronounced in Latin America, the Caribbean, the Middle East and Eastern Europe.
- 'Depression is the leading cause of years lost due to disability'; the burden is 50 per cent higher for females than males. At all income levels, 'alcohol dependence and problem use is in the ten leading causes of disability'.

(Source: Based on WHO, 2009a, p. 8)

- a potential for modification;
- being neither too broad (e.g. diet) nor too specific (e.g. lack of broccoli); and
- reasonably complete data being available for that risk.

The risk transition, across places and age groups (discussed in Chapter 6), is also relevant to this discussion.

Grand challenges in health today: Millennium Development Goals (MDGs)

What are the MDGs? The basics

The Millennium Development Goals, as seen in Chapter 1, are in many ways 'quantified' types of broad challenges, a number of which are specific to long- or short-term health status. Adopted by some 190 United Nations member states and at least 23 international organizations in 2000 and set mainly to be achieved by 2015, the MDGs have provided numerical benchmarks for tackling the many dimensions of extreme poverty (UNDP, 2010). Eight MDGs are divided into 21 quantifiable, time-bound targets measured by 60 indicators. The MDGs also provide a framework within which the international community can work towards a common end, ensuring that human development reaches all people in all places. If these goals were to be achieved, world poverty would be reduced by half, tens of millions of lives would be saved, and billions more people would have the chance of benefiting from the global economy. Clearly, many of the goals have very wide ramifications but, as noted in Chapter 1, equally clearly, many feel these goals were always unattainable, especially in their entirety (Waage *et al.*, 2010).

Taken collectively, all MDGs have either direct or indirect implications for global health, given their focus on environmental safety, access to safe water, education, especially of young girls, and the like. While the MDGs have their specific aims, they are inherently interlinked. Three goals focus explicitly on health (Goals 4, 5 and 6, shown in Box 7.2) – reducing child mortality, improving maternal health and combating specific diseases such as HIV/AIDS and malaria – but all goals potentially contribute towards health improvements or lack of progress. Goal 1, for example, on eradication of extreme poverty and hunger, has obvious health outcomes, as does Goal 2 – the achievement of universal primary education. Promotion of gender equality is also likely to be essential to the achievement of Goals 4 and 5, while Goals 7 and 8 are essential for health improvements and well-being in a globalizing world. The specific health goals are mainly orientated to infectious and nutritional conditions, but many of the other MDGs will be very relevant for conditions that can lead to NCDs (see below).

BOX 7.2 The MDGs and principal targets

The 8 MDGs break down into 21 quantifiable targets, measured by 60 indicators of progress (details shown only for explicitly health-related goals):

Goal 1: Eradicate extreme poverty and hunger.
Goal 2: Achieve universal primary education.
Goal 3: Promote gender equality and empower women.
Goal 4: Reduce child mortality:

- Target 4A: Reduce by two-thirds, between 1990 and 2015, the under-5 mortality rate. Indicators: under-5 mortality rate; infant (under 1 year old) mortality rate; proportion of 1-year-old children immunized against measles.

Goal 5: Improve maternal health:

- Target 5A: Reduce by three-quarters, between 1990 and 2015, the maternal mortality ratio. Indicators: maternal mortality ratio; proportion of births attended by skilled health personnel.
- Target 5B (added in 2005): Achieve, by 2015, universal access to reproductive health. Indicators: contraceptive prevalence rate; adolescent birth rate; antenatal care coverage (at least one visit and at least four visits); unmet need for family planning.

Goal 6: Combat HIV/AIDS, malaria and other diseases:

- Target 6A: Have halted, by 2015, and begun to reverse spread of HIV/AIDS. Indicators: HIV prevalence among population aged 15–24 years; condom use at last high-risk sex; proportion of population aged 15–24 years with comprehensive correct knowledge of HIV/AIDS; ratio of school attendance of orphans to school attendance of non-orphans aged 10–14 years.

continued

- Target 6B: Achieve, by 2010, universal access to treatment for HIV/AIDS for all those who need it. Indicator: proportion of population with advanced HIV infection with access to antiretroviral drugs.
- Target 6C: Have halted, by 2015, and begun to reverse incidence of malaria and other major diseases. Indicators: prevalence and death rates associated with malaria; proportion of children under 5 sleeping under insecticide-treated bed-nets; proportion of children under 5 with fever who are treated with appropriate anti-malarial drugs; prevalence and death rates associated with tuberculosis; proportion of tuberculosis cases detected and cured under DOTS (directly observed treatment short course)

Goal 7: Ensure environmental sustainability.
Goal 8: Develop a global partnership for development.
(Source: United Nations, *Millennium Development Goals Indicators* website)

Progress towards reaching the principal MDG goals and many of the specific targets is reported annually by the UN. This progress has been uneven (Box 7.3). In the decade to 2010, definite progress was seen on some MDGs in many countries, such as reductions in poverty globally, significant improvements in enrolment and gender parity in schools, reductions in child and maternal mortality and increasing HIV treatments. However, while the proportion of poor people is declining, the absolute number of poor in South Asia and sub-Saharan Africa has been increasing. The reductions in poverty have not necessarily addressed gender inequality and environmental sustainability and a lack of progress in reducing HIV has been hindering improvements in both maternal and child mortality. The expansion of health and education services has not always been matched by their quality.

BOX 7.3 Progress to the health-related goals, 2009, 2010

Goal 4: Reduce child mortality

In 2006, for the first time since mortality data have been gathered, annual deaths among children under 5 dipped below 10 million to 7.6 million in 2010, but it is unacceptable that millions of children still die from preventable causes each year. A child born in a developing country is over thirteen times more likely to die within the first five years of life than a child born in an industrialized country.

Sub-Saharan Africa accounts for about half the deaths of children under five in the developing world. In 2010, 24 of 26 countries with the highest under-5 mortality rates were in sub-Saharan Africa, but 6 of 14 countries with 50 per cent reduction in child deaths were also in this region. Disparities remain in all regions: mortality rates are higher for children from rural and poor families and whose mothers lack a basic education.

Goal 5: Improve maternal health

Maternal mortality remains unacceptably high across much of the developing world. Progress has been made but more than 350,000 women died from complications of pregnancy and childbirth. Ninety-nine per cent of these deaths occurred in the developing regions, with sub-Saharan Africa and South Asia accounting for 87 per cent of them. In sub-Saharan Africa, a woman's risk of dying from treatable or preventable complications of pregnancy and childbirth over the course of her lifetime is 1 in 22, compared to 1 in 7,300 in the developed regions.

Goal 6: Combat HIV/AIDS, malaria and other diseases

Every day, nearly 7,500 people become infected with HIV and 5,500 die from AIDS, mostly due to a lack of HIV prevention and treatment services. Nevertheless, some encouraging developments have been seen. Following improvements in prevention programmes, the number of people newly infected with HIV declined from 3 million in 2001 to 2.6 million in 2008. With the expansion of antiretroviral treatment services, numbers of people dying from AIDS have started to decline, from 2.2 million in 2005 to 2 million in 2008. With longer survival, the number of people living with HIV rose from an estimated 29.5 million in 2001 to 33 million in 2008. Infection rates have stabilized in most regions but are rising in Eastern Europe and Central Asia.

(Sources: Based on UNDESA, 2011 and UNDP, 2010)

Global economic circumstances have inevitably had an impact. Progress on the MDGs is threatened by the fallout of international financial and economic crisis combined with the high food prices discussed in Chapter 10. Indeed, economic crisis may mean that over 50 million more people are likely to remain in extreme poverty between 2010 and 2015 than might otherwise have been the case. Some projections do remain relatively optimistic – for example, that the number of extreme poor could total no more than 920 million in 2015, a decline of almost 50 per cent from the 1.8 billion people in 1990. Nevertheless, it seems inevitable that the crisis will impact seriously on global health, especially if it deepens. Richer countries may be less willing and/or able to assist poorer countries, and the health and welfare of many people in the rich countries themselves may be damaged by unemployment and poverty. Some estimate that globally 1.2 million more children under 5 and 265,000 more infants will die between 2009 and 2015. The crisis, through its impact on broader human development indicators, will likely affect other targets, too. For example, 50,000 more children will not complete primary education and 100 million fewer people will have access to safe drinking water in 2015 (World Bank, 2010).

Some countries have achieved many of the goals but others are unlikely to realize any within the time frame. Major countries achieving some goals include China, for example in poverty and hunger reduction, if not poverty eradication, and India, due to robust internal and external factors of population and economic development, though it is slipping on child health goals. However, many countries with the greatest need for action, including many in sub-Saharan Africa, have not yet made substantial changes or progress towards the targets, as we saw in Chapter 6 for MDG Goal 4 – the aim of reducing child mortality (see also below). Most sub-Saharan countries are unlikely to meet many, if any, of the MDGs by 2015. Crucial issues also persist of geographical and socio-spatial differences in well-being, gender differences, poor governance, corruption, insecurity, widespread poverty and a lack of basic services that would contribute to achieving the later development-related goals. Weak institutional capacity and corruption especially in many conflict and post-conflict countries, have hindered progress. In many places, rapid and often uncontrolled urbanization has been placing unmanageable strains on social services.

Millennium Development Goals on maternal and child health (MCH)

MDG 4 is to reduce child mortality, with a target to reduce by two-thirds mortality of children younger than 5 between 1990 and 2015. However, in spite of achievements, many countries and regions have made insufficient progress towards this goal since 1990, including sub-Saharan Africa and South Asia (see Table 6.2). Child mortality has been declining worldwide as a result of socio-economic development and implementation of child survival interventions, yet, as was seen in Chapter 6, 8.8 million children under 5 die every year (Black *et al.*, 2008, 2010; Figure 7.1). An acceleration of the decline in mortality is considered possible by expanding interventions targeting the important causes of death. An addendum on child mortality to the *MDG Report 2011* (UNDESA, 2011) states that evidence is building that Target 4 can be reached but, while the rate of decline in child mortality has accelerated, it is currently insufficient to reach the goal and time is now short.

A major benefit is access to good healthcare during pregnancy, as it is increasingly evident that lifetime health is influenced by the health of the mother and her well-being during pregnancy. Crucially, access to safe delivery, by qualified staff, for mothers and good post-natal care, and feeding plus care for infants, are integral to the achievement of MDG 4 and MDG 5 (to improve maternal health). However, global research by Save the Children (2011) indicates that one-third of mothers give birth without the attendance of a trained person. One thousand mothers and two thousand children die daily, almost all from relatively easily avoidable causes should trained birth attendants and basic facilities have been available. Of the ten most risky countries to give birth, nine are in Africa.

Infectious challenges: not yet 'on the retreat'?

It is tempting to think that infections are no longer a widespread cause of death and morbidity. In some places and for some groups, this belief is reasonably valid but elsewhere, despite many advances in infection control and treatment, infectious diseases remain a major threat. They often hinder the attainment of many MDGs and also hamper wider economic and social development. New antibiotics are being developed for some conditions, but new and some resurgent viral conditions (such as avian and swine flu, SARS, viral encephalitis, and several others) are of course not amenable to antibiotics, and antivirals are rarely very effective. Moreover, certain 'superbugs', such as MRSAs, are emerging in both hospitals and the community, raising the real threat that antibiotic resistance will become ever more common (discussed in Chapter 11). Infectious diseases continue to be a particular threat to children and in certain regions and countries, causing almost 9 million childhood deaths worldwide in 2008 (Black *et al.*, 2010; Figures 6.2 and 7.1). Three infectious diseases alone – HIV/AIDS, malaria and tuberculosis – pose a huge burden, principally on developing countries. They cause enormous family misery and hold up local and national economic and social development. The bulk of people who had HIV in 2011 lived in poorer countries, where the majority of morbidity and mortality from the condition occurred. However, even in rich countries, a million Americans live with HIV/AIDS. It is no longer a condition without hope and, with access to the appropriate drug combinations, it can become a chronic, but manageable, condition. Such treatment also dramatically slows or prevents

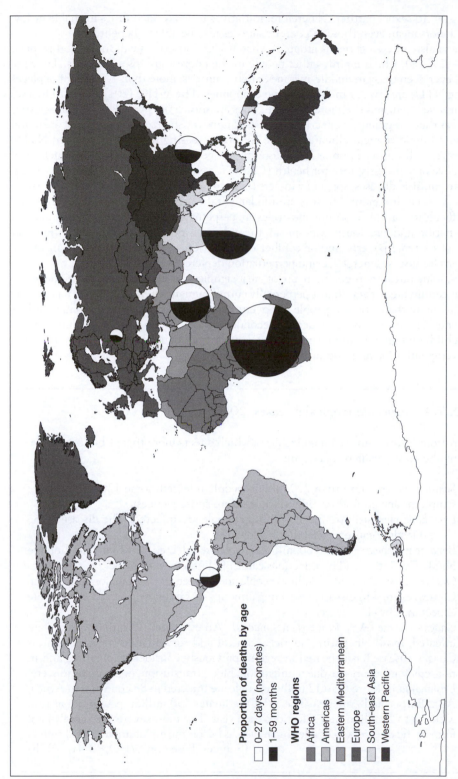

Figure 7.1 Distribution of 8.8 million child deaths 2008, by WHO region

Source: Black *et al.*, 2010. Reprinted from *The Lancet*, 375 Black, R.E., *et al.*, for the Child Health Epidemiology Reference Group of WHO and UNICEF (2010). "Global, regional, and national causes of child mortality in 2008: a systematic analysis", pp. 1969–1987. Copyright (2010) with permission from Elsevier.

transmission to sexual partners. Therefore, initiatives to make such drugs available at low cost by donors mean even those in poorer countries may be able to benefit.

There is also a heterogeneous group of what WHO and others call 'neglected tropical diseases' (NTDs), which mainly afflict people in the poorest groups and places. They are rarely, if ever, seen today in middle-income or rich countries: more than 70 per cent of places reporting NTDs are low- or middle-income economies. The WHO (2011i, 2012b) focuses on about seventeen, and the more prevalent ones are shown in Box 7.4. These diseases are *neglected* as they are primarily infectious diseases of impoverished settings and most are found in hot and humid tropical climates. There is now increasing research interest in NTDs, though they still impact upon as many as a billion people and receive a tiny fraction of official development assistance for health (Centre for Neglected Tropical Diseases, 2012). Many are parasitic diseases, spread by insects (mosquitoes, blackflies, snails, sandflies, tsetse flies, etc.), so environmental factors are fundamental to their distribution, and these are often difficult to control. Transmission cycles are perpetuated where there is environmental contamination and, previously widespread, these diseases now tend to be concentrated in settings of extreme poverty and/or conflict or disruption. They reflect almost all of the conditions for disease emergence and perpetuation depicted in Figure 3.1.

NTDs, some rare, others common, are of great significance in global health and development. In certain areas, they almost perpetually curtail human potential, playing a large part in keeping more than a billion people in poverty and placing enormous economic burdens on endemic countries. Some reduce the economic productivity of young adults, others impair childhood growth and cognitive development; all cause human misery and often result in stigmatization and discrimination.

BOX 7.4 Neglected tropical diseases, 2010

Apart from soil-transmitted helminthiasis, which affects more than 1 billion people, among the most prevalent NTDs are:

- *Schistosomiasis:* More than 200 million people infected; some 120 million have symptoms and around 20 million show severe consequences.
- *Lymphatic filariasis:* Around 120 million people are infected. The disease is the second leading cause of disability worldwide.
- *Blinding trachoma:* Around 80 million people are infected, of whom 6 million are blind. This is the leading infectious cause of blindness worldwide.
- *Onchocerciasis:* Around 37 million people are infected, the vast majority in Africa. Causes severe skin disease, visual impairment and blindness, and can shorten life expectancy by up to fifteen years.
- *Chagas' disease (American trypanosomiasis):* An estimated 13 million people are infected, mostly in Latin America. Control and surveillance are important as Chagas' disease has appeared in regions previously considered to be free and in non-epidemic countries due to migration, blood transfusion, organ donation, etc.
- *Leishmaniasis:* More than 12 million people are infected in 88 countries in Africa, Asia, Europe and America. The WHO estimates 350 million people are at risk, with 1.5 to 2 million new infections each year. The most severe and rapidly fatal form of the disease, visceral leishmaniasis, is becoming an 'ominous global trend'.

(Sources: Based on WHO, 2011i, 2012b)

In Chapter 6, we discussed other major infectious diseases, such as measles, which principally affects children. An even more important and more widespread infectious disease which affects all age groups in widespread geographical areas, and often youngsters in particular, is malaria – an example of an ongoing high-prevalence, multifactorial condition.

Malaria

Almost half of the world's population (about 3.3 of 7 billion) is at risk from malaria. Despite many decades of research into prophylaxis, including vaccines, and effective cures, malaria remains one of the biggest killers, especially of children, particularly in sub-Saharan Africa. It also causes substantial acute and chronic adult ill-health and loss of economic productivity (see Box 7.1). News and research on malaria can be very confusing, although the WHO does report that some good progress is being made and as many as one-third of countries at risk may be on course to eliminate the disease in the next decade (WHO, 2011e; see Box 7.5). Other research points to a longer time scale to achieve substantial reductions (Murray *et al.*, 2012; Schlein, 2012).

Malaria is a parasitic disease transmitted from person to person through the bite of a female *Anopheles* mosquito. Some 60 types of the 400 mosquitoes in this sub-group can transmit malaria, and the keys to prevention are avoidance of their habitats and especially avoidance of being bitten. This is easier said than done, as these vectors are potentially very widespread and habitats easily created, especially in warm climates. The mosquito has been called the 'innocent postman' in transmitting the disease to humans during its blood meal. The illness itself is caused by the *plasmodium* parasite, which reproduces in a complex cycle in the mosquito and human as alternate hosts. In spite of the complexity of the malaria cycle, the disease is extremely common, especially in some areas of the tropics. The *plasmodium* is an efficient parasite that overcomes many obstacles and adapts effectively to its ecosystem. It hides in liver and blood cells, avoiding the immune system. Fever is caused when it breaks out into the bloodstream, causing several variants depending on the duration of the fever, which tends to be regular, occurring every 48 hours, 72 hours, etc. The forms vary in severity, with one of the most dangerous, especially for children, being the cerebral type.

As indicated, data on malaria cases and deaths are a matter of considerable debate. There are over 200 million cases of malaria each year and it is a leading cause of death in young children (Chapter 6). Between one in four and one in five childhood deaths in Africa are from the effects of malaria, depending on methodologies of different studies. Pregnant women have generally been identified as the main adult risk group in most endemic areas of the world, though new research indicates that malaria may be an under-recognized cause of other adult mortality (Murray *et al.*, 2012). The disease remains widespread in many parts of Asia, Latin and Central America, Africa and Asia-Pacific. Endemic malaria has been eradicated in almost all of Europe although it is seen sporadically in imported cases. Like HIV, malaria exerts its heaviest toll in Africa, with some 90 per cent of global malarial deaths, especially among children (Box 7.1). It constitutes 10 per cent of the continent's overall disease burden, although some 40 per cent of episodes of malaria occur in Asia.

Malaria is acknowledged as a major public health challenge which is eroding development in the poorest countries, though the WHO's most recent *Malaria Reports* and *MDG Report* (WHO, *World Malaria Report 2010* and 2011 websites and UNDESA, 2011) show good progress towards targets (see Box 7.5). Data from these reports indicate global declines in deaths from malaria from 985,000 to 655,000 between 2000 and 2010. However, using different sources and estimates, Murray *et al.* (2012) found much higher death rates. They estimated a decline from a peak of 1.82 million deaths in 2004 to 1.24 million in 2010, almost twice the WHO's figure. By these estimates, malaria is a much bigger risk than previously thought to both child and adult health. All estimates of malaria cases and deaths have considerable ranges in terms of statistical uncertainty. However, they all agree that there have been considerable declines in morbidity and mortality this century as a result of the strategies mentioned below. The recent estimates do, nevertheless, shed considerable doubt on whether the MDG goals and other revised targets for reduction and elimination of malaria will be met by 2015, and suggest a much longer horizon is more likely. As well as its direct human health impacts, malaria costs Africa more than 12 billion dollars annually and may have slowed economic growth in some African countries by 1.3 per cent annually. Estimates suggest the compounded effects give a gross domestic product level as much as one-third lower now than it would have been had malaria been eradicated from Africa in 1960.

BOX 7.5 Malaria: progress towards targets, 2010

Positive news emerged after increased malaria control programmes between 2008 and 2010. Lower rates were seen after using insecticide-treated mosquito nets (ITNs) to protect more than 578 million people at risk in sub-Saharan Africa, and indoor residual spraying protected 75 million people, 10 per cent of the population at risk in 2009.

A downward trend in malaria

- Deaths due to malaria were estimated reduced by 20–30 per cent globally, from 985,000 to 781,000 (2000–09), and to 655,000 (2010).
- The estimated incidence of malaria globally has declined by 17 per cent since 2000 and malaria-specific mortality rates have declined by 26 per cent (2010).
- Decreases have been observed in all WHO regions; largest proportional decreases in deaths seen in the European Region; largest absolute decreases in Africa.
- In Africa, eleven countries have shown a greater than 50 per cent reduction in confirmed malaria cases or malaria admissions and deaths over the past decade.
- Decrease of more than 50 per cent in the number of confirmed cases of malaria have been found in 32 of the 56 malaria-endemic countries outside Africa in this period. A downward trend of 25–50 per cent has been seen in eight other countries.
- In 2009, the WHO European Region reported no cases of *Plasmodium falciparum* malaria for the first time.

The WHO sees these as the best results in decades, indicating current strategies are working. Roll Back Malaria targets were updated in 2011 to: (i) reduce global malaria deaths to near zero by the end of 2015; (ii) reduce global malaria cases by 75 per cent from 2000 levels by the end of 2015; and (iii) eliminate malaria by the end of 2015 in ten new countries since 2008, including in the WHO's European Region.

Strategies to fight malaria evolve:

- In 2010, the WHO recommended the confirmation of suspected cases by a diagnostic test before antimalarial drugs are administered.
- It should not be assumed every person with a fever has malaria and needs antimalarial treatment. Reliable cheap diagnostic tests are available for healthcare workers in the community.

- Increased access to insecticide-treated mosquito nets (ITNs); and protection by indoor residual spraying (IRS).
- Use of tests improves care for patients and reduces over-prescribing of artemisinin-based combination therapies (ACTs), reducing build up of drug resistance.

However, malaria control can be fragile

Resurgences were observed in parts of some African countries, so gains can be fragile, and momentum must be maintained. Resistance to artemisinins was reported in a growing number of countries in South-east Asia; resistance to pyrethroids (insecticides in ITNs) was reported widely.

(Source: Based on WHO, *World Malaria Report 2010* and *2011* websites and UNDESA, 2011)

Control, containment or eradication?

A problem in combating malaria has been not only its different forms but its changing epidemiology. In South-east Asia, in particular, drug-resistant strains of the parasite have emerged and spread, posing great difficulties in regional elimination of an effectively 'evolving target'. Resistance to and growing ineffectiveness of many insecticides for spraying mosquitoes has been recognized for seventy years or more, and many sprays are environmentally toxic. Vaccines against malaria have been sought for years but (perhaps as it is mainly a tropical disease) these have yet to be successful, although optimism surfaces regularly. Trials of a vaccine on children in Africa in 2011 showed promising results, with up to 50 per cent reduction in chances of contracting malaria for at least a year. The ultimate, currently elusive, aim is eradication; an updated goal, formulated in 2011, is near-zero deaths globally by the end of 2015, although, as noted above, this is likely to be highly elusive, too (see Box 7.5). Huge financial resources are needed for the goal of malaria control and reduction, as much as 4–5 billion dollars annually and, crucially, this must be sustained over the next three decades, if not indefinitely. Many forms of control and avoidance have been suggested over the years but almost all have some sort of shortcoming or limited duration of effectiveness (Box 7.6). Many similar controls are also needed for other mosquito-borne diseases, such as dengue fever and Japanese encephalitis.

The WHO recommends reduction of malaria mortality and morbidity through improved 'prevention, diagnosis and treatment'. To have any chance, these need to be supported by effective and low-cost interventions:

- Prompt parasitological confirmation is recommended for suspected malaria, before treatment is started (for example, by rapid diagnostic tests, RDT).
- To reduce resistance developing, oral artemisinin-based monotherapies are discouraged and should be replaced with artemisinin-based combination therapy (ACT) for *P. falciparum* malaria, in various suitable combinations.
- Intermittent preventive treatment (IPT) is recommended for population groups in areas of high transmission who are particularly vulnerable to contracting malaria or suffering its consequences, especially pregnant women and infants.
- Especially important is vector control, with the prediction and containment of epidemics.

BOX 7.6 Factors in the control of malaria

- *Vector control (control of mosquitoes)*: Kill mosquito larvae via water drainage, emptying small receptacles of water, spraying, indoor residual spraying of walls of dwellings; care in settling newly cleared forest areas, etc.
- *Avoid being bitten*: By using, for example, DEET screens, insecticide impregnated bed-nets; avoid biting times of day; use sprays, creams, long sleeves, etc.
- *Local environment*: Knowledge of environmental requirements and the malaria cycle; maintenance of drainage systems, water tanks; avoid stagnant water; caution when extending settlement into new areas in tropics (especially agriculture and housing in former forest areas).
- *Social factors*: Spread knowledge of careful use and storgage of water; regular use of anti-malarial drugs (costs and acceptability); insecticidal spraying; careful agricultural and urban practices; mosquito surveillance.
- *Preventing the disease with drugs*: Prophylactic tablets advised for visitors to endemic areas. Costs of, resistance to and side-effects of cheaper drugs such as chloroquine mean continuous drug prophylaxis is not always practical for long-term populations, so avoidance of biting is crucial. Some effective drugs are potentially toxic – e.g. fansodar. An effective vaccine, though promised, remains some years away.
- *Treatment*: Generally effective if given early, so early detection is crucial. However, in endemic areas, treatment of adults and children can be problematic due to drug resistance and toxicity building up.

Field research shows that these approaches, alone or in combination, can be effective. They are usually targeted at the most vulnerable: young children and pregnant women, but, as a rule, the whole community needs to be involved, to make environmental and other controls effective and durable. Unfortunately, it can be difficult to sustain efforts when the immediate risks subside, but all populations locally will benefit from a combination of personal and community protective measures. Malaria is a disease for which prevention is definitely better than cure.

Therefore, known, existing interventions need to be used to the fullest extent possible. Sustained local vigilance is very important and intersectoral efforts – such as between farmers, local engineers and the health sector – are essential. For example, studies in Brazil around 2010 emphasize that malaria is not always going away, and newly cleared forest areas for cultivation and residences are particularly risky, as they expose many new people to mosquitoes.

Non-communicable diseases and global health

NCDs are not explicitly among the Millennium Development Goals but for all nations, and increasingly for poorer countries, they are hugely costly in human and financial terms. They can restrict socio-economic development and many are, perhaps surprisingly, associated with poverty. NCDs – mainly heart disease, strokes, cancer, chronic obstructive pulmonary disease and diabetes – were responsible for an estimated 35 million deaths in 2005. They are often thought of as a 'rich country' health issue but, as noted earlier, 80 per cent of NCD deaths occurred in low- and middle-income countries (LAMICs) and they are certainly a growing global challenge (Alwan and Maclean, 2009). By 2030, it is likely that eight of ten leading causes of death will be linked to these types of conditions. As we saw in Table 4.5, for a variety of reasons, many NCDs have median mortality rates at younger ages in the LAMICs than in high-income countries.

The burden of NCDs thus has serious implications for social and economic development worldwide, and for LAMICs in particular (Abegunde *et al.*, 2007; WHO, 2008a). As we shall discuss below with respect to cancers, these poorer countries almost invariably have few resources to devote to NCDs in the face of ongoing acute and infectious conditions and lack of finances. The WHO and its members have developed the Global Strategy for the Prevention and Control of Noncommunicable Diseases (WHO, 2008a), advocating an integrated approach to NCD prevention and control, emphasizing the role of primary healthcare, based on current scientific knowledge and evidence, and taking account of international experience (Box 7.7). It comprises a set of actions to tackle the growing public-health burden imposed by NCDs, requiring high-level political commitment and the concerted involvement of all parties, governments, communities and healthcare providers. Longer-term public-health policies will need to be reoriented and resource allocation

---

BOX 7.7 NCD strategies in low- and middle-income countries

Any strategy to prevent and control NCDs aims 'to reduce the level of exposure of individuals and populations to the common risk factors and their determinants' (p. 4); *early intervention for prevention of NCDs* has been advocated for some time. Thirty years' experience has demonstrated that primary prevention and promotion policies and programmes need to be community-based and intersectoral, involving many sectors with an interest in and influence on health and development.

- *Tobacco use:* More than a billion people smoke tobacco, the majority in LAMICs. Education and control of use are essential. Only about 5 per cent of the world's population is covered by comprehensive tobacco controls.
- *Targets:* Salt reduction in diets; cholesterol, blood pressure; use of aspirins; increase fruit and vegetable intake; reduce excessive alcohol intake; cooking; clean water for hepatitis A avoidance; sexual behaviour and practices for hepatitis B avoidance (reduce risk of liver cancer); primary healthcare interventions.
- *Overweight, obesity, diabetes:* Interventions on diet and physical activity can be effective for resource-constrained settings. Inactivity is contributing to the rise in obesity prevalence: 'around 40 per cent of people worldwide are not participating in sufficient physical activity to benefit their health' (p. 5).
- *Harmful use of alcohol:* The fifth leading risk factor for premature death and disability worldwide, estimated to cause about 2.3 million premature deaths. Programmes are needed to educate people on the risks of drinking.
- *Social targets:* Increase exercise; reduce exposure to indoor smoke from solid fuels and urban air pollution.

Delivery of low-cost, effective interventions targeting high-risk populations and individuals can have substantial, fairly quick, benefits. Tobacco, salt and multi-drug measures 'have a potential saving of over 32 million lives in ten years' (p. 7).

(Sources: Based on Alwan and Maclean, 2009, pp. 4, 5, 7 and WHO, 2008a)

improved. However, for controlling obesity, a major risk factor for some NCDs, as we shall see later, effective strategies have yet to be devised.

Disabilities: the global picture

Disabilities are a major and growing factor affecting the quality of life and life opportunities of almost 15 per cent of the world's population: an estimated 1 billion people had a disability in 2011. The first official global report on disabilities was published by the WHO and World Bank (WHO, 2011c) and provides overwhelming evidence that disability affects people in all countries, at all ages, and impacts on well-being, education, employment and health. The scale and nature of disabilities are great, though they tend to differ by age and by country groupings (Table 7.1; Box 7.8). Population ageing is often held to increase disabling NCDs and chronic health conditions, such as cardiovascular and respiratory diseases. Indeed, as populations have aged, the proportion of people with disabilities has grown from around 10 per cent in the 1970s. Disabilities affect all ages, though some, such as hearing loss, vision problems, arthritis and dementias, affect older groups much more than younger. Other forms, such as alcohol and drug dependencies, depression amd some psychiatric conditions, affect younger ages in greater numbers. There are also considerable variations in prevalence and types between rich and poorer countries (Table 7.1)

Many richer and some middle-income countries have introduced legislation and pro- grammes which attempt to improve inclusion and opportunities for people with disabilities, but they have not been totally effective. Disabled people often remain effectively second- class citizens and as many as one in five experiences 'significant difficulties'. Even in richer countries, disabled people are three times more likely to be denied healthcare than others. Employment rates are much lower and, in some Eastern European countries with high primary school enrolment rates, rates for children with disabilites can be 50 per cent lower than those without. Many barriers have been identified to the participation of people with

---

BOX 7.8 Disability and the emphasis on environmental factors

The new International Classification of Functioning, Disability and Health (ICF) emphasizes environmental factors in creating disability, a difference from the previous International Classification. ICF recognizes problems with human functioning cate- gorized in three interconnected areas:

- *impairments*: problems in body function, alterations in body structure, e.g. paral- ysis or blindness;
- *activity limitations*: difficulties in executing activities, e.g. walking or eating; and
- *participation restrictions*: problems with involvement, such as discrimination in employment or transportation.

Disability refers to difficulties met in any or all three areas of functioning. The ICF uses neutral language and does not distinguish between the type and cause of disability (such as 'physical' and 'mental' health). *Health conditions* are diseases, injuries, and disorders; *impairments* are specific decrements in body functions and structures.

In the ICF, disability arises from the interaction of health conditions with *contextual factors* – environmental and personal factors:

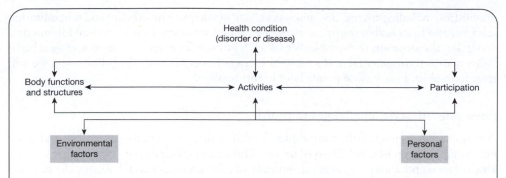

The ICF classifies **environmental factors** affecting people with different levels of functioning as either facilitators or barriers. These include products and technology, the built and natural environments, support and relationships, attitudes, and services, systems and policies.

The ICF regards disability as a continuum rather than categorizing people with disabilities as a separate group; disability is a matter of 'more or less', not 'yes or no'.

(Source: Based on WHO, 2011c, Box 1.1)

Table 7.1 Prevalence of moderate and severe disability, by leading health condition associated with disability, by age and income status of country, c. 2004

Health condition	High-income countries (with a total population of 977 million)		Low-income and middle-income countries (with a total population of 5,460 million)		World (population 6,437 million)
	0–59	*60 years and over*	*0–59 years*	*60 years and over*	*All ages*
1 Hearing loss	7.4	18.5	54.3	43.9	124.2
2 Refractive errors	7.7	6.4	68.1	39.8	121.9
3 Depression	15.8	0.5	77.6	4.8	98.7
4 Cataracts	0.5	1.1	20.8	31.4	53.8
5 Unintentional injuries	2.8	1.1	35.4	5.7	45.0
6 Osteoarthritis	1.9	8.1	14.1	19.4	43.4
7 Alcohol dependence and problem use	7.3	0.4	31.0	1.8	40.5
8 Infertility (unsafe abortion, maternal sepsis)	0.8	0.0	32.5	0.0	33.4
9 Macular degeneration	1.8	6.0	9.0	15.1	31.9
10 COPD*	3.2	4.5	10.9	8.0	26.6
11 Ischaemic heart disease	1.0	2.2	8.1	11.9	23.2
12 Bipolar disorder	3.3	0.4	17.6	0.8	22.2
13 Asthma	2.9	0.5	15.1	0.9	19.4
14 Schizophrenia	2.2	0.4	13.1	1.0	16.7
15 Glaucoma	0.4	1.5	5.7	7.9	15.5
16 Alzheimers and other dementias	0.4	6.2	1.3	7.0	14.9
17 Panic disorder	1.9	0.1	11.4	0.3	13.8
18 Cerebrovascular disease	1.4	2.2	4.0	4.9	12.6
19 Rheumatoid arthritis	1.3	1.7	5.9	3.0	11.9
20 Drug dependence and problem use	3.7	0.1	8.0	0.1	11.8

Note: * Chronic obstructive pulmonary disease.
Source: WHO, 2011c, p. 297

disabilities, including stigma, discrimination, lack of adequate healthcare and rehabilitation services, and inaccessible transport, buildings and information. In low- and middle-income countries, the situation is often bleaker (WHO, 2011c). The report is important as it highlights many environmental and structural barriers to people with disabilities, and we will refer to disabilities at several points later in this book.

Emerging 'lifestyle' challenges to health

A very extensive group of often interlinked health challenges related to individual and group behaviour has been labelled 'lifestyle' factors. These can include excess consumption of some kinds of food and drink; excessive use or intake of substances such as tobacco or alcohol; and legal or illicit drug use. These are known or suspected to be implicated, to a greater or lesser extent, in a wide range of NCDs and some disabilities discussed above. We turn now to other conditions in which at least some of the risk is likely to be related to lifestyle factors.

Behavioural factors such as diet, eating habits, exercise and occupational and recreational variables are considered in the cases of obesity, diabetes and impaired glucose tolerance. Increasingly, it is appreciated that behaviour and wide-ranging socio-economic factors may well be affected by individual and geographical variations in immutable factors, such as genetics. A further group of health challenges relates to socio-environmental development and occupational factors, such as accidents in the home, at work and on the road; and occupational- and industrial-related health impacts, including workplace violence and stress.

However, the whole area of 'lifestyle research' sometimes needs to come with a 'health warning'. Readers will be aware of some tendency for moral judgement and even of a moral panic approach in many areas of alleged lifestyle diseases or predisposing conditions. Anti-drink, anti-drugs and anti-tobacco lobbyists are almost global; they and health zealots, religious groups and others can sometimes exhibit considerable intolerance and moral indignation. Research findings can be definitive or contradictory (especially with respect to diet) and hyped concern is sometimes promulgated in the media and sometimes even extends into health establishments. This has the potential to exaggerate the real extent of some problems or the significance of some research findings. More problematic for health policy development, such attitudes can instigate a blame culture. So, real or apparent statistical trends need to be presented and judged as objectively as possible.

Recent trends in childhood and adult obesity

The increase in childhood obesity in most countries is one area of growing concern (see Chapter 6). Not only can it potentially affect a child's behaviour and development but obese youngsters are increasingly identified as likely to be at early risk of a number of 'adult' chronic conditions, which may emerge at a far younger age than would be expected. However, even in countries with reasonably good data, there are problems in comparing trends over time, as studies have often used different definitions, such as of obesity and overweight. Recent rapid rises in obesity affect many adults as well as children. Until recently, the tendency has been to regard obesity as mainly a rich-country problem, almost quintessentially an American phenomenon, but it is increasingly becoming almost universal. Global estimates for 2008 clasified 1.46 billion adults and 170 million children as overweight or obese (Swinburn *et al.*, 2011).

A group studying the 'global burden of metabolic risk factors of chronic diseases' has been investigating trends in weight, blood pressure and cholesterol, all important risk factors for a number of conditions and premature death (see Finucane *et al.*, 2011; Danaei *et al.*, 2011). Its papers show that the worldwide prevalence of obesity has nearly doubled since 1980.

However, there have also been impressive reductions in mean blood pressure and cholesterol levels in high-income countries, although some countries have done better than others. Looking specifically at overweight, data for 199 countries showed mean Body Mass Index (BMI) among adults aged over 20 had increased since 1980 by 0.4 kg/m² per decade for men and 0.5 kg/m² per decade for women. By 2008, about 1.5 billion adults globally were estimated to be overweight, with BMI of 25 kg/m² or greater. Of these, about half a billion were obese, an estimated 205 million men and 297 million women. Trends over the three decades and mean population BMI in 2008 varied considerably between countries. BMI was highest in some Oceania countries for males and females; it tended to be lower (less than 21.5 kg/m² for men and women) in a few countries in sub-Saharan Africa, and East, South and South-east Asia. The USA had the highest BMI among wealthy countries (Finucane *et al.*, 2011). Interventions and policies to help reduce BMI and mitigate the effects of high BMI are therefore needed in the majority of countries.

Similar increases in adults' weight have also been seen in many other countries. The OECD (2010a) found that just over half (50.1 per cent) of adults in the European Union were overweight or obese, compared with 68 per cent in the United States. As in the USA, obesity had increased, with the EU rate of obesity more than doubling over the previous twenty years. Among youngsters, one in seven EU children was overweight or obese, with numbers expected to rise further. The consequences are likely to be even more severe in some of the poorer regions and especially among the most obese nations noted above. As much as absolute levels of overweight, concern focuses on the rapidity of recent increases, and, in the USA and elsewhere, the term 'epidemic' is often used to describe these trends. Between 1960 and 1980, there was only a minor increase in the number of overweight or obese Americans. Thereafter, not only did the percentage increase, but much was concentrated in the 'obese' category, which grew by 60 per cent in the decade to 2000.

In gender terms, there does not seem to be a clear or uniform pattern of obesity across countries (OECD, 2010b). Worldwide, and in OECD countries, obesity rates may tend to be higher in women than men, on average. However, male obesity rates have been growing faster than female rates in most OECD countries. The gender dimension may prove important given its interactions with other social, economic and employment characteristics. Indeed, the OECD notes a complex relationship between socio-economic condition and obesity, which changes as economies become more developed. For example, poorer people are more likely to be affected by obesity in rich countries.

Causes, consequences and dealing with obesity

In Chapter 6, we discussed some possible causes of the obesity among children. Similar reasons seem to obtain among adults: individuals taking in more energy than they expend; possibly some genetic susceptibility; changing eating habits; and reduced levels of physical activity. Among adults, there may be work–life balance issues as many are involved in sedentary jobs, based in offices or working at computer screens. It has been suggested that a wider acceptance of being overweight may permit people to become heavier and eventually obese. UK research suggests that individuals have less choice in the matter of their weight than might be assumed and

> the present epidemic of obesity is not really down to laziness or overeating . . . [Rather,] our biology has stepped out of kilter with society. As a result, most adults in the UK are already overweight and modern living ensures every generation is heavier than the last. This is known as passive obesity.
>
> (King, 2011, p. 743)

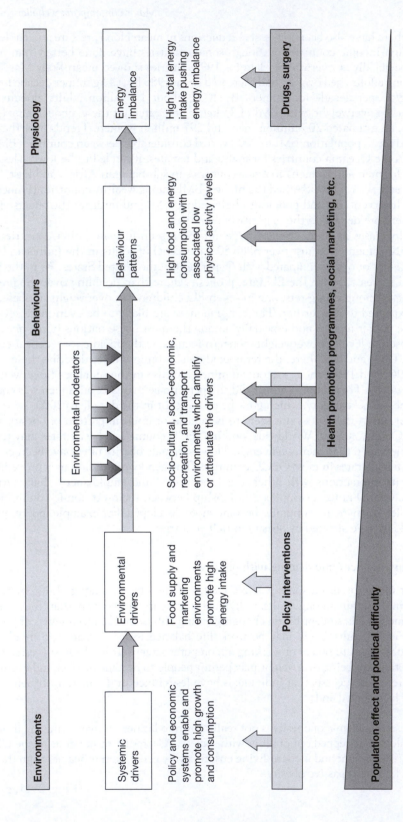

Figure 7.2 A framework to categorize obesity determinants and solutions

Source: Swinburn *et al.*, 2011. Reprinted from *The Lancet*, *278*, Swinburn, B.A., *et al.* "The global obesity pandemic: shaped by global drivers and local environments", pp. 804–814. Copyright (2011) with permission from Elsevier.

Swinburn *et al.* (2011) suggest an important explanation for the increases in obesity occurring in most countries may be changes in global food production and distribution. More processed, affordable and well-marketed food leads to passive overconsumption of energy and therefore to obesity. However, the consumption and marketing of foods interact with local environmental factors, giving variations in obesity between and within populations. 'Within populations', in particular, 'interactions between environmental and individual factors', including genetics, can help explain considerable 'variability in body size between individuals' (Swinburn *et al.*, 2011, p. 804).

Figure 7.2 provides a framework of obesity determinants and solutions, including environment, behaviours and physiology (food supply, consumption and energy imbalance). Some interventions can be policy based, while health promotion programmes can affect environments and behaviours. On the left, 'upstream' interventions targeting the systemic drivers can have larger effects, but political implementation is more difficult than for health promotion programmes and medical services (Swinburn *et al.*, 2011).

Consequences have health, social, emotional and economic–healthcare system aspects. Health risks are associated with both childhood obesity and adult overweight and especially extreme overweight: raised blood pressure, increased risk of diabetes, associated with cardiovascular disease, heightened risk of stroke; mobility and joint problems; associations with a number of digestive and other cancers; and, for both males and females, fertility problems. Some specific conditions, such as type 2 (adult-onset) diabetes (discussed below), are strongly associated with obesity. For example, women who are obese are twelve times more likely to develop type 2 diabetes than women of a healthy weight. As mentioned in Chapter 6, overweight children (and adults) may have poorer self-images and may interact less with others, especially in terms of sports and physical activities, possibly a cause-and-effect relationship in many cases.

Obesity appears to have more negative health consequences than smoking, drinking or poverty, and it also affects more people. Many of the risks of being overweight are exacerbated if a person drinks to excess and, especially, if they smoke. Obesity has, however, been linked to very high rates of chronic illnesses, higher than living in poverty, and much higher than smoking or drinking. It was the equivalent in terms of chronic conditions of ageing from 30 to 50 (Sturm, 2002). British research data suggest that 'being overweight during at least one time period in adult life was associated with an increased risk of diabetes', with the risk from being overweight cumulative across the lifecourse. This cumulative association highlights the need for health practices to avoid the development of 'excess weight at a young age, and so possibly reduce future diabetes prevalence' (Jeffreys *et al.*, 2006, p. 507), as well as other weight-related problems. However, many popular 'treatments' for overweight tend to emphasize one-off weight loss. It seeems better to regard obesity, like diabetes (discussed below), as a chronic condition. It builds over a long time and consequently requires long-term support and treatment to maintain more reasonable weight over the lifecourse.

Other social consequences of obesity include potential direct and indirect impacts on employment, which the OECD (2010b) calls 'labour market outcomes', in which obese individuals are less likely to be part of the labour force and to be in employment. Possible discrimination in hiring, possibly due to expectations of lower productivity, contributes to the employment gap, and white women were especially disadvantaged in this respect. Moreover, obese employees were likely to earn less than people of normal weight, with wage penalties of up to 18 per cent associated with obesity. Obese individuals tend to have more time off work, lower work productivity and a greater access to disability benefits than people of normal weight. The OECD (2010b) points to a need for government intervention to protect obese people in labour markets and ensure they enjoy the same opportunities as others in employment types and terms.

Looking forward, it seems that obesity is very likely to increase globally. It is estimated that, by 2050, as many as 60 per cent of men and 50 per cent of women in the UK could be clinically obese, with very considerable costs in health and financial terms (King, 2011). Similar data are seen in many other countries. There are numerous projected increases in healthcare costs associated with the current and forthcoming obesity epidemic. Costs and outcomes are ever more important concerns given the pressures on health and welfare budgets everywhere, and obesity may become a major contributor to health and welfare increases. In England, it was predicted that about one in four adults would be obese by 2010, with overall costs to the National Health Service and the wider economy of around £3.6 billion (UK Parliamentary Office of Science and Technology, 2003). Research in England forecast total costs linked to excessive weight could increase by as much as 70 per cent between 2007 and 2015 (OECD, 2010c). *The Lancet* (2011) notes projections for 2030 indicate 65 million more obese adults in the USA and 11 million more in the UK, with a large number of additional people with diabetes, heart disease and stroke, and cancer. The projected costs to treat these additional preventable diseases were an increase of some 48–66 billion dollars per year in the USA and around 2 billion pounds per year in the UK.

As discussed in Chapter 6, and as with diabetes discussed below, it is probably best to address overweight and obesity as a long-term rather than as a potentially quickly fixed condition, and one demanding continuing support and back-up. Unfortunately, unlike some other causes of preventable death and disability, such as tobacco and accidents, as Swinburn *et al.* (2011) note, there are as yet no 'exemplar populations' where public health measures have helped reverse the obesity epidemic. This adds urgency to the need for research, policy and action, perhaps with a focus on the control or reduction of supply-side drivers that permit and encourage passive overconsumption of energy and passsive obesity. At the moment, in most places, self-regulation of the food and beverage industry is the norm and generally has little effect – indeed, the number of adverts for fast-food increases.

Diabetes – the 'global pandemic' and increasingly earlier onset

Diabetes mellitus (DM) is one of the most common NCDs worldwide, on the increase and becoming evident at ever-younger ages (as noted in Chapter 6). It is linked with a number of risk factors, including the almost global increase in both childhood and adult obesity, discussed above. DM ranks as the fourth or fifth leading cause of death or DALYs in most high-income countries (see Table 4.10) and there is evidence that it is of growing significance in many middle-income, newly industrialized nations and poorer nations.

Diabetes is not a single disorder but a group of heterogeneous disorders with the common elements of hyperglycemia (excess of glucose in the bloodstream) and glucose intolerance, due to deficiency and/or impaired effectiveness of the action of the pancreatic hormone insulin, important for regulating the amount of sugar in the blood (Box 7.9). DM is classified as an endocrine or nutritional/metabolic disorder, a disorder of carbohydrate metabolism in which sugars in the body are not oxidized to produce energy because of lack of the pancreatic hormone insulin. Accumulation of sugar leads to its appearance in blood and then urine. Symptoms include thirst, loss of weight, excessive urine production, fatigue and sometimes susceptibility to some yeast and other infections. Diabetes has also been linked to depression.

If untreated, prolonged high blood glucose levels can cause many problems, such as heart disease, eye problems and blindness, reduced blood supply to the limbs and extremities, possibly leading to amputation, nerve damage, erectile dysfunction and stroke. Metabolic changes using fats as alternative sources or energy lead to acid-base imbalance and accumulation of keytones, eventually to convulsions and diabetic coma.

BOX 7.9   Diabetes types and treatments

Diabetes mellitus (DM) often exists for some time before being recognized. It is often treatable or manageable but not strictly curable. Three main types of DM exist, excluding a rarer form diabetes insipidus that is due to a pituitary hormone deficiency.

- Type 1 generally starts in childhood or adolescence and is usually more severe as the patient's body makes little or no insulin. It is sometimes called juvenile or insulin-dependent diabetes, as it is normally treated through insulin therapy (injections), which has been known for almost a century.
- Type 2 (non-insulin-dependent) diabetes was previously said to occur usually after age 40. The pancreas retains some ability to make insulin but inadequately or it cannot be used properly. Patients may require treatment from oral hypogly-caemic drugs, although it is often controllable, especially in earlier stages, by exercise, lifestyle and diet modifications. This is the increasingly common form of the condition. Type 2 diabetes is often, though not always, associated with obesity, which itself can cause insulin resistance and lead to elevated blood glucose levels. It runs in families, though major susceptibility genes have not yet been identified.
- Gestational diabetes (GDM) affects pregnant women and usually disappears after childbirth, though a woman who has had GDM faces a higher risk of developing Type 2 diabetes later in life. GDM can pose a danger to the unborn child and mother: the child may be born severely obese, at higher risk of dangerously low blood glucose levels and/or of severe breathing problems. As with type 2 diabetes, gestational diabetes is usually controlled through diet.

(Source: Based on International Diabetes Federation, 2009)

Risk factors for diabetes

The reasons for developing type 1 diabetes have not been identified, although some suggest interaction of dietary factors during pregnancy and early neonatal life. Research is suggested on diet, genetic susceptibility and early onset of type 1 diabetes (Muntoni *et al.*, 2000). By contrast, risk factors for type 2 diabetes are well recognized and include:

- Age (mostly occurs in people aged over 40, although childhood incidence is increasing).
- Overweight, especially obesity, particularly with a body shape that carries extra weight around the middle.
- A low-activity or sedentary lifestyle.
- High cholesterol, high blood pressure and a high-fat diet.
- Having a family member who has diabetes.
- Gestational diabetes gives a 40 per cent risk of developing type 2 diabetes.
- Having given birth to a baby weighing more than four kilos may give higher risk.
- Ethnic factors: some ethnic groups have higher risk than others (e.g. aboriginal people in Canada have three–five times greater risk than other Canadians; people of Hispanic, Asian, South Asian or African descent are also at greater risk). The 'thrifty gene', which hoards calories in poor food times, has been implicated in obesity and diabetes when such populations are exposed to modern diets.

Some of the above risk factors are not modifiable but others do fall into the lifestyle category and are amenable to action. Health and education policies therefore increasingly emphasize exercise, avoiding overweight/obesity, limiting fat and sugar intake and not smoking. Maintenance of cholesterol levels within low-healthy ranges and normal blood pressure are also important, especially for people with confirmed or 'borderline' diabetes. These are very similar approaches to maintaining cardiovascular health. It is of course impossible to avoid genetic risk factors but understanding these – such as the thrifty gene – can encourage people to pay special attention to their modifiable risk factors and undertake regular monitoring when growing older.

Successful campaigns try to get diabetes under control as a 'manageable wellness' issue rather than as an illness. Finland, where there is a high genetic predisposition to type 1 in particular, has been one of the first countries to mount large-scale and successful diabetes prevention strategies (International Diabetes Federation, 2010). This was based partly on earlier experience in heart disease management, and achieved reductions of almost 60 per cent. The campaigns involve aiming for modest weight reduction and thirty minutes' moderate exercise five times a week, particularly targeting pre-diabetic people. Education, linked with community encouragement and changing the environment for overweight, with easy access to preventive services, has made Finnish diabetes prevention world famous.

The impacts of diabetes

From the global health perspective, the most important features are huge recent increases in incidence and prevalence of type 2 DM and its increasingly younger age of onset in almost all countries. Excellent overviews and the regional distributions can be found in the International Diabetes Federation *Diabetes Atlas* (International Diabetes Federation, 2009, 2011). The Federation notes that the consequences of diabetes increases are varied and sometimes severe. Diabetes ranks among the leading causes of blindness, renal failure and limb amputation in almost every high-income country. It is now also one of the leading causes of death (Table 7.2), mainly because of a marked increase in risk of coronary heart disease and cardiovascular disease/stroke. As noted, DM places high economic costs on healthcare systems and economies, as well as the suffering of individuals from diabetes-related complications, and the huge burdens they can place on families and carers. Global healthcare expenditures to treat and prevent diabetes and its complications were expected to total at least 376 billion dollars in 2010. By 2030, they are projected to exceed 490 billion dollars. However, DM is often avoidable and, when detected, with care and sometimes with medication, it can be well managed for many years. Hence, there is great need for avoidance, early detection, advice and treatment.

It may surprise many to learn that diabetes, or complications arising from it, now accounts for almost 7 per cent of all mortality in the 20–79 age group (over 3 million deaths), more than the number from HIV/AIDS. To the International Diabetes Federation, Rand and others, it is *the* epidemic of the twenty-first century. The Federation notes that, only twenty years ago, the best information suggested that 30 million people around the world had the disease. By contrast, it now expects that the number of people living with diabetes could be over 400 million by 2030 if nothing is done. This could even be an underestimate (see below).

Diabetes on the increase worldwide

The International Diabetes Federation (2009) notes the global prevalence of all types of diabetes increased considerably from an estimated 151 million in 2000 (the first edition of

Table 7.2 Regional estimates for diabetes and comparative prevalence, population aged 20–79, 2010–30

Region	2010				2030			
	% of region's deaths attributable to diabetes 2010	Pop. aged 20–79 (millions)	No. with diabetes (millions)	Comparative prevalence %	Pop. aged 20–79 (millions)	No. with diabetes (millions)	Comparative prevalence %	% Increase 2010–30 in no. with diabetes
North America & Caribbean	15.7	320	37.4	10.2	390	53.2	12.1	42.4
Middle East & North Africa	11.5	344	26.6	9.3	533	51.7	10.8	94.0
South-east Asia	14.3	838	58.7	7.6	1,200	101.0	9.1	72.1
Europe	11.0	646	55.4	6.9	659	66.5	8.1	20.0
South & Central America	9.5	287	18.0	6.6	382	29.6	7.8	64.5
Western Pacific	10.0	1,531	76.7	4.7	1,772	112.8	5.7	47.0
Africa	6.0	379	12.1	3.8	653	23.9	4.7	97.5
Total		4,345	284.6	6.4	5,589	438.4	7.7	54.0

Source: Based on data in International Diabetes Federation, 2009

the Federation's *Atlas*) to an estimated 285 million when the fourth edition appeared in late 2009. This represents 6.4 per cent of the world's adult population. However, data vary; research reported in *The Lancet* in 2011 found fasting plasma glucose levels had risen each decade and so had numbers with diabetes. It suggested 347 million adults globally had diabetes in 2008, well over double the 1980 figure (138 million were in China and India), and there were 3 million deaths worldwide. While rates have been relatively stable in Europe, Latin America and rich Asian countries, they rose fastest in countries such as Cape Verde, Samoa Saudi Arabia, Papua New Guinea and the United States. Danaei *et al.* (2011) note that these global rises are driven by population growth and ageing, and by increasing age-specific prevalences.

The International Diabetes Federation (2009) projections to 2030 suggest as many as 438 million people globally will have diabetes. In global health terms, the 2009 *Atlas* emphasizes that, far from being a disease of the wealthy nations, diabetes is increasingly associated with poverty. Indeed, the major burden of diabetes is being borne by low- and middle-income countries while, in the wealthier countries, it disproportionately affects lower socio-economic groups, disadvantaged and minority groups (see Table 7.2, but note there is considerable intra-regional variation in most regions). Similar to a disease such as malaria, the potential impacts of diabetes in development terms have been recognized. The UN, in Resolution 61/225 from 2006, stated, 'diabetes is a chronic, debilitating and costly disease associated with severe complications, which poses severe risks for families, Member States and the entire world and serious challenges to the achievement of internationally agreed development goals including the Millennium Development Goals' (cited in International Diabetes Federation, 2009).

Diabetes and national development status

The WHO estimates that in 2005 some 80 per cent of diabetes-related deaths occurred in LAMICs (Alwan and Maclean, 2009). Table 7.3 shows high-prevalence diabetes countries, which are not surprising, since these are mainly where many of the most rapid and extreme changes in lifestyles, work patterns and living conditions are found. More refined methods suggest there are about 3 million deaths globally attributable to diabetes every year, close to the IDF estimates above.

Projected increases are likely to be relatively highest in the Middle East, sub-Saharan Africa and India, as well as China. The prevalence of diabetes in such countries appears to be increasing faster than in high-income countries and, while increasing, urban–rural differences are also emerging. In the urban population of Chennai in India, the prevalence is reported to have increased by 72 per cent in only fourteen years. Prevalence of diabetes in China was previously thought to be considerably lower than in India, but it has risen substantially within a relatively short period of time.

A major study in China in 2007–08 (Box 7.10) suggests the disease has become an increasing public health problem, affecting as many as 10 per cent of adults with diabetes and a further 15.5 per cent with pre-diabetes (Yang *et al.*, 2010). Given China's population, this equates to an enormous number of affected people, so strategies aimed at the prevention and treatment of diabetes are urgently needed. This is a very important conclusion for a fast-modernizing country in which modern lifestyles, overweight and obesity are becoming quite common.

Table 7.3 'Top ten' in comparative prevalence and rank of diabetes and impaired glucose tolerance (IGT), age 20–79 years, 2010 and projections for 2030

2010 rank			2030 rank		
Diabetes	*Diabetes prevalence %*	*IGT prevalence (rank) %*	*Diabetes*	*Diabetes prevalence %*	*IGT prevalence (rank) %*
1 Nauru	30.9	(1) 20.4	1 Nauru	33.4	(1) 21.5
2 United Arab Emirates	18.7	(4) 18.8	2 United Arab Emirates	21.4	(3) 20.1
3 Saudi Arabia	16.8	–	3 Mauritius	19.8	(8) 14.0
4 Mauritius	16.2	(8) 13.5	4 Saudi Arabia	18.4	–
5 Bahrain	15.4	(3) 18.8	5 Réunion	18.1	–
6 Réunion	15.3	–	6 Bahrain	17.3	(2) 20.1
7 Kuwait	14.6	–	7 Kuwait	16.9	–
8 Oman	13.4	–	8 Tonga	15.7	(9) 14.0
9 Tonga	13.4	(9) 13.1	9 Oman	14.9	–
10 Malaysia	11.6	–	10 Malaysia	13.8	–
Singapore	–	(2) 18.8	Singapore	–	(4) 19.8
Kiribati	–	(5) 17.3	Kiribati	–	(5) 18.3
Poland	–	(6) 15.3	Poland	–	(6) 16.5
Ghana		(7) 14.1	Syrian Arab Republic		(7) 15.3
Syrian Arab Republic		(10) 13.0	Denmark		(10) 13.8

Note: Only includes countries where surveys with glucose testing undertaken.
Source: Based on data in International Diabetes Federation, 2009

BOX 7.10 Prevalence of diabetes and impaired glucose tolerance (IGT) in China

Like many rapidly modernizing countries, China has noted considerable increase in diabetes and IGT. Given its size and rapidly changing lifestyles, China may have the largest disease burden related to diabetes.

Earlier prevalence studies among adults age in China had found 2.5% diabetes and 3.2% IGT (1994) and, in 2001–1, 5.5% and 7.3%, though findings are not exactly comparable due to different methods. In 2007–2008, a national study tested 46,239 adults aged 20-plus from 14 provinces and municipalities for previously undiagnosed diabetes and pre-diabetes (impaired fasting glucose or IGT). Participants also self-reported previously diagnosed diabetes.

Even higher rates of diabetes and IGT were found than earlier. Age-standardized prevalences of total diabetes and pre-diabetes were 9.7% (10.6% in men, 8.8% in women) and 15.5% (16.1% M, 14.9% F). Interestingly, urban-rural differences emerged, perhaps lifestyle-associated. Diabetes prevalence was significantly higher among urban (11.4%) than rural residents (8.2%), although pre-diabetes was slightly lower among rural residents. Prevalence increased with age and with increasing weight/BMI.

continued

The detailed study suggests that China may have 92.4 million adults with diabetes and even more, 148.2 million, with pre-diabetes, an important risk factor for developing diabetes and cardiovascular disease. The figures suggest diagnosed and undiagnosed diabetes at epidemic levels, representing a major public health challenge, calling for national prevention, detection and treatment strategies in China.

(Source: Based on Yang *et al.*, 2010)

Other international impacts of diabetes

Diabetes, and related overweight, may challenge the achievement of some MDGs, especially those related to child health. If current trends prevail, diabetes prevalence is expected to rise even in countries where the young adult population is currently impacted by the AIDS epidemic. The link between diabetes and tuberculosis has been long recognized and DM prevalence is increasing globally, fuelled by obesity. About 15 per cent of new tuberculosis cases in India can be attributed to diabetes. There is increasing evidence that DM is an important risk factor in tuberculosis, and could affect presentation and response to treatment. It is also possible that tuberculosis might induce glucose intolerance, worsening glycaemic control in people with diabetes, so this will be even more important in poorer countries where tuberculosis is serious (and among ageing populations) (Dye *et al.*, 2011; Dooley and Chaisson, 2009). In many places, as diabetes onset moves into younger age groups, more pregnancies are likely to be associated with the condition, prejudicing the health of mother and child during pregnancy and birth, as well as the long-term risk of diabetes and cardiovascular diseases in babies. Another UN resolution on diabetes (UN General Assembly at its 65th session in 2010: agenda item 113) called for increased awareness of the condition and related complications. It encourages countries to develop prevention and control programmes, very similar to the subsequent calls in China and many other countries.

Impaired glucose tolerance (IGT)

Given the large numbers identified with pre-diabetes and predisposition to diabetes in many countries, IGT is becoming a key indicator as it can represent a stage in the transition from normality to diabetes. Many people with IGT are at high risk of progressing to type 2 diabetes, though this is not inevitable, as over 30 per cent of individuals with IGT return to normal glucose tolerance over a period of several years. Nevertheless, IGT greatly increases the risk of developing diabetes and it is also associated with the development of cardiovascular disease. Importantly, some of the best evidence on the prevention of type 2 diabetes derives from studies involving IGT. This status is clearly a huge challenge, as there were an estimated 344 million people worldwide (7.9 per cent in the age group 20–79) with IGT in 2010. Like diabetes itself, the vast majority are in low- and middle-income countries. By 2030, the number of people with IGT is projected to increase to 472 million, 8.4 per cent of the adult population (International Diabetes Federation, 2009). The comparative prevalence of diabetes 'top ten' countries is remarkably similar from 2010 to 2030, though in terms of the precursor risk condition IGT, a number of new countries appear, such as Singapore, Poland, the Syrian Arab Republic and Denmark (see Table 7.3).

Tobacco consumption, substance misuse and related disorders

Smoking of tobacco is associated with many types of chronic ill-health. Smoking is generally declining in industrialized countries, especially among educated people (though some groups, particularly young girls, are sometimes seeing an increase). Against a trend elsewhere, smoking is on the increase in many poor and middle-income countries. Nevertheless, even in developed regions, in such countries as England, smoking causes or is associated with as many as a third of cancer deaths, a quarter of heart disease and four-fifths of deaths from bronchitis and emphysema. Diseases such as lung cancers are often multi-causal but over three-quarters of lung cancer cases are related to smoking. Smoking is also a major risk factor for 80–90 per cent of the chronic lung condition COPD (chronic obstructive pulmonary disease). COPD increases with age, with over 5 million cases globally in 2002, and 3 million deaths in 2004, projected to reach almost 6 million by 2030 (Chau *et al.*, 2011). Lung cancer and other disease trends are greatly predicted by past cigarette consumption patterns in the population and these are expected to continue to increase globally. This is especially so in low and middle-income countries, where heavy marketing and consumption of tobacco products persists. As noted with respect to NCDs, tobacco remains a risk factor for six of the eight leading causes of death, and is top in high- and second in middle-income countries (see Table 4.10). More than a billion people globally use tobacco and it contributes to killing up to half the people who use it, as many as 5 million people worldwide each year (Alwan and Maclean, 2009).

Previously, many governments have apparently had a love–hate relationship with tobacco, as sales often generate substantial tax revenues, but these have almost always been shown to be outweighed by the costs of smoking-related disease treatment as well as misery of sufferers. While developed world smoking rates may generally be falling, decreases in deaths will take more time to evolve. As the WHO map shows (Figure 7.3), in 2004 there were still high rates of deaths in the 30-plus age group caused by tobacco in many developed countries and fewer, relatively speaking, in many African and Latin American countries.

Smoking by individuals – and societies – has both health and economic costs. Increasingly, attention is focusing on its effects on others, and the risks of *passive smoking* ('second-hand smoke') have been under scrutiny for some time. In the 1990s, some argued that cancer rates were not raised by passive smoking but that exposure increased the risk of coronary heart disease (Macdonald, 1998). Comparative data have been rare but a major international study published in 2010 found that passive smoking accounted for 600,000 deaths per year worldwide, 1 per cent of overall mortality. Of major concern was that almost one-third were deaths of children (Öberg *et al.*, 2011). This backs up other studies in the UK and elsewhere (Royal College of Physicians, 2010). So, passive smoking is confirmed as a major public health risk, exacerbated because, unlike personal tobacco consumption, those exposed to second-hand smoke have no choice. Adults and children exposed to passive smoking are at risk from all the problems associated with tobacco smoke. The risk of lung cancer among non-smokers living with smokers is estimated to be increased by up to 30 per cent. Exposure can occur at home, at work or in the general environment and may be more serious for certain sub-groups, such as asthma sufferers and those with lung disease. It may also be a danger for women who take the oral contraceptive pill and could be at higher risk of heart disease and stroke.

Policies to restrict and discourage smoking are well known and widespread in most developed countries, involving education, bans on tobacco advertising and sponsorship, and graphic health warnings on cigarette packages. Combined with regulations limiting smoking in public and workplaces, and higher taxes on cigarettes and tobacco, these have helped reduce overall smoking. By contrast, smoking or tobacco consumption is often increasing in

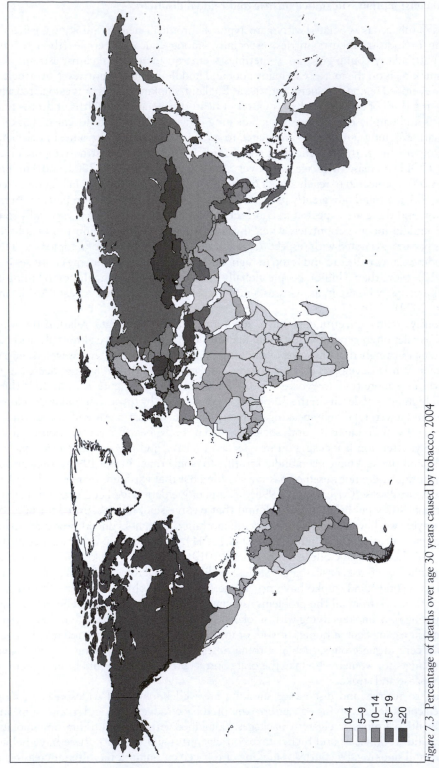

Figure 7.3 Percentage of deaths over age 30 years caused by tobacco, 2004

Source: WHO, 2009a, Fig. 11, p. 22

0–4
5–9
10–14
15–19
≥20

many other regions, where it is poorly controlled and even facilitated by low taxes and cheap tobacco. Most worryingly, it is often taken up at a very young age in some developing countries. Research in Indonesia found that one-third of adult smokers started before the age of 10. Thun *et al.* (2009) see the need to strengthen international tobacco control as one of the major priorities to mitigate the anticipated increase in global cancer (especially in poorer countries). This is not happening in some major tobacco markets. In China, for example, there were an estimated 673,000 tobacco-related deaths in 2005 (Alwan and Maclean, 2009). China is a major country in need of tobacco control, and Hong Kong is suggested as a model for this (Koplan *et al.*, 2010). China has actually started to focus public policy and start controls. A ban was introduced in May 2011 on smoking in 'enclosed public places', such as hotels, restaurants, theaters and public transport waiting rooms, but not in offices or factories. It is hoped this partial ban, whether successfully enforced or not, will raise some awareness of the risks of smoking. We return to this topic in Chapter 8 (Box 8.6), when we discuss innovations and impacts of public policies.

Injury, accidents and road traffic accidents

Worldwide, but especially in the developing world, injury and/or accidents are a very important, varied and growing cause of mortality and long-term disability (Figure 7.4). Injuries cause some 12 per cent of the global burden of disease, and are the third leading cause of overall mortality. They are especially important in middle-income countries (see Table 4.9). Some 5 million people die annually from injury worldwide, almost 16,000 every day, with almost 25 per cent of these from road traffic injuries, which leave a further 50 million people injured. These deaths, and the people who are hurt and need long- or short-term care, place huge strains on healthcare systems and cause much human misery. However, the nature and scope, and treatment potential, of injuries vary hugely inter-nationally. For example, more than 90 per cent of deaths due to injuries occur in the

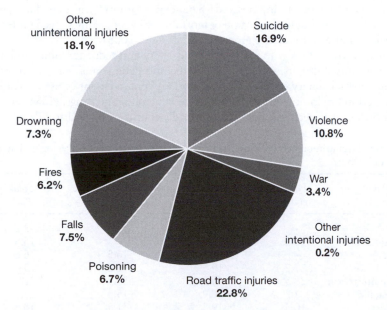

Figure 7.4 Global injury mortality by cause, 2002
Source: WHO, 2004, Fig. 2.1, p. 34

low- and middle-income countries. Male injury mortality is twice the rate of that for females. Males in Africa have the highest rates of injury mortality and women in the Americas the lowest. The age group 15–44 accounts for almost 50 per cent of global injury mortality (McKinzie, 2007). Accidents are the third leading cause of mortality among males in the USA and in some lower-income countries, and they are the leading cause among those under 40 worldwide. As we discuss in Chapter 9, there are also large numbers of people living and existing near industries that are often poorly sited or regulated, giving rise to many actual and potential industrial and environmental accidents, especially but not exclusively in poor and middle-income countries.

As the WHO (2004, 2011b) notes, road traffic injuries are a major but neglected public health challenge, affecting disproportionately the poorest and especially the middle-income countries (Table 7.4). Accidents and injuries are common, because road traffic systems are the most complex and dangerous of all the systems and environments with which people interact daily. Worldwide, road traffic injuries alone are predicted to rise from the ninth major cause of death in 2004 to fifth by 2030 (WHO, 2011b) and they have already become the leading cause of death for the 15–29 age group, the economically active. Over 90 per cent of road traffic deaths and injuries occur in low- and middle-income countries, where there are only 48 per cent of the world's registered vehicles, indicating combinations of deficient road, vehicle, training and regulation systems. In terms of burden of disease, an estimated 1.3 million people are killed in road crashes each year and as many as 50 million injured. As noted, these figures are projected to increase by about 65 per cent over the next twenty years unless there is new commitment to prevention. While many accidents involve cars, caused by combinations of road conditions, unsafe driving and vehicles, (often large) commercial vehicles are frequently a major cause of death and serious injury in many poorer countries (Nzegwu *et al.*, 2008).

In traffic accidents, head and spinal injuries are very common, and the variety of two- and four-wheeled transport on the roads, and high-density pedestrian and vehicular traffic, mean injuries and deaths are very common. Indeed, in India, it is estimated that 11 per cent of deaths from NCDs are due to injuries and 78 per cent of injury deaths are due to road traffic accidents. These form the leading cause of mortality for young adults (aged under 45) and a major burden of disease for all age groups (Pathak *et al.*, 2008).

In many countries, the key to improving road safety and reducing injury and deaths will be better training of drivers, separation of traffic and pedestrians, serious enforcement of speed limits, vehicle safety checks and provision and enforcement of use of seat belts, plus concerted action on driving under the influence of alcohol and drugs. However, the WHO (2009c) notes that fewer than half of the world's countries have drink-driving limits on

Table 7.4 Road traffic injury fatality rates per 100,000 population, by WHO region and income group, c. 2008

Region (WHO)	High-income countries	Middle-income countries	Low-income countries	Total
African	–	32.2	32.3	32.2
The Americas	13.4	17.3	–	15.8
South-east Asia	–	16.7	16.5	16.6
European	7.9	19.3	12.2	13.4
Eastern Mediterranean	28.5	35.8	27.5	32.2
Western Pacific	7.2	16.9	15.6	15.7
Global rates	10.3	19.5	21.5	18.8

Source: Data from WHO, 2009c

blood alcohol levels equal to or less than 0.05g/dl. Moreover, in many countries, even the traffic regulations that do exist are routinely ignored, or police are routinely bribed to overlook offences.

There is widespread need to reduce the carnage witnessed daily on many roads and in workplaces and homes in many countries; there is room for improvement even in the richest countries. To promote this, data on the epidemiology of injury from accidents, road and industrial safety, and violence, are of great importance. In policy terms, the WHO's Department for Injury and Violence Prevention promotes global initiatives on injury prevention and control. Injuries are classified into intentional (suicide, interpersonal violence and war-related violence) and unintentional, including road traffic accidents, falls, fires and drownings. In richer countries, there is an interest in minimizing accidents for public health, legal and financial reasons. In many poorer countries, there is often less interest in, or incentives for, accident prevention: reduced regulation and the pursuit of profit or simply making a living take priority. Consequently, environmental, workplace and road conditions are often very dangerous and even lethal.

Worldwide chronic disease: the challenge of cancer

Cancer causes around 7.6 million deaths worldwide each year (WHO, *Cancer* website, 2011h), the third leading cause of death, with 13 million or more new cases occurring. The *World Cancer Report* (Boyle and Levin, 2008) estimates the global cancer burden doubled over the last thirty years, may double again between 2000 and 2020, and may almost triple by 2030. By then, deaths from cancer are projected to have risen to around 17 million worldwide, alongside population increase and demographic ageing. However, as noted in Chapter 4 and below, there are great international variations in the burden and types of cancer. Low- and middle-income countries accounted for just over half (51 per cent) of all cancers worldwide in 1975, and 55 per cent in 2007. However, this is projected to reach 61 per cent by 2050 (Thun *et al.*, 2009).

There have been considerable advances in early cancer detection, treatment and even prevention over recent years, but access to diagnosis and treatment varies greatly both internationally and between different groups and locations within individual countries. The incidence, prevalence and sometimes mortality rates for all types of cancer have increased worldwide. Not only do individuals and families suffer, but there are enormous overall medical and non-medical costs and lost productivity, estimated to total 286 billion dollars in 2009 (Global Health Council, 2010). Indeed, the American Cancer Society (2010) estimated the global economic impact of premature death and disability from cancer in 2008 to be as much as 895 billion dollars, or 1.5 per cent of global GDP, almost 20 per cent higher than heart disease, the second-greatest cause of economic loss.

What is cancer?

Cancer is not a single disease but involves a group of diseases in which abnormal cells divide in an uncontrolled manner, and it can occur in different parts of the body (Kumar and Clark, 2009). Some cancer cells can spread (metastasize) to nearby tissues and to more distant parts of the body via the bloodstream and lymphatic system; there are also cancers of the blood, such as leukaemias, and lymphomas involving the lymphatic system itself. The seriousness and speed of metastasis vary considerably, according to cell type. Many tumours are benign, not cancerous, and do not spread to other parts of the body, although they too can sometimes be life-threatening or cause problems by putting pressure on other organs. Cancers are often named after their main (primary) site, such as lung, breast, stomach, prostate or brain. Many cancers can occur at any age, although some types tend to affect children and younger groups more, while others tend to predominate in older people. By and large, cancers tend to increase with age. Some, such as ovarian, uterine, prostate and testicular, are specific to females or males.

The causes of many types of cancer are unknown but many have distinctive lifestyle and dietary associations, or even direct causes. Each type arises in a different cell, so each tends to require different approaches to prevention and treatment. Most cancer types also tend to have different sets of causes and predisposing factors, although some factors, such as tobacco and exposure to radiation, are relevant in the causation of several cancers. Overall, the WHO estimates that up to 40 per cent of all cancer cases could be prevented by changes in lifestyle and improved prevention and screening. Cancer risk can be significantly reduced by avoiding recognized risk factors such as tobacco use, heavy alcohol consumption, excessive sun exposure and obesity, and adopting healthier diets, lifestyles and exercise. Despite better education in many countries, cancer incidence continues to rise and, like some other conditions, such as dementias and obesity, this is often called an 'epidemic'. Governments have a crucial role to play in raising awareness and supporting comprehensive early detection measures, and many are doing so, at many levels. However, in many poorer countries, it is often difficult to prioritize such cancer-awareness education and detection, or to afford treatment and follow-up cancer services. Nevertheless, well-conceived and continuing national cancer control programmes are essential to fight the disease and improve quality of life for cancer patients. There is a huge demand for the four basic components of cancer control: prevention, early detection, diagnosis and treatment, and palliative care (Boyle and Levin, 2008; WHO, *Cancer* website, 2011h).

Treatment for cancers varies greatly with type and even among different medical systems. Outcomes are usually improved by early detection, and treatments may involve simple procedures, surgery, chemotherapy and/or radiation therapy. Some types of cancer, such as early non-melanoma skin cancers, respond well to treatment, while others, such as lung cancer, tend to do less well; for some types, survival rates have not improved significantly over the years. 'Silent' types, such as pancreatic and ovarian cancers, frequently give symptoms late, by which time they are often advanced or have spread, making treatment more difficult and generally less effective. Survival and cure rates vary greatly for different cancers, their clinical stage of development and the treatment options available to people (see, for example, Tracey *et al.*, 2007).

The WHO and others note that the rapid increase in the cancer burden represents a real crisis for public health and health systems almost everywhere. How to raise sufficient funds to treat all cancer patients effectively and provide palliative, supportive and terminal care for the large numbers of patients who will be diagnosed in the coming years, and their relatives, will be a major challenge even for resource-rich countries (Boyle and Levin, 2008). Nevertheless, prevention, diagnosis, survival rates and access to sophisticated and effective cancer treatment are generally improving in most wealthy countries. Unfortunately, most low- and middle-income nations are facing increasing cancer caseloads with little or no access to prevention, treatment and care, or even basic palliative pain relief. All these are very limited because of costs, lack of technology, inaccessibility, and unavailability of specialist staff, and there are consequently considerable differences between and within poorer countries in survival rates (Sankaranarayanan *et al.* 2010; Sankaranarayanan and Swaminathan, 2011). Cancers can require technical equipment for initial diagnosis and treatment, often prolonged and involving regular attention and follow-ups (see also Chapter 11). The availability of diagnostic and treatment facilities varies greatly geographically and, being a particularly complex health problem that involves extensive human and financial health resources, cancer has generally been relatively neglected in most developing countries, especially for the majority of their populations.

National policy-makers and international donor and health agencies, especially in the poorest countries, find this situation very difficult to address. Resources in many poor and middle-income countries are often insufficient to deal with even the most basic immediate public health issues, such as clean water, nutrition and infectious disease control. Therefore, providing the sophisticated systems needed for dealing with many of the commoner cancers is just not considered affordable or a priority (International Network for Cancer Treatment and Research, 2010). Unfortunately, there is double jeopardy: low-income and disadvantaged groups are often particularly exposed, by residence or work, to risk factors and infectious agents which can lead to avoidable cancers, yet they have the poorest access to healthcare. These groups face extra dangers, as they are generally less aware of risk factors, especially environmental risk factors; and, even if recognized, they have little chance to avoid them or deal with the health outcomes.

Therefore, priorities for global cancer control must include a focus on low- and medium-resource countries and the identification, delivery and evaluation of effective cancer control measures. Prevention research is of utmost importance, as is translational research – translating scientific discovery into new approaches to cancer treatment – and increasing knowledge of cancer risk factors in order to change people's behaviour (Boyle and Levin, 2008).

International variations in cancer incidence, prevalence and survival

Great disparities exist globally, and even locally, in the burden of cancer (incidence and prevalence) and in outcomes (Mackay *et al.*, 2006; Thun *et al.*, 2009; see Table 4.8). Until relatively recently, cancers were considered mainly diseases of the rich Western world but, as mentioned above, the real picture is very different (see Table 4.9) and cancer is recognized as 'globalizing' (Boyle, 2006; Boyle and Howell, 2010). The developing world accounted for only 15 per cent of newly reported cancers in 1970. In 2007, more than 72 per cent of cancer-related deaths occurred in low- and middle-income countries. By 2020, some 60 per cent of all new cancer cases are likely to occur in the least developed, poorest nations (Global Health Council, 2010, citing WHO). This is a 'looming public health crisis'. There is certainly a growing health gap in cancers between rich and poor countries (Axios, 2010).

In detail, of the WHO's estimated 14.5 million new cancer cases in 2004, approximately 66 per cent occurred in LAMICs. By cancer type, 64 per cent of lung cancer (12.7 per cent of the total), 82 per cent of stomach cancer (8.2 per cent of the total), 56 per cent of breast cancer (7.6 per cent of the total), 52 per cent of colon and rectal cancer (9.5 per cent of the total), 47 per cent of prostate cancer (5.3 per cent of the total) and over 90 per cent of cervical cancer (3.6 per cent of the total) occurred in LAMICs in 2004 (Alwan and Maclean, 2009). This increase probably represents a combination of real increases in cancers and their better recognition and reporting, but estimates rely very heavily on local data availability and reliability.

The types of cancers, and hence their aetiology, tend to vary regionally and even locally. For example, the WHO (*Cancer* website, 2011h) and the Global Health Council (2010) and others estimate that infections (such as by viruses, bacteria and other pathogens) caused some 20–26 per cent of cancers in low- and middle-income countries but only 6–10 per cent in developed countries. Lung cancer is expected to keep killing more people than any other type, unless efforts for global tobacco control are greatly intensified. However, as discussed, many developing countries, such as China, have increasing smoking populations. Some cancers, such as of the prostate, breast and colon, are more common in developed countries;

others, such as cancer of the liver, stomach and cervix, are more common in developing countries. This can relate to many factors: infections, dietary behaviour, social behaviour (including sexual practices), and environmental conditions, such as heavy pollution in some poorer and middle-income countries. Indeed, migrant studies indicate that cancer rates in successive generations tend to shift in the direction of the rates prevailing in the host country. This suggests international variations in cancer rates for most cancers reflect differences in environmental risk factors rather than genetic differences (Jemal *et al.*, 2010). A significant portion of cancers worldwide are also associated with reproductive health. Unfortunately, this problem has been neglected by the scientific community until recently, resulting in limited data on the epidemiology of reproductive health cancers in developing countries.

Research on the fifty-three countries in the WHO's European region showed skewed regional distributions (see also Table 4.7). For example, Hungary had the highest cancer mortality rate (458 per 100,000 population), followed by the Russian Federation and Ukraine (347 per 100,000), likely due to high smoking rates. Breast cancer caused the most cancer-related deaths in women (17.2 per cent of the total), while lung cancer was a leading killer among men (26.9 per cent of the total). Importantly, outcomes can also differ internationally for the same conditions. For example, lung cancer mortality rates per 100,000 were highest in Hungary (135), followed by Poland (93) and Croatia (86). Romania had the highest cervical cancer deaths (21 per 100,000 population), while breast cancer deaths were highest in Belgium and Armenia (37). The picture is complex, and studies have shown considerable sub-national, sub-regional and even social variations in cancer incidence and survival after treatment, even within relatively small nations.

Data on incidence of cancers internationally have been collected since the early 1960s and published periodically in *CI5: Cancer Incidence in Five Continents* (IARC, *CI5* website). Using *CI5* data and WHO mortality data available for some national registries, Jemal *et al.* (2010) have analysed global patterns and trends in cancer incidence and mortality. Based on their very useful paper, which also explains issues of age standardization of incidence and mortality rates, some selected examples of global patterns of cancer incidence and mortality trends are given below.

- *Lung cancer:* Worldwide, this is the leading cause of cancer deaths in men and second in women. For males, the highest incidence rates are reported in the United States (among blacks) and in Eastern European countries. The lowest rates are found in Africa, Central and South America and South Central Asia. Among females, the highest rates are reported in North America and parts of Europe, including the United Kingdom and Denmark. The lowest are in Africa, South Central Asia and Latin America. These international variations in lung cancer largely reflect different stages and amounts of smoking, which accounts for some 80 per cent of global lung cancer deaths in men and half of the deaths in women.
- *Colon and rectum cancer:* This, the third most common cancer in men and the second in women, shows a more than tenfold difference in regional incidence rates among both men and women. The highest rates among both men and women are in Eastern European countries (e.g. Czech Republic and Slovakia), Japan (Miyagi), New Zealand, Australia, Germany and US blacks; the lowest rates are in Africa, Central and South America and South Central Asia (India and Pakistan). There are also ethnic group differences within countries such as the USA. Colorectal cancer incidence rates are stabilizing or even declining in previously high-risk areas, but they are increasing rapidly in several former low-risk countries, such as Japan, Korea, China and Eastern European countries. The increase in incidence rates in some Asian and Eastern European

countries (and Spain) probably reflects diet and lifestyle changes, plus smoking and obesity. In some places, while incidence may have been increasing, colorectal cancer death rates have been decreasing at least in part due to better treatment, increased awareness and early detection. In this cancer, as in others, mortality rates are often increasing in countries with limited resources and health infrastructure, but where need is growing.

- *Stomach cancer:* This, the fourth most commonly diagnosed cancer and the second leading cause of cancer death globally, has incidence rates ranging from 3.3 per 100,000 in men and 2.0 in women in Egypt to 65.9 in men and 25.9 in women in Korea. Large regional variations reflect differences in *H. pylori* infection (which accounts for more than 60 per cent of gastric cancers), and in part differences in smoking, nitrate intake and possibly dietary sodium. Incidence rates in a number of Western countries have steadily declined over the past half-century, and in some countries with previously high rates, such as China, Japan and others. This important global decrease in incidence and mortality rates may be associated with better diets, more fresh fruits and vegetables, treatment of *H. pylori*, screening, probably decreased use of salted and preserved food, and reduced smoking in most Western countries.
- *Liver cancer:* This is the sixth most commonly diagnosed cancer, and the third leading cause of cancer death worldwide. There is a twenty- to forty-fold difference in international variations in liver cancer rates, and nearly 85 per cent of the cases occur in less developed countries, with more than 50 per cent occurring in China. Highest rates are in Asia and West and Central Africa, and lowest in Europe, Oceania and North America. The international variations in liver cancer rates are largely explained by chronic hepatitis B and C virus infections, which together account for almost 80 per cent of global liver cancer deaths, and as high as 90 per cent in Japan and Singapore. Other dietary factors, cirrhosis and obesity probably act as cofactors with existing chronic viral infections.

Jemal *et al.*'s analysis also covered breast cancer in females and prostate cancers in men. Both are common and leading causes of death globally. Breast cancer incidence and mortality rates vary internationally more than fivefold, with highest incidence rates found in Switzerland, US whites, Italy and many other European countries. Low rates tend to be seen in Africa, Asia and South America. The high incidence rates in white women in the USA and most European countries are thought to be due to established reproductive factors associated with increased breast cancer risk, such as early menarche, late childbearing, fewer pregnancies and hormone replacement therapy, plus increased detection through mammography. Despite these international variations, nowhere is 'safe' from a globalized disease (Boyle and Howell, 2010). Incidence rates of prostate cancer also vary greatly, by nearly fiftyfold: from 3.9 per 100,000 in India to 178.8 in US blacks. More than half of cases and deaths are expected to occur in more developed countries; in general, highest rates are in North America, Oceania and Northern and Western Europe, with lowest rates in Asia and North Africa.

Other studies have focused on *childhood cancers*, which are often among the most curable, yet survival rates show the starkest differences between rich and poor countries. Children in rich countries diagnosed with many common forms of childhood cancer, often probably embryonic in origin, have 75–80 per cent chance of a cure (Hammond, 2011). But this falls to as low as 10–30 per cent for the same cancers in poor countries, where over 100,000 children are estimated to die annually with little or no treatment or pain relief. Over 100 poor countries lack specialist staff, diagnostics and treatment, which is further hindered by the costs of drugs and the logistical difficulties of patients and their parents accessing care and following rigorous treatment regimes. Childhood cancers represent one area of global health in which assistance, international partnerships for specialist knowledge, use of simple remote technology links and low-cost drugs may bring about substantial improvements in survival rates in coming decades (see Chapter 11).

Challenges from global ageing: dementias and impaired ADLs (activities of daily living)

Dementias

Like many other conditions, there is an increasing tendency to identify a worldwide 'epidemic' of dementias in recent decades, and especially when looking to the future (see also Chapter 8 about growing costs). Even more than the epidemics of cancers, widespread increases in numbers with dementias are related strongly to global ageing, as the older population is statistically at far higher risk than young and middle-aged populations. The prevalence of dementia nearly doubles for every five years after age 65 (see Box 7.11). As discussed in Chapter 4, many countries now have life expectancies well over 70 and into the eighties (see Figure 4.8). Alzheimer's disease and other dementias (see Table 7.5) are already the fourth leading cause of moderate–severe disability in the high-income countries among the 60-plus age group, following hearing problems, refractive errors and osteoarthritis (WHO, 2011c; see Table 7.1). They are also a growing cause of disability in middle- and low-income countries.

Strictly speaking, dementia is a condition or symptoms, rather than an illness. The symptoms involve progressive, irreversible loss of cognitive and intellectual ability caused by cerebral (brain) disease or damage. Dementia also tends to be used as a general term for the loss of memory and other intellectual abilities serious enough to interfere with daily life. It can manifest in many ways, including as impaired cognitive functioning, impaired behaviour and personality changes in later stages. Most importantly, it is degenerative, although the speed and course vary considerably among individuals.

People with dementias tend to show memory impairment (such as difficulty in learning new material, short-term memory loss or recalling previously known material), difficulty working things out, and difficulty with at least one cognitive capacity, such as language, recognition, and organization and/or performance of motor (movement) activities. In spite of popular images of memory failing in old age, dementias are definitely not part of normal ageing, even though the incidence increases with age. It can be called a psycho-pathology as it is abnormal though increasingly common in ageing populations. Everywhere, policies need to recognize

---

BOX 7.11 What is dementia?

'Dementia is a syndrome that can be caused by a number of progressive illnesses that affect memory, thinking, behaviour and the ability to perform everyday activities. Alzheimer's disease is the most common type of dementia. Other types include vascular dementia, dementia with Lewy bodies and frontotemporal dementia. The boundaries between the types are not clear, and a mixture of more than one type is common. Dementia mainly affects older people, although there is a growing awareness of cases that start before the age of 65. After age 65, the likelihood of developing dementia roughly doubles every five years.'

(Source: Alzheimer's Disease International, 2010, p. 8; see also Alzheimer's Disease International, 2009 for detailed information on dementia)

Table 7.5 Characteristics of sub-types of dementia

Dementia subtype	Early, characteristic symptoms	Neuropathology	Proportion of dementia cases
Alzheimer's disease (AD)*	Impaired memory, apathy and depression Gradual onset	Cortical amyloid plaques and neurofibrillary tangles	50–75%
Vascular dementia (VaD)*	Smiliar to AD, but memory less affected, and mood fluctuations more prominent Physical fraility Stepwise onset	Cerebrovascular disease Single infarcts in critical regions, or more diffuse multi-infarct disease	20–30%
Dementia with Lewy bodies (DLB)	Marked fluctuation in cognitive ability Visual hallucinations Parkinsonism (tremor and rigidity)	Cortical Lewy bodies (alpha-synuclein)	<5%
Frontotemporal dementia (FTD)	Personality changes Mood changes Disinhibition Language difficulties	No single pathology – damage limited to frontal and temporal lobes	5–10%

Note: * Post-mortem studies suggest that many people with dementia have mixed Alzheimer's disease and vascular dementia pathology, and that this 'mixed dementia' is underdiagnosed.

Source: Alzheimer's Disease International, 2009, p. 14

that dementia is not a normal part of ageing and to overcome the myth that 'nothing can be done about it'. In the UK, for example, only 31 per cent of primary-care doctors believed they had adequate training to diagnose and manage dementia. Sufferers tend to present to doctors late, on average three years after the onset of their symptoms, as more than half of caregivers believe the symptoms are a normal part of ageing (Alzheimer's Disease International, 2010).

Table 7.5 summarizes the major dementia sub-types. The majority of dementias from Alzheimer's disease (up to 70 per cent of dementias) are associated with distinct patterns of change and damage within the brain. Vascular dementia is another common type, responsible for 20–30 per cent of dementias, caused by reduced blood flow to parts of the brain. There are also other less common causes. As vascular dementia can be caused by strokes or disruption of blood supply to the brain, it may be related to lifestyle factors. The symptoms of dementia tend to vary depending on the cause, the exact area of the brain affected and how it has come about (especially if disease, stroke or perhaps substance misuse are involved). While memory loss is often the earliest and most noticeable symptom, other key symptoms of dementia can include:

- Difficulty in recognizing familiar people and places.
- Difficulties in finding the right words to express thoughts or name familiar objects.
- Problems planning and carrying out tasks, especially IADLs (such as balancing household accounts, dealing with figures, performing calculations, following a recipe, or writing a letter).
- Trouble exercising judgement, such as knowing what to do in an emergency.
- Difficulty controlling moods or behaviour.
- Depression, which is common; apathy, agitation or aggression may also occur.
- Not maintaining personal care (ADLs), such as grooming or washing and toileting.

- Not eating properly, so some people lose weight unless encouraged to eat regularly.
- Sleep disturbance and other behavioural problems.

Dementias often follow a three-stage progress, which can be variable over as long as ten–fifteen years or a much shorter time. Death often results from an associated cause, rather than the dementia itself (see Box 7.12). These stages often involve sets of symptoms, although everyone is affected differently (Alzheimer's Disease International 2009):

1   In the early stages, the first year or two, symptoms are often vague (memory disturbances, visual and spatial functioning, language and concentration). Sufferers forget recent events, words, time or day, and may become lost in familiar places.
2   In the second to fourth or fifth years, people may have more serious difficulties in daily living, with sensory and visual disturbances, become very forgetful, especially of recent events, and find it difficult to express themselves. They are often unable to cook, clean or shop and need help with personal hygiene, dressing and toileting. Wandering may occur and there may be behavioural problems, such as sleep disturbance, annoying repetitive behaviour, delusions, hallucinations and often more severe agitation.
3   In the later stage, perhaps the fifth year and later, people have near total dependency, with difficulties eating and inability to communicate. Many clinical and social problems occur, including incontinence and inappropriate behaviour in public, and dementia patients may be confined to a wheelchair or even a bed.

BOX 7.12 Why do people die from Alzheimer's and other dementias?

Why do people die from 'memory loss'? Dementias are more than this and involve progressive decline affecting behaviour; they are essentially life-shortening diseases. Another condition or illness (such as bronchopneumonia or a heart attack) may be identified as the cause of death on the death certificate. However, sometimes no specific cause of death is found, other than dementia. A major problem is that many people become unable to look after themselves, unable to eat properly, and often lose weight (this was previously thought a diagnostic feature but resulted from lack of eating) and condition as a result. As the disease progresses, patients become less able to coordinate basic motor skills, such as swallowing, walking, bladder and bowel control. Hygiene becomes a problem. Difficulty in swallowing can cause food to be inhaled, which can result in pneumonia. Inability to walk can lead to bedsores. Incontinence can result in bladder infections.

Infections can become very difficult to deal with because dementia and Alzheimer's patients lose the ability to understand and participate in their own treatment. People can fall, which may result in injury and fractures – difficult to avoid and treat among most older people and especially in people with Alzheimer's disease/dementias. Such incapacitation sets the stage for deadly infections. Clinicians say that an Alzheimer's patient could progress so that damage from the disease to the areas of the brain that control breathing could cause death, but patients rarely get that far without an infection setting in. Pneumonia and dehydration are frequent immediate causes of death. Early diagnosis is now called for to help deal as effectively as possible with these aspects and prepare for better care.

(Sources: Based on Slate, 2001; Alzheimer's Disease
International, 2009, 2011; Alzheimer's Society, 2011)

How many people are affected by dementias?

As noted in Chapter 6, dementias are now openly acknowledged in many regions as one of the major current health and social care challenges and one likely to grow hugely over the next few decades (Access Economics, 2006, 2009; Global Action on Aging, 2010a, Alzheimer's Disease International, 2010, 2011; Table 7.6). The WHO's *Global Burden of Disease* report identifies dementias as accounting for 4.1 per cent of total disease burden (DALYs) among people aged over 60, as well as 11.3 per cent of years lived with disability and 0.9 per cent of years of life lost. Dementias form the second most burdensome chronic condition of the 'other chronic non-communicable diseases', accounting for 11.9 per cent of years lived with disability and 1.1 per cent of years of life lost. Dementias may not be among the top causes of death – heart disease (32.9 per cent of years of life lost) and cancer (22.5 per cent) are ranked higher – but these rank only eighth and ninth as disabling conditions (Alzheimer's Disease International, 2009). Dementias also have huge and growing cost implications, as discussed in Chapter 8.

Alzheimer's Disease International (2009) recently estimated 35.6 million people with dementia in 2010, with numbers likely almost to double every twenty years – to 65.7 million in 2030 and 115.4 million in 2050. They now feel their previous estimates, published in *The Lancet* in 2005, were too low. New studies, particularly from low- and middle-income countries, have provided probably more reliable estimates that are 10 per cent higher than the 2005 figures (Alzheimer's Disease International, 2009). Crucially, well over half (58 per cent) of all people with dementia worldwide now live in low- and middle-income countries, and this is likely to rise to 71 per cent by 2050. Future increases are clearly going to be proportionately much greater in low- and middle-income countries within the broad regions shown in Table 7.6, and the main regions hide considerable sub-regional differences. In the Americas, for example, North America will see a 63 per cent proportionate increase in dementia between 2010 and 2030, and 150 per cent by 2050, whereas Central, Andean and Tropical Latin America regions will all see increases of over 130 per cent by 2030, and over 400 per cent by 2050. Similar differences are seen elsewhere, with Australasia having similar proportionate increases to North America, but Oceania, for example, having 100 and 400 per cent increases by 2030 and 2050, respectively (Alzheimer's Disease International, 2009).

Uncertainty about the numbers of people currently affected and the incidence of dementias is exacerbated by difficulties of diagnosis, recognition and reluctant acknowledgement. Data are often unreliable or even non-existent in poorer countries, where people with dementia may never be officially assessed. Epidemiological studies show a range of dementia typically of 3–39 per cent in elderly populations and perhaps 5 per cent of adults over 65 and 30 per cent aged over 85 have some type of dementia. Usually, however, far fewer have severe cognitive impairment caused by dementia.

Table 7.6 Dementia estimates for 2010–50, by Global Burden of Disease main regions

Region	Population over 60 (millions) 2010	Estimated prevalence (%) 2010	No. with dementia (millions)			Proportionate increase (%)	
			2010	2030	2050	2010–30	2010–50
Asia	406.55	3.9	15.94	33.04	60.92	107	282
Europe	160.18	6.2	9.95	13.95	18.65	40	87
The Americas	120.74	6.5	7.82	14.78	27.08	89	246
Africa	71.07	2.6	1.86	3.92	8.74	111	370
World	758.54	4.7	35.56	65.69	115.38	85	225

Source: Alzheimer's Disease International, 2009

Social impacts of dementias: what can be done?

While such estimates as those given in Table 7.6 show the numbers of people who have dementia now and probably future increases, we ask: how many people are *affected* by dementia? This will be much larger as dementia impacts on all the family and carers, especially when people are living at home. Later, if they move into residential accommodation, round-the-clock care is often needed. Families may wish to visit and may feel guilt about institutionalizing a spouse or parent who may no longer recognize them, so the impacts of dementias are very far reaching.

Social and medical impacts are considerable as, unfortunately, there are currently no curative treatments, nor even any that significantly alter the progressive course of dementia and Alzheimer's. The presently available drugs may work best in the early stages, for a short period, so early diagnosis is important (Alzheimer's Disease International, 2011). Moreover, disability in older age often involves many interacting factors, so dementias frequently overlap with other co-morbidities and general frailty (Vellas and Aisen, 2010). Individuals with early dementias are thus decreasingly able to deal with what gerontologists call instrumental activities of daily living (IADLs): household management, cooking, cleaning, budgets and accounts, and shopping (Hooyman and Kiyak, 2010). As dementia symptoms progress, people with dementia lose their ability to perform activities of daily living (ADLs), the most basic personal care tasks, such as washing, dressing, eating, toileting and moving around. Therefore, in early stages, people may need help to exist at home. Later, they often need specialist dementia care in institutions. With early diagnosis and early recognition, people may be maintained in better health for longer and have the benefit of support put in place for them, though sadly this often does not happen.

Practically, there is great need for information, education and support for carers, especially information, choice of services and respite care. Simple design and layout improvements can be made within houses (labelling kichen cupboards, doors and rooms, safety items and the like) so that people can live at home for longer, so community care support and help for carers are essential. However, ultimately, many people may have to move to specialized accommodation, so maintaining the quality of such care is essential. Unfortunately, almost everywhere, capacity for this form of care is inadequate and threatens to become more expensive and even less adequate in the future. Specialist care facilities are expensive, with high staffing ratios in nursing homes, to give long-term personal and medical care. In many of the more ageing countries, such as parts of Europe and Japan, expenses are already very great and it is often difficult to find suitable staff to help with dementia patients, especially those still living in the community.

Moreover, home care is becoming difficult as the pool of informal carers is shrinking in many countries, due to smaller family sizes and many traditional female carers now working outside the home. Maintaining the levels of care necessary for people with dementias is therefore a huge challenge. Many sufferers are older women, often widows with few if any relatives living with or near them, especially those able and willing to provide round-the-clock help. In the USA, the Alzheimer's Association (2012, p. 27) note that 'eighty percent of care is produced by family caregivers', and 'over 15 million Americans provide unpaid care for a person with Alzheimer's disease or other dementias.' Dementias therefore not only cause considerable disability and reduced quality of life for individuals but impact very heavily on their families and, of course, on social care systems. Moreover, dementias can be very disruptive and distressing to family life and relationships. As the condition can last several years, children, spouses and relatives grieve and often feel anger as they see their loved relations inexorably change in personality and become increasingly frail.

Research continues and a number of conventional and alternative therapies are at various stages of clinical trials. One potential, though difficult, approach is looking at individuals before neuropathy has become symptomatic dementia, the 'pre-dementia' or 'early dementia' stages (Vellas and Aisen, 2010) and initiating drug treatment early on. Moreover, given the high incidence and probable very high future prevalence of dementias worldwide, if effective new therapies or interventions were to be developed, there will inevitably be enormous ethical and practical challenges in making them widely and equitably available. Particularly, would they reach the two-thirds of people with dementia who live in low- and middle-income countries? (See Chapters 8 and 11.)

Dementia care and management may be complex and expensive but they are not hopeless. The latest *World Alzheimer Report* report focuses on the benefits of early diagnosis and intervention and offers recommendations to governments globally (Alzheimer's Disease International, 2011). This emphasizes the importance of planning for what will become a major future global challenge. We look at various other issues concerning health and social care costs and strategies for dementias in Chapter 8 and future scenarios in Chapter 11.

Discussion topics

1   Do you feel the Millennium Development Goals are reasonable targets or unachievable rhetoric?
2   'Far from being "on the retreat", infectious conditions are becoming ever more of a threat in all parts of the world.' How far do you agree?
3   Discuss the likely global social and health impacts of dementias (also refer to Chapters 8 and 11).

Part III

Global health futures

Future transitions and health planning

8 Health systems, finance and planning

An understanding of trends in global health and the sub-concept of health transition is essential to anticipating possible future health scenarios and planning challenges. These can then be based on knowledge of current patterns and the trends that have influenced them. Clearly, many health transitions are slow and long term but some, such as population ageing, chronic disease emergence and infectious disease resurgence, are having fairly obvious short-term and near-future effects, as well as long-term effects. Taken together, many trends, such as the movement towards NCDs, have enormous long-term implications and confront those involved in the planning and financing of health at all scales. An understanding of global health and transitions can assist policy-makers and providers through the quagmire of such issues as health services reform, universality of care, prioritization, privatization versus public sector, future costs and the like. Here, we introduce a number of these to highlight existing and forthcoming international changes and challenges.

Health sector reform and health sector strengthening: an ongoing dilemma?

Health sector reform does not have, or need, a single agreed definition, but it is generally considered to be a continuing, sustained process of fundamental change in policies and institutional arrangements within individual nations' health sectors. Reform could result in large-scale or relatively minor changes, but the key seems to be an aim of achieving some sort of sustainable 'improvement'. Depending on the national system, such reform would usually be guided by the gvernment, but it often also involves private sector actors and perhaps a range of external international organizations. Moreover, not all changes in health systems would automatically class as health sector reform, as they may not be specifically designed to improve the health system or, indeed, health (Berman and Bossert, 2000). Health sector reform encompasses a wide variety of features, revolving around efficient use of resources, distribution, access and broad quality. A common factor should be that any meaningful reform process would be based on evidence and information about the current state of affairs, and potential effects of alternative policy choices. However, in many health-care systems, from the most to the least sophisticated, detailed data are lacking. As a result, many participants locally and globally become involved in an industry-within-an-industry, of generating such evidence and information, and evaluation, for health policy.

Health sector reform, in various guises, has been around as a concept for two decades or more. Today, it is less commonly used as a shorthand but it lives on directly or indirectly in many approaches to achieving health sector administrative and funding improvement, quality concerns, or health sector coverage problems. The concept has evolved somewhat over time (see, e.g., Cassels, 1995; Peters *et al.*, 2009). Initially, it was applied mainly to developing country systems and was associated with a variety of related aims, such as improving governance in all sectors, avoidance of corruption and, more generally, trying to achieve greater equity or at least better use of limited resources. However, it can apply anywhere, as all health systems are undergoing more or less constant 'reform' and evolution, regardless of any nation's economic development. Today, there is increasingly an emphasis on *strengthening* health services, in terms of their quality and ability to meet needs (Peters *et al.*, 2009). A number of highly interrelated issues have been involved in, or targets of, health sector reform in various places (Cassels, 1995; Mills *et al.*, 2001):

- inefficient use, or improving efficiency of use, of scarce health resources, so the aim is to improve resource allocation and management;
- service availability and affordability;
- systemic factors, such as lack of access to health services because of socio-economic, institutional and geographic barriers; decentralization of services and decisions often sought;
- services that are unresponsive to people's needs (lack of consumer orientation);
- services that are of poor or uneven quality, including for reasons of incompetence and corruption;
- perhaps making health deliverers and systems run more like private enterprises, and attempting to make systems more responsive to, or inclusive of, consumers; and
- broadening the sources and increasing funds for health services, often to include user fees, the private sector, etc. (see below).

Health systems: aims and objectives

Agreeing and establishing the objectives of any healthcare system, and the means by which the system will deliver 'improved health' to its population, are major questions that have to be addressed to make reform in any health system practical. While general objectives are identifiable (see Box 8.1), each health system exists in its own unique historical, political, economic and social contexts. Any system will have a given level of technical and human resources which it can utilize more or less effectively. Generally, unless major new resources become available (for example, through reallocation from other sectors, from new sources of revenue or from donor aid), health sector reform or improvement generally involves *redistribution* – or rationing – hopefully to achieve more equitable use of what is available. To do this requires considerable political determination and the ability to agree reasonable prioritization, so governance and control are crucial. Achieving social policy objectives, such as tackling the issues above, usually requires data and organizational management research that often do not exist, even in the most advanced systems. In many countries, too, the health sector and healthcare professions have enormous political and economic power. Their cooperation is essential as they can stall the most determined efforts of politicians and management to implement changes.

In recent years, for numerous political and economic reasons, health sector reform has emerged as a major issue in richer economies as well as lower- and middle-income countries. The United States under President Obama, for example, faced enormous political and professional group opposition in the attempt to address several of these issues, especially the lack of coverage for the poor and for people in some areas, as well as spiralling costs of health-care which had been impacting on the whole economy. In practice, however, meaningful health sector reform has become bogged down in the USA in the face of many entrenched commercial, professional and political interests. Similarly, one of the oldest national health services, the United Kingdom's National Health Service (NHS), while in practice already addressing the five 'distributional' issues outlined above, has been in an almost constant state

BOX 8.1 The WHO and health systems

Health systems provide the interface between life-saving, life-enhancing interventions and the people who need them. If health systems are weak, these interventions will also be weak, less effective or non-existent.

> Health systems are defined as comprising all the organizations, institutions and resources that are devoted to producing health actions . . . The objective of good health itself is really twofold: the best attainable average level – *goodness* – and the smallest feasible differences among individuals and groups – *fairness*.

Their very complexity means it is difficult to identify exactly what a health system is, what it consists of, and where it begins and ends. The WHO (2000) defines a health system to include *all the activities whose primary purpose is to promote, restore or maintain health*. So:

> Formal health services, including the professional delivery of personal medical attention, are clearly within these boundaries. So are actions by traditional healers, and all use of medication, whether prescribed by a provider or not.

Goals of a health system: i. Better health (the primary goal); ii. fairness in financial contribution (sharing of risk); iii. responsiveness to expectations with regard to non-health matters, reflecting 'the importance of respecting people's dignity, autonomy and the confidentiality of information'.

(Source: WHO, 2000; extracts from pp. xi, 5, 21)

of evolutionary spin over the decades since its inception in 1948, constantly trying to address many internal, structural, training and cost-funding problems, under constant political pressure from the various administrations.

Health sector reform is frequently further quagmired by highly dubious dogma such as 'value for money' (VFM) approaches. VFM in health services naturally begs many questions, the most basic being: how do we value and put a price on people *not* having good health? How do we *cost* the effects of children whose entire lives are blighted because of avoidable childhood illnesses or lost opportunities? How do we cost the effects of miserable health in later life? How can economies prosper with unhealthy populations? Other common approaches have involved ideologies such as decentralization and disaggregation of decisions and resources to local levels, and 'governance'. Achieving any rationalization or reform often demands a commonsense approach, but this is not easily achievable when local systems (of many types) either do not exist or do not function as they should. Political and management ideologies are rife in the health sector and impact on any changes within it, with examples including private–public partnerships, cost recovery, neo-liberal approaches, 'new public management', sustainability, and many others, which have been, and continue to be, focused on the sector (Berman and Bossett, 2000; Mills *et al.*, 2001).

Any changes – reform, redirecting or strengthening – in the health sector are clearly also highly influenced, and in many ways determined, by broader developments in related public and private sectors, notably education, welfare, housing and environment, but also many others. They inevitably run alongside many other areas of real and attempted reforms, including decentralization and financial reforms in these sectors, and changes are readily encouraged or derailed by financial crises or booms. In the earlier days, health reform attempts tended to be focused on countries with extremely limited resources and they sometimes came along faster than similar processes in many richer countries. Common targets included many that we have touched on elsewhere, such as increasing emphasis on primary healthcare, priority setting in resource allocation, public accountability, monitoring and evaluation, and better accessibility to needed services (physical, economic and social).

We can ask why health sector reform (generally defined) has been relatively unsuccessful despite huge efforts, yet why it is so crucial in tomorrow's global health. Health services, for most countries, are either already or are becoming the major sources of national expenditure. This is especially true when health expenditure is expanded to encompass related services, such as welfare, social and long-term care, and education (both for health personnel and more broadly as part of modern public health and national development). Especially in times of economic crisis (and when has there *not* been economic crisis in the past few decades?), health expenditure comes under constant political scrutiny. However, even in manifestly inefficient systems, root and branch changes have generally been impossible to effect, so minor budget shifting (for example, causing the public to pay for insurance cover, or to pay co-charges for medicines) are all that can be achieved.

Reform or changes in health services operate at different levels: the political, the conceptual and the practical. Instead of reforming entire systems, many of the more achievable efforts tend to focus on specific targets – often development goals that may be related to the MDGs: childhood vaccinations, reproductive health services and campaigns against specific infectious diseases. Parties involved include the major international organizations, such as the World Bank and the WHO, individual country donor organizations, such as USAID, NGOs and charitable organizations and, of course, national and local health and welfare authorities and numerous other 'stakeholders'. Health sector reform increasingly also takes place in post-conflict situations, so huge, urgent decisions are needed on which reforms to focus on and the potential effects of such policies. Indeed, as a study in Kosovo (Percival and Sondorp, 2010) illustrates, post-conflict health reform is relatively under-researched. It lacks established frameworks for examining how health interventions interact with the post-conflict social, political and economic environment, and health and welfare services are clearly major components of successful restoration of peace and well-being.

Where are we now in terms of health financing?

Closely interrelated with any consideration of healthcare delivery and health sector reform are the sources and application of funds and resources for health. This is hugely complex and often controversial. A 2005 World Health Assembly resolution states (optimistically) that everyone should be able to access health services and not be subject to financial hardship when doing so. Globally, we are still very far from achieving this, often to extreme extents. For example, in service coverage, in some countries, as discussed later, as few as 10 per cent of births may be attended by a skilled health worker, whereas this is almost 100 per cent for countries with the lowest maternal mortality. Within countries, great variations in resourcing often exist, even within rich countries, though these discrepancies are almost always smaller than in poorer countries. Social and gender gaps are commonplace. For example, in many poor countries, wealthy women generally obtain similar good levels of health coverage and often as good as those in rich economies, whereas poor women miss out. Women in the richest 20 per cent of the population are up to twenty times more likely than poor women to have a birth attended by a skilled health worker. Internationally, the WHO talks of 'closing the gap' between rich countries and some fifty poor countries which, in this example, would potentially save more than 700,000 women between 2010 and 2015. Similarly, rich children live longer than poor children, and closing the gap for a range of services for children under the age of 5 could save more than 16 million lives (WHO, 2010a).

However, resources as well as organization are needed. Money can be the main factor (though not invariably), so healthcare funding is crucial. However, there have always been many other social, physical and systemic variables affecting access to and use of health services (Joseph and Phillips, 1984). Costs are nevertheless one major barrier to use of services and many people simply cannot afford healthcare. Even if care is cheap, many cannot afford to access it and, when ill, they may lose any meagre income they have. Ill-health and the system can therefore inadvertently push many into poverty, whereupon they have to rely on relatives or charity or otherwise obtain no healthcare or other welfare services. Formal financial transfers to protect those too ill to work are familiar in some richer countries, usually welfare state-based, but their availability is far from universal. Indeed, it is estimated that only one in five people in the world has broad-based social security protection that also includes cover for lost wages in the event of illness. The ILO estimates that more than half of the world's population lacks any formal social protection. There are the expected regional variations, for example, only 5 to 10 per cent of people are covered in sub-Saharan Africa and South Asia, while in middle-income countries coverage rates range from 20 to 60 per cent.

Countries achieving the closest to universal coverage generally have more to spend on health. For example, OECD countries, including only 18 per cent of the world's population, spend 86 per cent of the world's expenditure on health, and almost all of them spend at least 2,900 dollars per person annually. However, some lower- and middle-income countries have achieved reasonable broad-based coverage, a good example being Thailand. It has considerably improved service coverage and protection against the financial risks of ill-health despite spending much less on health than higher-income countries. It has done this by changing the way it raises funds for health and moving away from direct payments, such as user fees (WHO, 2010a). Many countries still rely heavily on direct payments from individuals to health service providers and these, with associated costs, can be major disincentives to using health services. The nature, sources and security of health financing are thus crucial. The WHO encourages countries to develop a comprehensive 'social protection floor' for income replacement and social support in the event of illness.

The *personal* costs of healthcare can be direct or indirect. Direct payment may be obvious: paying *directly* for the costs of a consultation, medicines or treatment at the time received (see Box 8.2). Costs can also be indirect, less obvious, through payments for insurance schemes (even if provided, say, by an employer, forming a part of someone's remuneration) or as co-payments shared between the person receiving care and an insurance or reimbursement scheme (public or private). Payments for *public* health are yet broader, as they are usually intended for community benefit, such as health promotion, public sanitation or broad-based immunization programmes, or developing networks of clinics feeding more specialized hospitals. Within any health system, as the WHO (2010a) suggests, basic questions can be raised about the nature of funding (see Box 8.3).

Distribution of resources in healthcare planning, reform and strengthening

Improvement of healthcare planning is arguably the 'fundamental step' in any reform or strengthening. At a basic level, planning can be about arranging the distribution of resources, personnel and facilities to cover a given population. However, this is complicated by many factors, notably the underlying nature of the healthcare system in any place: is it

BOX 8.2 What are direct payments?

Healthcare services often levy charges or fees for consultations, medical or investigative procedures, medicines and other supplies, and for laboratory tests. They may be total costs or partial costs. Many people have to pay these 'out of pocket'.

These costs may be charged by government, NGOs, faith-based and private health facilities. Some are officially approved charges but many can be unofficial and in the nature of 'supplements' or bribes (e.g. in China). Even when covered by insurance, patients usually share such costs, via co-insurance, co-payments and/or deductibles (excess or uncovered costs, paid by the patient at the time they use services). One issue is that such payments may cause people to use health services only when they are ill, and not for health promotion or preventive care. Direct payments at the time when care is needed can be a barrier to universal coverage and may hinder millions from seeking care.

The WHO uses *direct payments* and *out-of-pocket payments* interchangeably.

(Source: After WHO, 2010a, p. 5)

BOX 8.3 The WHO: key components of a situation analysis for health financing

Financial risk protection

- What funds are available, from what sources?
- What spending priority does government give to health?
- How much do people have to pay out of pocket for health services (direct payments)?
- What financial risk protection is available for financial catastrophe and impoverishment?
- Who pays what in other contributions to the health system (perceived fairness)?
- Who is covered from pooled funds, for what services and for what proportion of costs?

Access to needed services

- How to measure financial access to services directly? Can be difficult, so analysis generally focuses on coverage for key interventions and may assess reasons for apparent low coverage, especially for vulnerable groups.
- Considers how changes to the financing system could improve access.

Efficiency

- Identify main efficiency problems in the system, their consequences and their causes.

Health system characteristics and capacities

- Description and quantification of fundraising and pooling, and use of funds.

- Need to understand how funds are used in the system, from source to use (internal and external funds); look for policy fragmentation and misalignment.
- Governance arrangements also must be scrutinized.
- Availability, distribution and patterns of use of all health facilities, personnel and key inputs (medicines and technologies) must be analysed.

Factors outside the health system

- Demographic variables (population growth rates, age structure, geographical distribution, migration, labour force, etc.).
- Main disease problems and their likely changes (implications for costs of extending future coverage).
- Existing social safety nets for long-term illness, and financial barriers to accessing services.
- Public sector administration, legal framework, and scope for changes within existing rules and laws, such as: how are health workers paid? What are the rules? Decision-making on financial resources allocated across levels? (Centralization–decentralization issues.)
- How are public sector budgets drawn up and how far can state bodies (such as public hospitals) redistribute funds?

(Source: Based on WHO, 2010a, p. 93)

public, private or some mixture? Then, does it provide free universal access, or is care rationed by some means (pricing and/or 'gatekeepers')? What is the geographical distribution of healthcare resources and are they located appropriately for demand? However, almost immediately, healthcare planning tends to focus on systems and costs. It is difficult to generalize thereafter, as costs vary enormously internationally, even between systems that appear philosophically similar, and between countries of similar levels of income. Moreover, healthcare costs can be almost infinite and they are very subject to inflation (see Chapter 11). Increasingly, in an attempt to generate new funds, it is being asked whether funds from certain sources should be earmarked ('hypothecated') for health. Health ministries often desire earmarked funds, while national treasuries often resist hypothecation as it affects their ability to adjust funding between sectors. Moreover, even hypothecated funds for any given purpose (for example, tobacco taxes earmarked for healthcare) are rarely stable or guaranteed (WHO, 2010a).

Can health services obtain greater 'value for money'?

The costs of healthcare are increasing for almost everyone on the planet. Costs come in many forms, not just the direct and indirect costs discussed above, and paying for costs impacts individuals, communities and whole economies. For example, having a poor health system and an unhealthy population will affect the whole economy and society, and the future of all citizens. Huge amounts are spent on health, in relative and absolute terms, and much effort is devoted to attempting to achieve the best from it (or at least to deter waste and diversion of funds). The WHO's *World Health Report* for 2010 focused on health systems' financing and identified many areas for potential improvements and for research on inefficient expenditure. For instance, estimates suggest that between a third and more than half of the $2 trillion-plus that the USA spends annually on health is wasted. The European

Health Care Fraud and Corruption Network calculated that, of the global annual health expenditure of about $5.3 trillion, some 6 per cent (about $300 billion) is lost because of mistakes or corruption alone. Losses may be greater in some places than others, but nowhere appears immune.

Given their scale, the majority of health systems do not make the best use of their resources and many seem to provide very poor value, given the amounts provided to them. This happens for numerous, often intercorrelated, reasons: procedural, misallocation, mismanagement and pure irrationality. The WHO report says bluntly, 'there is nothing inevitable about this and there are many shades of inefficiency' (WHO, 2010a, p. 61). The WHO has identified the 'top ten' reasons for financial inefficiencies globally, many of which can be avoided or at least mitigated (see Box 8.4). It also notes that many countries obtain better coverage and health outcomes for their expenditure than others and that there can be a huge gap between what many countries achieve and what they could potentially achieve with the same resources. Raising funds for basic care is often crucial for the poorest countries but, everywhere, getting the most out of what is available is also paramount. Almost all high-income countries are facing enormous pressures to rein in health and other cost increases and, increasingly, to cut overall expenditures. Everywhere, too, there are many opportunities for efficiency gains, which does not simply mean cutting costs but implies improving outputs or quality. For example, health outcomes or services may be improved for a given input (cost), providing an efficiency gain, which can then help to contain subsequent costs.

Cost containment pressures are almost universal but so, too, opportunities to do more with the same resources exist almost everywhere. Given that (conservatively) 20–40 per cent of resources spent on health are wasted or very ineffectively used, there should be ample scope to improve what is done with any given expenditure. Inefficient health spending is often exemplified in the use of expensive medicines when cheaper, effective options are available. Another example is misuse and overprescribing of antibiotics and other drugs, contributing to antibiotic resistance and subsequent need for more expensive medicines (discussed in Chapters 7 and 11). Many systems undertake excessive and often unnecessary procedures and tests. Admittedly, health systems are generally huge and complex, so carelessness, poor practices, poor price negotiations, various forms of pilfering and poor storage can thrive and all lead to wastage. It is suggested that just controlling unnecessary expenditure on

---

BOX 8.4   The WHO's ten leading causes of financial inefficiency in health services

1   Medicines: underuse of generics and higher than necessary prices for medicines.
2   Medicines: use of substandard and counterfeit medicines.
3   Medicines: inappropriate and ineffective use.
4   Healthcare products and services: overuse or supply of equipment, investigations and procedures.
5   Health workers: inappropriate or costly staff mix, unmotivated workers.
6   Healthcare services: inappropriate hospital admissions and length of stay.
7   Healthcare services: inappropriate hospital size (low use of infrastructure).
8   Healthcare services: medical errors and poor quality of care.
9   Health system leakages: waste, corruption and fraud.
10   Health interventions: inefficient mix/inappropriate level of strategies.

(Source: WHO, 2010a, Table 4.1, p. 63)

medicines, with more appropriate use and quality control, could save many countries up to 5 per cent of their health expenditure. Indeed, the WHO (2010a) notes that medicines account for three of the most common causes of inefficiency identified (see Box 8.4). Suggested solutions for inefficiencies include:

- getting the most from available technologies and health services;
- motivating health workers to perform better;
- improving hospital efficiency;
- getting initial care right by reducing medical errors;
- elimination of waste and corruption; and
- critical assessment of what services are needed.

All systems of payments to healthcare providers have strengths and weaknesses, but fee-for-service payments can be particularly problematic (WHO, 2010a). Fees can encourage health providers to 'overprovide' services to those who can pay or are covered from various funds, but to underserve those who cannot pay. Increasingly, too, there is little evidence that private sector health facilities are more or less efficient than government facilities, and this depends very much on the context. Private sector systems may be better at delivering some specific types of service, especially one-off services, whereas it often falls to public services to provide unglamorous and ongoing long-term care, especially for the poor or for chronic conditions, and services requiring widespread education, environmental and infrastructural actions. Whatever the health system, improving governance is almost universally hailed as one key to improving efficiency and equity, but many also argue for the reduction of 'red tape' and bureaucracy. In particular, where countries are in receipt of health sector assistance, donors can make their contributions more efficient and effective. They can help countries to develop domestic financing institutions, reduce the fragmented delivery of many donor funds, rigorously monitor their use and try to reduce duplication of aid at the global level (WHO, 2010a). Various ways of reducing financial barriers to better care and use of resources are given in Box 8.5.

BOX 8.5 The WHO: core ideas for reducing financial barriers

Key question: how might existing health financing systems be adjusted to take advantage of strength in numbers and/or protect gains achieved? Core considerations are suggested for policy-makers seeking to increase their populations' financial protection while reducing barriers to use of services.

- *Pooling pays:* Move towards universal coverage by introducing forms of prepayment and pooling (take advantage of the strength in numbers).
- *Consolidate or compensate:* Cover can be improved by consolidating fragmented pools, or helping transfer of funds between them.
- *Combine tax and social health insurance:* Taxes and insurance contributions can be combined to cover the population as a whole, rather than being kept separate.
- *Compulsory contribution helps:* Universal coverage appears best achieved by some form of compulsory contribution arrangement, from general government revenues or mandatory insurance contributions. Pooled funds can cover people, found everywhere, who cannot pay.

continued

- *Voluntary schemes are a useful first step:* If the economy or financial circumstances enable only low tax collection or compulsory insurance contributions, voluntary schemes can provide some protection against the financial risks of ill-health, though their potential seems limited.
- *Drop direct payment.*

(Source: Based on WHO, 2010a, p. 53)

International assistance, financial crisis and the health sector

This is a very significant topic in the context of global health, but it is complex and evolving. International health assistance – for general and specific health purposes – may be long term, short term, regular or unsteady, and subject to the aims, scrutiny and varying generosity of donors, and it may be affected by factors such as political alliances. Official development assistance (ODA) comes from official sectors, with other sources of health aid including charities, private foundations and NGOs. Some operate country-to-country, other forms come as part of wider multi-nation packages; some ODA goes to multilateral health organizations such as the WHO, the UNFPA and the GAVI, and to cross-sectoral organizations with partial interests in health (e.g. UNICEF, UNDP, the World Bank). Some sources of assistance are more or less continuous, while other assistance is given in response to specific appeals or following events such as natural disasters or disease outbreaks (see Chapters 9 and 10). Whatever the source, we should note that there is a considerable potential for aid being squeezed when donor sources come under domestic pressure due to financial exigencies. Unfavourable economic conditions 'at home' have the potential to be a brake on donations when there is some growing global recognition that external financial support for health needs to rise, though this is not a universal view. Bilateral development assistance in general tends to reflect economic conditions in the donor countries. However, for the health sector in particular, this is not always the case and many donor sources do their best to protect and maintain health-related assistance even when faced with domestic economic crises.

The OECD tracks aid to health in statistics and charts (OECD, 2009, 2011a). It notes that prioritization of aid to health actually increased to 18 per cent of total DAC countries' bilateral sector-allocable aid dedicated to health in 2006–07, compared with 12 per cent in 2001–02. Donors providing the highest proportions of their aid to the health sector were Ireland and the United Kingdom (40 per cent each), Luxembourg (36 per cent), the USA (28 per cent) and Canada (25 per cent). However, in the subsequent downturn, some donors pledged to maintain their commitments but other large donors felt obliged to reduce or postpone their contributions (WHO, 2010a).

Whether the general maintenance of health aid will continue is not clear. The WHO (2010a) feels the effects of economic downturn (especially after 2008) on development assistance are unclear. However, many potential bilateral donor countries in the richer groups (such as Greece, Ireland, Portugal and others in the EU) were around 2010–12 being beset by exceptional financial challenges and budgetary debt crises, meaning future assistance is uncertain. It can be politically difficult for some Western governments in particular to maintain international health aid while drastically cutting their own health, welfare and social security services, especially pensions, whilst often raising taxes.

International assistance – aid – is by no means ideologically neutral or free from criticism. Moyo (2009) provides an insightful critique of aid, the corruption, disease, poverty and dependency it has engendered, and its discouragement of free enterprise. She offers practical alternative modes of financing development (with respect to Africa in particular). Health sector assistance may be less criticized than many trade and military aid agreements yet, as in other sectors, there are many problems and it is always possible that health aid will be subject to the whims of fashion. For example, it may be focused on popular or high-profile health initiatives or 'high-profile' diseases, while other more basic, ongoing, essential requirements are neglected (see, for example, Table 8.1). Given the criticism that aid leads to dependency and undermines the fostering of local talent, some technical assistance has often focused on in-country capacity building, skills training and facility improvement.

A related criticism of assistance is that it can reinforce longstanding unequal power relationships with poorer countries, the infamous North–South divide: the rich are the helpers, the poor are the helpless. It is clear that twenty-first-century development assistance must be alert to these and perform better. However, it seems equally clear that many countries have not been moving towards supporting themselves or even devoting serious proportions of their own resources to health. In the Abuja Declaration of April 2001, subsequent to the adoption of the MDGs in 2000, heads of African Union countries pledged to set a target of allocating at least 15 per cent of their annual budgets to improving the health sector. They also urged donor nations to meet the target of 0.7 per cent of GNP as official development assistance. A WHO (2011g) review found that, over the decade since 2001, twenty-six countries had increased the proportion of total government expenditures allocated to health but only one, Tanzania, had achieved Abuja's 15 per cent target. Eleven countries had *reduced* their relative contributions of government expenditures to health and there was no obvious trend in the other nine. The median level of real per capita government spending from domestic resources on health had increased slightly from $9.4 to $13.4, although the lowest remained very low ($0.47); thirty-three governments spent less than $33 per capita on health. As we note elsewhere, most African Union countries are not on track to achieve the health MDGs, and the WHO states part of the explanation lies in the lack of financial resources (international and domestic) that are available. The failure of almost all states to meet their Abuja Declaration domestic funding pledge is often seen by commentators as symbolic of lack of commitment and a reliance on aid. Moreover, the lack of domestic funding for health – even for cheap vaccines, as some countries rely on the GAVI to provide them – is serious in terms of sustainability or continuation of health improvements, if ODA declines because of ongoing international financial problems. Moreover, many feel that aid recipient countries must try to avoid continuing aid dependency and be prepared for the time aid finally falls away.

In terms of aid to health sub-sectors, it is probably inevitable that high prevalence and serious conditions, or major disasters, will attract the greatest amounts from donor sources, so this factor will surely affect how much aid is raised and the conditions or purposes to which it is allocated (see, for example, Table 8.1). Allocations can change over time, so aid to health sub-sectors between 2000 and 2006 changed in favour of reproductive health, especially HIV/AIDS control (a growing priority in many donor programmes), while aid to tuberculosis, malaria and other infectious disease control increased modestly (OECD, 2009). The WHO (2010a) notes that, between 2002 and 2006, MDG 6 (HIV/AIDS, malaria, other diseases, tuberculosis; see Box 7.2) accounted for 46.8 per cent of total external assistance for health. However, consequently, little was left for the other goals, such as MDGs 1, 4 and 5 (nutrition, child mortality reduction, and maternal health), or for other areas, such as NCDs and strengthening health systems. Indeed, more funds were needed for strengthening health systems alone. The distributional picture is somewhat brighter, however, if we consider efforts by some initiatives, such as the GAVI Alliance (especially its successes in fundraising in 2011) and some other fundraising by global health alliances on AIDS, tuberculosis and malaria to support health systems development and capacity building.

Table 8.1 Bilateral aid to health, commitments by sub-sectors, 2007

Health sub-sector	Percentage commitments
HIV/AIDS control	39
TB, malaria, other infectious disease control	18
Other basic health	16
Health, general	14
Other reproductive health	13

Source: Based on data in OECD, 2009

Nevertheless, considerable concerns remain that 'Cinderella' conditions and diseases which do not make headlines can be neglected by donors, especially support for less visible areas such as management, logistics, procurement, infrastructure and workforce development, the essential if unglamorous areas which keep health services working (WHO, 2010a). There are also very important questions as to whether donor funds for health should be additional to or replace domestic spending, then allowing this to be redirected to other sectors (perhaps to allied areas, such as education). Taking a broad view of development, it can be sensible for a country to substitute donor funds to allow them to divert their own resources to other priorities, but health sector specialists tend to feel health funds should stay within the health sector.

Costs and health conditions: some examples

Innovative policies to improve global health?

In every health system, as we have seen, there are inefficient uses of funds and physical and human resources more generally. But, likewise, everywhere there are 'high-cost' conditions and priorities, which it makes financial and epidemiological sense to target. Many places attempt to target direct and indirect causes of either ill-health or behaviour linked to ill-health, such as consumption of alcohol, tobacco and illegal drugs. Such public health initiatives are often linked with education or general advertisements and aim to improve health and reduce costs by making people less likely to use health services, thus reducing demand. Direct examples include tobacco-control legislation (see Box 8.6) in an attempt to reduce a huge range of possible illnesses; and, on the roads, seat-belt and drink-driving legislation and campaigns. 'Indirect approaches' tend to adopt more subtle behaviour-modification strategies, though their effects tend to take much longer and can be very difficult to evaluate directly: for example, can we pay people to stay healthy (see Box 8.7)? Similarly, campaigns to promote healthy eating, exercise or avoidance of various forms of risk taking may take years or decades to show effects. Some campaigns may be aimed at the general public, while others target specific 'risk groups', such as teenage girls in pregnancy-avoidance schemes, drug users, or workers in specific occupations.

Targeting the financial and human consequences and costs of some conditions

Avoidable mortality

For decades, since Thomas McKeown and before, healthcare planners have been asking whether healthcare saves lives. Many causes of death are unavoidable and, of course, everyone dies from something. Many increasingly feel a focus should be on how well services

BOX 8.6 Can smoking bans improve public health?

Yes, it seems so: bans on smoking in public places appear effective but impacts may vary according to location of smoking and types of health conditions. Bans in the United States, Canada, Ireland and elsewhere have shown impressive effects in reducing acute myocardial infarctions (AMI) in particular. This is attributed to a near elimination of rapid, harmful effects of second-hand smoke on blood platelets and arteries supplying blood to the heart. Canadian research has also found reductions in respiratory conditions (bans effective in restaurant settings).

Short-term impact of smoke-free legislation in England

Research in England (2010) showed a small but significant reduction in emergency admissions for myocardial infarction after implementation of legislation banning smoking in public places (July 2007). Retrospective analysis of hospital admissions suggested 1,200 fewer admissions (1,600 including readmissions) in the first year. The main benefit may be from avoidance of passive smoking, a recognized risk for coronary heart disease, heart attack and stroke.

In England, research suggests that smoking bans reduce passive smoking, especially for people working in the hospitality trade, restaurants and pubs. Bans may cut the numbers of people having heart attacks. However, many studies suggest it is less clear whether fewer people smoke as a result of smoking bans.

(Sources: Sargent *et al.*, 2004; Naiman *et al.*, 2010; Sims *et al.*, 2010)

BOX 8.7 Can we pay people to stay healthy?

Financial incentives (in forms such as cash or food and/or shopping vouchers) have been tried in several countries to encourage people to behave more healthily. The concept involves behavioural modifications via rewards, social protection and investment in human capital.

A well-known initiative is the Progresa-Oportunidades scheme in Mexico, a government social assistance programme founded in 2002 and based on an earlier (1997) programme.

- The scheme targets poverty by providing cash payments to families on condition of regular school attendance, health clinic visits and nutritional support.
- It links income transfers with interventions in health, education, nutrition and attempts to tackle intergenerational poverty transmission mechanisms.
- It is credited with decreasing poverty and improving health and educational attainment in regions where it has been deployed.
- As of 2006, around one-quarter of Mexico's population participated in the scheme.
- Programme requirements target measures considered likely to lift families out of poverty, focusing on health, nutrition and children's education.

continued

- Oportunidades has become a model for programmes instituted elsewhere, including New York City, Nicaragua, Brazil, Honduras, Jamaica, Chile, Malawi and Zambia.
- However, in some countries, such as Bangladesh, food vouchers in such programmes did not work very well, so there appear to be situational and socio-economic conditions.

(Sources: Levy, 2006; Niño-Zarazú, 2010)

perform with respect to things that can be avoided, so the concept of avoidable – or 'amenable' – mortality has emerged. This involves deaths that should not occur given effective and timely healthcare, and it is interesting to consider this issue alongside the discussion in Chapter 5 on the difference between health inequities and health inequalities (see Box 5.1). Much initial research on avoidable mortality was undertaken in the 1980 and 1990s and, even in the few years since, many advances in healthcare have been made that may have affected the outcomes. Nolte and McKee (2004) have pointed out that 'avoidable' mortality was never intended as more than an indicator of potential weaknesses in health-care, which could then be investigated more specifically. It is almost certainly a useful indicator of how things are going. Looking at deaths in the European Union, they found that causes of death amenable to prevention by timely and effective healthcare were relatively common in many countries in 1980. Reductions in these more common causes, especially via declining infant mortality, boosted the increases in life expectancy between birth and age 75 during the 1980s. In addition, in some countries, such as Denmark, the Netherlands, the United Kingdom, France (among males) and Sweden (among women), reductions in deaths among middle-aged people were very important. By contrast, in the 1990s, reductions in amenable mortality contributed less to life expectancy increases, especially in the Northern European countries, though they remained important in Southern Europe, where initial death rates were higher. These authors feel such data illustrate that improvements in access to effective healthcare did have demonstrable impacts in many countries, especially in the 1980s and 1990s, mainly through lower death rates among infants, middle-aged and older people.

However, the use of avoidable/amenable mortality as a 'performance' indicator may be time-limited since many health improvements are time-specific and reflect starting conditions. Moreover, these days, differentials may be too small to show much variation. For example, Nolte and McKee (2004) argue that, where infant mortality was relatively high in Europe, such as Greece and Portugal, there was the greatest potential for improvement, and the greatest reductions in amenable infant mortality were therefore noted. By contrast, in countries like Sweden, infant mortality was already so low by the 1990s that there was little room for improvement. Likewise, there was much greater potential for improvement in amenable adult deaths where the rates were initially the highest. As rates fall – converging, in similar countries – so variation concomitantly decreases. Therefore, Nolte and McKee feel that, this century, in more developed countries in particular, we may not learn much by comparing health system performance using aggregate mortality data, purely because differences and outcomes will be small. They feel that amenable mortality rates may remain useful as a tool to indicate potential problems for further examination and to study inequalities in access to care or outcomes *within* populations, when suitable data are available (see, for example, Chau *et al.*, 2011). This may be useful in systems where inequalities are widening, or in poorer countries which, as noted, often have substantial socio-economic differentials in many indicators, including access to healthcare, health status and health outcomes.

Accidents, especially road accidents and injuries

In Chapter 7, we noted substantial global differences in the incidence, causes and consequences of accidents. Accidents and injury place huge burdens, though internationally variable, on almost all health systems and communities, on many families and, of course, on the injured individuals through direct costs and also DALYs lost. Cost reduction and lessening of burdens on health systems provide one impetus for the focus on accidents and injuries; improved development, human rights and increasing expectations form another. We noted earlier that some groups, such as older people, have a higher risk of injury from falls and relatively minor accidents. Another major focus is workplace and industrial accidents which, especially in some heavy and primary industries, have increasingly been under scrutiny because of productivity losses and economic impacts. In richer countries, legislation has for decades (and even centuries) attempted to improve industrial and occupational safety. Globalization spreads some elements of this, for example by locating the factories and production units of multinational corporations in newly industrializing locations (even if compliance may sometimes be lower).

Other major sources of injury and stress are workplace violence, disruption and aggression, increasingly recognized as causes of physical and psychological ill-health and as direct costs to the health sector. Industrial accidents can impact on wider communities and environments. We only have to think of the problems caused by nuclear accidents due to poor design or practices (as at Chernobyl in 1986) or natural disasters (as at Fukushima in 2011) (see IAEA, 2011). In central India, many families and the wider community are still feeling the health impacts of the Bhopal industrial disaster of 1984 (see Box 8.8).

In recognition of the crucial importance of just one area – traffic and transport – 2011–20 has been designated the Decade of Action for Road Safety (see Figure 8.1). The global plan seeks to save millions of lives by a multi-target strategy: improving the safety of roads and vehicles; enhancing the behaviour of road users; and improving post-crash response by emergency services, health and rehabilitative systems.

BOX 8.8 Bhopal – a major environmental health tragedy

In 1984, one of the world's largest industrial accidents to date occurred. A gas chemical leak at the Union Carbide India pesticide plant in Bhopal, central India, killed 2,259 immediately, as many as 3,000 within weeks, and 8,000 subsequently. A government affidavit in 2006 stated the leak caused over 500,000 injuries, including over 38,000 temporary partial injuries and about 3,900 severely and permanently disabling injuries.

This tragedy illustrates many issues: the wider community risk of some industrial undertakings located near to mass slum dwellings, maintenance and safety issues, plus the length and difficulty of getting legal redress for environmental health and of obtaining data for accidents, especially in some countries.

In 2010, seven local executives were fined and sentenced to two years' imprisonment. Directors could not be held to account as they fled and escaped extradition, which is still sought.

(Sources: Phillips, 1990; BBC, 2010)

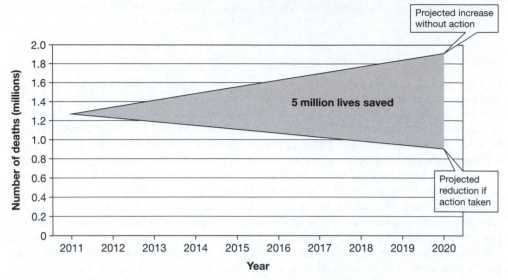

Figure 8.1 Decade of Action for Road Safety, 2011–20: saving millions of lives

Source: WHO, 2011b, p.5

The avoidance of road accidents and injuries has become a major aim in many countries and many studies and data on accidents focus on this area. In Chapter 7, we noted that these accidents kill as many as 1.3 million people each year and injure 20–50 million more, many of them young and vulnerable road users. It is predicted that, without action, road traffic crashes will result in the deaths of around 1.9 million people annually by 2020. In addition to the sorrow and pain they cause, road traffic crashes result in considerable economic losses to victims, families and national economies, costing many countries between 1 and 3 per cent of their gross national product. Action is desperately needed, as only 15 per cent of countries have comprehensive laws relating to five key risk areas: speeding; drinking and driving; and non-use of helmets, seat-belts and child restraints (WHO, 2011b).

Thailand provides an example. Research from 2005–07 estimated that road accidents cost a cumulative 232.8 billion baht (about $7.2 billion) in financial terms in 2007. This was about 2.8 per cent of the country's GDP, or some 60 per cent more than the amount the Thai government spent that year on health service delivery (World Bank, 2007). Clearly, this illustrates the advantages to the nation of accident reduction, meaning the combined strategy outlined is crucial.

Changing sources of future healthcare demands: costs and planning implications

As healthcare needs from many conditions increase globally (especially needs arising from NCDs, ageing and rehabilitation), there is an ever-greater blurring of the boundaries between health and social care. This makes the demarcation of budgets into, say, those for health, welfare and social care ever more difficult and even unrealistic. This particularly affects budgets involving long-term care, which often have substantial 'social' as well as medical components. Nevertheless, many administrations like to have clearly defined budgetary areas – health, pensions, education, housing, etc. – even if this sort of boundary demarcation is becoming less useful and, perhaps, less meaningful. For example, if older people need some personal support to enable them to live alone or in their community because of failing physical or mental faculties, how could they manage if their pensions were calculated purely in terms of 'basic needs' with no element for care? 'No-care' financial support might mean they might have to leave their own homes and move into more expensive residential care.

Another example is that, almost everywhere, it now has to be recognized that cost shifting by moving patients from, say, the hospital sector to primary care and then on to a welfare budget is purely that: cost shifting. It is perhaps a less critical issue within fully state-funded welfare systems (a limited, decreasing number, to be sure). However, in mixed systems, private funding of, say, healthcare may pay for immediate curative care and perhaps for short-term rehabilitation but rarely will privately funded or private insurance-based systems pay for extensive long-term care for people after catastrophic illness or during old age. Today, de-institutionalization, care in the community and 'normalization' are trends that are too big to stem, even if this were desirable. However, they do necessitate a total rethink of the financial boundaries for the funding of health and welfare. Globally, to succeed, these trends require more intersectoral collaboration than ever before in both funding and caring systems – the famous but rarely achieved 'seamless care'.

Costs of long-term care and therapies

Many conditions requiring long-term or expensive therapies, and the ever-longer survival of people with formerly life-threatening conditions, are major contributors to rising costs of healthcare. A particular characteristic of healthcare in general, and of many types of pharmaceuticals in particular, is that their costs tend to increase well ahead of the retail price index inflation in most countries. So, for example, annual healthcare inflation maybe in double digits while general inflation is less than 5 per cent. The global reach and demands for various forms of healthcare technology (both diagnostic and treatment) and for pharmaceuticals often lead to excessive rises in healthcare costs. This seems to happen even in countries that have developed indigenous pharmaceutical research and manufacturing capacity. Some conditions, such as those requiring intensive care and high levels of specialism, can be high cost because of their high-tech nature. Other, 'cheaper', conditions can cost a great deal *cumulatively* because of the large numbers of people affected. Of the latter, while older populations *per se* may not automatically be more expensive in terms of health, some aspects of long-term care for conditions principally affecting older people, such as dementias, can be costly because of the incremental costs involved in caring for growing numbers of people with a deteriorating condition. Below, as examples of increasing costs for long-term care and support, we consider dementias, for which there is currently no effective treatment, and disabilities more generally.

Dementias

Estimates of the total costs of dementias put them in the league of some national economies (see Table 8.2 and Figure 8.2) and generating greater costs than the revenues of major companies, such as Exxon and Wal-Mart.

If the overall costs are broken down into social, medical and informal (arising from losses in people's ability to perform ADLs), dementias may soon cost the higher-income countries in the Asia–Pacific, North America and Western Europe as much as 1.3 per cent of their annual GDP. In poorer countries, mainly because of the lack of care and lower social and medical costs, and smaller *current* numbers of people afflicted, costs may range from under 0.1 per cent to 0.4 per cent of GDP (Alzheimer's Disease International, 2010). Already, payments for care for people with dementias are estimated to cost the USA $200 billion in

Table 8.2 Annual costs per person with dementia

Project	Costs per person with dementia (US$ – all inflated to 2010)
USA	60,090
Sweden	49,413
Australia	34,552
EuroCoDe for EU27	31,939
Canada	30,812
UK	30,805
EuroCoDe for the whole of Europe	25,222
DWCD for Europe	24,850
Hungary	24,544
European Brain Council	16,585
Argentina	4,012
Turkey	3,393
China	2,641

Source: Alzheimer's Disease International, 2010, Table 22, p. 42

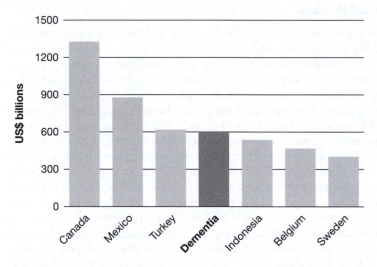

Figure 8.2 Costs of dementia compared to national economies, c. 2010

Source: Alzheimer's Disease International, 2010, Fig. 4, p. 38

2012 (Alzheimer's Association 2012). Looking to the future, in the USA alone, the overall costs of Alzheimer's disease to insurers, families and government will probably reach over a trillion dollars in current values by 2050 (see Figure 8.3). Unfortunately, in the poorer countries, these costs are also projected to burgeon over the next four decades, because of the growth in older populations and dementia cases worldwide, as we discuss further in Chapter 11. However, specialized care resources will be more limited in the majority of these countries.

Costs of disability

We have highlighted the global and local importance of disability as a health and welfare issue in many places throughout this book. Above, we considered the cost implications of

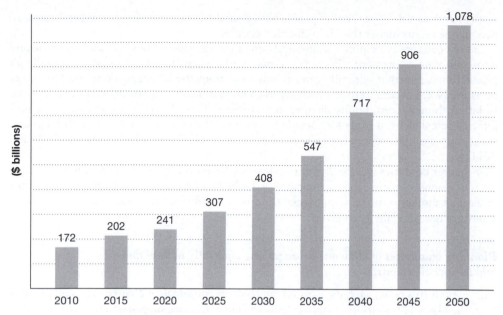

Figure 8.3 Projected costs of Alzheimer's disease for the USA, 2010–50 (in current dollar values)
Source: Alzheimer's Association, 2011, p.11

just one component (dementias, which principally affect older people). Looking more widely, as many as 15 per cent of the world's population have some sort of disability. This clearly has enormous planning and cost implications for health and welfare services, as well as for individuals and family long-term support. The costs of disability are definitely significant, but they are very difficult to calculate accurately, or compare, because of international data deficiencies, variable diagnoses, and the different sources, levels and costs of care and support in different countries.

The WHO (2011c) notes that disability can be thought of as having direct and indirect costs. *Direct costs* include the extra costs of living with disability and the costs of public spending on disability, both of which vary greatly. There is little agreement over how to measure the extra costs of living with disability, as these vary enormously by country and nature of individual circumstances. Research has found that there are indeed extra costs, ranging from around 10 per cent to over 50 per cent of income, to pay for such things as healthcare, personal care, food, mobility and specialized accommodation. Some may be purely private, out-of-pocket costs; others can be paid fully or partly by insurance or welfare systems. In many wealthier economies, costs tend to be supported by a mixture of personal and public (or shared) funds. In many poorer countries, by contrast, families and individuals have to meet almost all personal direct costs themselves. Similarly, there are wide ranges in international resourcing of public programmes for disability. For OECD countries, this can be 2 per cent of GDP (if sickness benefits are included) or higher in certain countries, and it is even greater than expenditure on unemployment in most of these countries. Indeed, disability benefit can cover 6–10 per cent of OECD populations, similar to the numbers covered by unemployment benefit (WHO, 2011c). Based on *World Health Survey* findings, the WHO (2011c, p. 67) also notes that 'disabled respondents in thirty-one low-income and low–middle-income countries spent 15 per cent of total household expenditure on out-of-pocket healthcare costs, compared with 11 per cent for non-disabled respondents'. Looking at all countries, 28–29 per cent of people with disabilities had catastrophic expenditures, 10 percentage points higher than non-disabled people.

Indirect costs are even more variable and difficult to calculate. They include economic and non-economic components. Economic costs involve such things as loss of an individual's productivity, plus that of family carers; early exits from the labour market; and loss of tax revenue. Non-economic costs, which are even more difficult to quantify, can include social isolation, human pain, family disruption and stress. Though indirect costs are extremely difficult to calculate, a study for Canada has estimated that loss of work through long- and short-term disability represented about 6.7 per cent of GDP (Health Canada, 2002; WHO, 2011b).

In poorer countries, where disability rates may be even higher, data are rarely available even to begin estimating the true impacts of disabilities on economies. However, they must at least be similar to and perhaps exceed the costs of infectious diseases, to which far greater attention has generally been given.

Planning challenges of epidemic polarization, especially in low- and middle-income countries

Throughout this book, we have pointed out that epidemiological change is less predictable than the classical transition model suggests. In Figure 4.11, we suggested a tripartite division into early-, mid- and late-transition countries can give a broad picture, but we recognize that this is overly simplistic, especially in terms of healthcare needs, planning and resource allocation. We emphasize that transition is very much *ongoing*, almost everywhere, often with different intra-country expressions regionally and locally. In many countries, right down to local communities, many epidemiological profiles exist, with 'old' and 'new' disease patterns coexisting alongside each other. This is true of causes of death, and, when morbidity is considered, the conditions making people unwell or, crucially, *predisposing* them to ill-health are very varied. The 'fifth' stage of epidemiological transition, with its re-emergence of infectious and parasitic diseases, is associated with many important characteristics. These include the increased use of immunosuppressive agents that leave individuals susceptible to many less serious infections, population ageing and malnutrition, combined with increasing examples of drug-resistant organisms (Cliff and Smallman-Raynor, 2009). We referred to this in Chapter 4 as the context of *epidemiological polarization*, but even this term appears almost too concise and implies a neatness in what is really often a very varied and differentiated epidemiological picture, even in the relatively short term.

Some of these issues are discussed further in Chapter 11, but here it is important to acknowledge the ways in which these aspects of health transition are making the identification of health service needs and health planning very complex in many places. Epidemiological polarization and variation provide huge challenges to health planners, giving a resource allocation conundrum, especially in the context of huge resource shortages and disparities, between and often within countries. This can be exacerbated by what we refer to below as a *technology divide* in the health sector. This can act as a sort of digital divide in access to healthcare information and technology, diagnostic imaging and treatment, and high-tech treatments between rich, middle-income and poorer countries, and especially between the haves and have-nots in specific places.

Health sector planning presents a special challenge in many 'early-transition' countries. As we noted in Chapter 4, as many as six out of every ten deaths are from communicable, maternal, perinatal and nutritional conditions, which have tended to be the major focus. Yet NCDs and injuries often also account for a third or more of deaths, giving a *double burden* of disease types, which is also clearly seen in some mid-transition states. The majority of the early-transition countries are in sub-Saharan Africa, so they are often resource poor and to a greater or lesser extent dependent on donor assistance for health, welfare and other human services. Therefore, proper needs identification is especially important. However, data and recording deficiencies are commonplace, often stemming from intermixed problems of accessibility, poor essential record maintenance and assorted local difficulties, so any well-informed, comprehensive and integrated health sector planning is very difficult. For the future, as age-standardized death rates from degenerative conditions in low-income countries might become even higher than in many richer countries, NCDs cannot be neglected (see Chapter 4).

Health sector planning, especially in epidemiologically varied countries, therefore needs to be ever better informed and based on reliable data: at present, this is an important short-coming. Planning also has to be integrated with education and lifestyle information and the availability of appropriate nutritional alternatives, especially in the mid-transition group. Death rates and morbidity from NCDs and degenerative conditions generally are often unnecessarily elevated in the group of lower- to middle-income developing countries, partic-ularly because of late identification and lack of treatment and support. However, these are the very places with the most rapidly changing lifestyles, moving away from the traditional and apparently readily adopting Westernized behaviour, increasing consumption of fats, sugars and salt-rich diets, and often high tobacco smoking (see Chapters 4 and 7). Stress is also a major factor affecting psychological well-being in counties where poverty, crowding and struggle, and the need to adjust to rapid development, are commonplace.

These countries often face major but undocumented burdens from psychological and psychiatric conditions, yet there is rarely any broad-based formal support for such illnesses in the poorest countries, except sometimes from traditional healers. As noted elsewhere, inadequate, or sometimes inappropriately targeted, health services may be another char-acteristic of many such nations. Richer groups and locations often display more 'modern' disease profiles and can consume Western-style health services fairly lavishly, while their poorer neighbours and places often suffer more from old-style diseases as well as emergent NCDs yet have little access to formal care. Such epidemiological admixtures and polariza-tion pose extremely difficult challenges for health resourcing priorities. For example, as discussed, the limited preventive, diagnostic and treatment services for cancer, heart disease, COPD and other degenerative disorders in much of the developing world are major factors behind these disparities at present, and this will probably exacerbate their impacts in the near future. We saw earlier, for example, that many African nations and several countries in Asia simply do not have sufficient, if any, radiation therapy devices for some types of cancers.

While, at present, the bulk of morbidity and deaths from NCDs still occur in late-transition countries, the richer intermediate countries are having to face the changing healthcare demands from ageing populations while also maintaining the quality of services for younger age groups that their population structures demand. As Chapter 4 reminded us, while the broad 'stage of transition' groupings shown in Figure 4.11 are useful for a general picture, information on detailed local situations is essential, too. Health service planning therefore has to use broad-brush allocation at national and regional levels, but then must refine this to reflect the detailed needs of local communities, which may be very varied socio-economically. Many countries and even localities with ostensibly similar epidemiological profiles can differ in important ways when refined needs assessment, resource availability and existing services are analysed.

Access to healthcare technology: international disparities – a technology divide?

One of the most marked features of modern healthcare, in both diagnosis and treatment, is an almost exponential reliance on technology. This technology comes in many forms: for instance, blood tests are routine in many medical spheres; and plain X-rays and more complex scans, including ultrasound, CT, PET and MRI, are increasingly relied on for diagnostic purposes and often to monitor the progress of treatments and the course of diseases. For almost all modern-trained health professionals, diagnostic imaging is now readily expected. Traditional forms of physical examination increasingly give way to highly informative technological diagnosis, leading hopefully to more effective, better-targeted therapies. Surgical interventions have also become ever more sophisticated, including 'standard' surgical techniques and newer, minimally invasive and micro-surgery methods. Gene therapies and gene prophylaxis are becoming available in many advanced systems and they are, of course, highly dependent on technology for diagnosis, assessment and application.

However, the enormous global and even local differences in the availability of almost all forms of technology form an important type of 'digital divide'. Cost, training preference, accessibility and many other factors mean that rich countries often now use a plethora of health tests, while middle-income and transitional economies have fewer, and health facilities in poor countries may often have almost no tests or technology available, even such basics as routine sterilization of medical equipment within hospitals and clinics. In terms of global health equity, this is perhaps one of the most glaring areas of excess versus disadvantage.

Differential access to technology is one feature of inequality, exacerbated by the problems of a lack of even the most essential healthcare in the poorest nations and for poorer groups in richer nations. This has been recognized for many years, but there is little evidence of a narrowing gap. Carr (2004) noted that more than a billion people worldwide were not receiving essential healthcare. To 'close the gap' between the world's wealthiest and poorest nations in health, as the WHO would wish, is almost overwhelming but can start with addressing a relatively small number of illnesses that disproportionately affect people in poorer countries (see Chapters 4, 6 and 7). Many of these conditions are MDG targets and hence will gain special attention: HIV/AIDS; malaria; tuberculosis; maternal and perinatal conditions; childhood diseases such as measles, tetanus, diphtheria, acute respiratory infection and diarrhoea; malnutrition; and tobacco-related diseases. These conditions are often responsible for the bulk of avoidable or excess deaths among the poor relative to the better-off. Sometimes environmental improvements will have as great an impact as technological interventions for many of them.

Yet major differentials often persist because of general environmental and socio-economic conditions. Economic conditions underpin this in part: global health spending ranges from as little as $11 per year per capita in many poor countries, mostly in sub-Saharan Africa and South Asia, to as much as 150 times more in rich countries. A major result of this is both poor environmental health and the lack of access to information, technology and quality basic care, which threatens to leave the global poor even further behind. Moreover, it fosters a divide in the *expectations* of the populations. Carr (2004) considered that the toll on families, communities and entire societies resulting from disparities in healthcare is not only rising steadily but could probably be avoided, perhaps at relatively little cost.

These global health differentials in access to services and technical healthcare are often interpreted as fundamentally unfair and reflecting global, regional and individual social and economic constraints, but they are very recalcitrant to resolution. Huge local, regional and international variations in distributions of, and access to, qualified healthcare professionals, such as doctors and nurses, have long been recognized. They are probably as great or even greater today than they were several decades ago (Joseph and Phillips, 1984; Phillips, 1990). Among the most serious manifestations are the marked differences in spending on healthcare and health research, education and training for health workers, inequalities in local capacity and unequal access to technology and information. This then also translates into differential global provision of, access to and use of healthcare technology.

Poor countries lag in technology: can simple technological linkages come to the rescue?

Dramatic advances in health and medical technology have been made in high-income and many middle-income countries, but these have generally not devolved to poor populations globally, or even to some disadvantaged groups within richer countries. Market forces have often meant the commonest diseases affecting poorer populations, especially those in tropical areas, have until recently remained neglected, as consumers cannot pay. It is hoped that this situation may change (Chapter 11). Private benefactor organizations, such as the Bill and Melinda Gates Foundation, have played a role in raising awareness of this and in some ways may slightly redress the balance (Jacobsen, 2008); they make strong political statements on the issue. The GAVI may gain cheaper medicines and vaccines due to the initiatives in 2011 of some multinational pharmaceutical companies. But, in the longer term, governments, communities and the wider international donor organizations have to continue addressing this issue.

However, to extend to the poorest countries what is now common or routine health technology in richer nations involves much more than merely providing 'hardware' (such as an MRI or CT scanner). It requires consistent technical and medical support for the technology's application, maintenance and interpretation of outputs; the equipment often needs a safe and stable location and, crucially, a reliable power supply. There is also the question of how to assure fair allocation and access locally once the technology is in place.

There are some glimmers of hope. As we explore further in Chapter 11, in the example of better care for childhood cancer, innovative international linkages and use of available, basic mobile communications technology may improve diagnosis and treatment. For example, links by mobile phone networks have leapfrogged the need for land telephone lines and have enabled advice on treatments from specialist international centres to be accessed in a number of remote locations in poor countries. Nevertheless, access to healthcare and especially to many forms of health technology often continue to be problematic in poorer countries (see Figure 8.4). Insufficient transport infrastructure compounds lack of access to services for people who already have limited availability of the fundamentals of healthy living, such as clean water, safe housing, education and public information. Governments may exacerbate distributional and access problems for the bulk of populations by allocating disproportionate amounts of limited health budgets to urban hospitals, rather than rural clinics. The very limited access to healthcare technology for rural residents in many low-income countries is often a stark contrast to that of many rural populations living in even more remote locations but in rich countries, such as Australia and Canada. There, special arrangements are often made to extend services to remote rural locations or to take isolated rural inhabitants to major service centres for assessment and treatment.

So, more comprehensive, often inter-sectoral, planning and policies are essential. They need to address often multiple social and economic causes of health disparities. Improving opportunities and reducing discrimination and isolation provide major social challenges; improving physical access to vital services is often a practical matter. They both demand a combination of reducing extreme poverty, improving education and employment training,

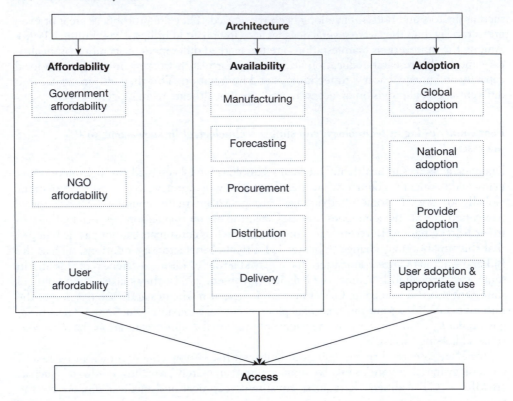

Figure 8.4 Factors affecting access to healthcare technologies for poor countries
Source: Frost and Reich, 2009

enhancing the position and status of women and other marginalized groups, promoting public health campaigns through a variety of media, reducing threats posed by environmental hazards and improving personal security. In many low- and middle-income countries, they also require huge improvements in transport and communications, to spread what is available more fairly.

It is an indictment that the health sector in many instances does not often succeed in making changes to serve the poor better. Yet, there are examples in which even the poorest countries have achieved substantial gains in the health of their most vulnerable citizens. This has often been by community empowerment, participation and forms of comprehensive primary healthcare, providing intensive training of community-based health workers, including traditional healers (discussed below). The avoidance of user-fees, previously fairly widely encouraged by donor pressure, may be one advance, as fees may discourage use of curative and preventive services by the poor (Carr, 2004). Successful examples include Thailand's fairly comprehensive thirty-baht (now free) system of care, originally provided at less than a dollar a time. Some countries, such as Kenya, have also started fee-reduction policies, although the long-term benefits remain unclear at present (Chuma *et al.*, 2009).

Traditional medicine in national health systems: a major resource

Traditional medicine (TM) exists in a huge range of forms and it is a major resource in many health systems globally. Indeed, in some systems, it is the first and often the only source of assistance, especially at the primary care level. There is, however, sometimes a tendency to consider TM as a purely a poor-country, untested substitute for 'reliable' Western allopathic healthcare. This is far from correct. First, in many poorer countries, traditional forms of healthcare are very culturally acceptable – especially for some conditions – and they are the first, and preferred, point of contact for many people, often the 'system of choice'. Second, traditional forms of healthcare are common and, indeed, have always been found in rich or developed countries. Here, alternative forms of practice – including herbalism, chiropractic, acupuncture and hypnotism – are often increasing in popularity today. In many places, they are formally licensed and included in some public and private health schemes. Outside the West, in many regions, such as South Asia and China, several well-established forms of TM are formally recognized, many with their own universities or training systems in addition to more common 'apprentice' systems. They usually operate alongside or even in conjunction with Western-style medicine; some are delivered by physicians and nurses with joint training in traditional and allopathic medicine. An earlier review (Phillips, 1990) notes that this does not merely reflect the maldistribution, expense or lack of access to 'modern' healthcare but, often, traditional, complementary or alternative medical (TCAM) practices represent a definite cultural preference, choice and belief, which extends to patients and practitioners (Phillips, 1990; Ong *et al.*, 2005). However, it is important to recognize that many Western scientists are concerned, sometimes justifiably, about a lack of research and evidence as to how and whether many aspects of TM/TCAM work and, equally importantly, whether they are safe.

Definitions of TM (and TCAM) vary, but a workable one by the WHO (2008e, p. 1) suggests, 'Traditional medicine is the sum total of knowledge, skills and practices based on the theories, beliefs and experiences indigenous to different cultures that are used to maintain health, as well as to prevent, diagnose, improve or treat physical and mental illnesses.' TM that has been adopted by populations outside the indigenous culture in which it developed is sometimes called 'alternative medicine' or, increasingly, 'complementary medicine'. Based on a classification by Neumann and Lauro (1982), Phillips (1990) notes at least four main types:

- spiritualists or magico-religious healers;
- herbalists;
- technical specialists, such as bone-setters; and
- traditional birth attendants (TBAs).

Medical pluralism, as it is sometimes known, is not only tolerated in many countries but may be actively encouraged (Phillips, 1990). In some systems, moreover, notably in China, traditional medicine coexists in many hospital and community settings alongside Western medicine. This is especially seen in two areas: diagnostic procedures and dispensing of medicines, where real alternatives are provided and different systems sometimes used in preference or in combination within the same settings.

In terms of health systems, national policies, legal status and regulation are important (Ong *et al.*, 2005). The WHO notes that not many countries have national policies for traditional medicine; however, many have some legislation or legislation pending (Ong *et al.*, 2005). Regulating TM products, practices and practitioners can be difficult in some places because of wide variations in definitions and categorizations of TM therapies. For example, a single herbal product could be defined as a food, a dietary supplement, a herbal medicine or even a poison, depending on the country. This disparity in regulations at the national level has implications for international access and distribution of products. Four broad categories of systems are still basically recognizable (Phillips, 1990):

- *Exclusive (monopolistic) systems*, in which only the practice of modern, scientific medicine is lawful. Other forms may be effectively illegal although rigour of enforcement and sanctions vary.
- *Tolerant systems*, in which, while formally recognizing only scientific medical activities, the practice of various forms of TM is more or less legally tolerated.
- *Inclusive systems*, which recognize and may even license systems other than scientific medicine.
- *Integrated systems*, which officially promote the integration and use of two or more systems, perhaps within a single recognizable service, and possibly with integrated training of various types of health practitioners.

A very useful *Global Atlas* has been compiled within the WHO (Ong *et al.*, 2005). This shows many examples of the range of legislation, education, funding and recognition of various forms of TM and TM practitioners internationally and gives considerable insights into the widespread nature of many forms of TM and their potential as a health resource within a huge number of health systems. It also maps the status of various types of TM, of which herbalists and practitioners of traditional Chinese medicine probably have the widest international legal recognition. Legal recognition of traditional medicine is shown to vary considerably in different countries, according to the exact type. For example, in South Asia, Unani and Ayurveda are legally recognized, whereas traditional birth attendants, herbalists, osteopaths, homeopaths, chiropractors and practitioners of traditional Chinese medicine are not (Ong *et al.*, 2005). In other countries and regions, patterns of legal recognition are very different.

Many monopolistic or exclusive systems, mainly but not always in the West and other richer countries, have previously tended to exclude TM, ostensibly to 'protect' the public from unsafe or untested practices, but sometimes an underlying reason is professional protectionism (and scepticism) from their medical establishments. One approach to overcoming such exclusion is to devise safety, effectiveness and quality standards, with scientific tests and evidence to evaluate the safety and effectiveness of TM products and practices. However, such evidence is generally limited. For example, while some evidence shows that acupuncture, some herbal medicines and some manual therapies can be effective for specific conditions, further study and published evidence are needed (WHO, 2008e). Moreover, consistent quality control and safety standards and guarantees are increasingly necessary in modern, litigious societies. If official licences are required for certain drugs or therapeutic practices, governments (or regulating agencies) are likely to be very wary unless there are evidence-based reasons for granting such approval. However, with many naturally based herbal products, for example, quality, safety, strength and effectiveness are highly dependent on the nature of the source materials (often natural constituents), and how these are handled, processed, stored, prepared and consumed. National and even supranational regulation (for example in member countries of the European Union) and insurance requirements can make the licensing of such products as medicines very problematic.

Long term, there are many issues associated with bringing TM (of various sorts) into formal healthcare systems. These include patient safety and use, training and licensing systems, knowledge and sustainability. In some places, opposition from formal medical representative groups and the scientific community can be difficult for governments or legislators to ignore. Increased patient awareness about safe usage of some TM products is important, especially if used in combination with Western medicines. Greater formalized training, collaboration and communication among providers of traditional and other medicines will also strengthen its international profile. Yet, locally, of course, many people are very happy with various traditional healers.

Who uses traditional medicine?

As the WHO (2008e) notes, in many countries, especially in some parts of Asia and Africa, up to 80 per cent of the population depend on traditional medicine for their primary health-care (see Box 8.9). This is also the case in some Latin American countries, although legal recognition tends to be lower in them. Moreover, even in some developed countries, as many as 70–80 per cent of the population have used some form of alternative or complementary medicine, such as acupuncture or, increasingly, chiropractic and osteopathy. In the West, these forms are increasingly recognized as reliable and are often included treatments even in some insurance schemes. The WHO states that, globally, herbal treatments are the most popular form of traditional medicine, and they are very lucrative financially. Annual revenues in Western Europe reached $5 billion in 2003–04. In China, sales of products totalled $14 billion in 2005. Herbal medicine revenue in Brazil was $160 million in 2007.

Traditional birth attendants (TBAs) and trained midwives

One of the most valuable and acknowledged traditional healthcare resources is often said to be birth attendants. Generically known as TBAs, or sometimes 'traditional midwives', they are known by such local terms as *hilots* (the Philippines), *dais* (India and Pakistan), and *comadronas* or *parteras* in various Latin American countries. They are almost ubiquitous in poorer countries, although legal recognition, training and status – and, hence, quality – are very variable. TBAs are regarded by the UN as persons who assist mothers during childbirth and who initially learned their skills through delivering babies themselves or via apprenticeship to other TBAs (Phillips, 1990; Ofili and Okojie, 2005). The vast majority of TBAs are older women, although in some countries male attendants exist. In many countries, especially in rural areas, they are either the only or the major source of advice during pregnancy and assistance during delivery, and they have sometimes been officially incorporated into health systems. In many poorer countries, between 60 and 80 per cent of deliveries occur outside modern healthcare. A significant proportion of these deliveries are attended by TBAs, with estimates suggesting between 50 and 65 per cent in Nigeria, 50 per cent in Zimbabwe, and 45 per cent in Sierra Leone and in Mexico (Ofili and Okojie, 2005; Sparks, 2004). Many mothers are confident in the ability of their TBAs, who are culturally acceptable, affordable and trusted. Moreover, they will attend home deliveries; without a TBA, many mothers would have to give birth alone or without any experienced person present.

BOX 8.9 The WHO's key facts on traditional medicine

- In some Asian and African countries, 80 per cent of the population depend on traditional medicine for primary healthcare.
- Herbal medicines are the most lucrative form of traditional medicine, generating billions of dollars in revenue.
- Traditional medicine can treat various infectious and chronic conditions, such as new antimalarial drugs developed from artemisinin from *Artemisia annua* L., a plant used in China for almost 2,000 years.
- Counterfeit, poor-quality or adulterated herbal products in international markets can pose serious patient safety threats.
- More than 100 countries have regulations for herbal medicines.

(Source: Based on WHO, 2008e, p. 1)

Criticism has sometimes focused on unsafe delivery practices. Indeed, a large proportion of perinatal mortality (around birth) occurs because of complications in deliveries and from neonatal tetanus. Many complications and deaths stem from poor hygiene and unsterile conditions, and there is a need to avoid other risks, such as HIV transmission. An important aim has therefore been to improve the practices of TBAs through training and incorporation, with proper reporting and record keeping. Unfortunately, research indicates that many of these older women are illiterate, which can make training and record keeping challenging, if not impossible.

TBAs have and will retain a strong potential role in reducing maternal and neonatal mortality, part of MDG 5 (see Chapter 7), the goal that is often the furthest from being attained. Targets for 2015 are to reduce by three-quarters the maternal mortality ratio, with a measure being the proportion of births attended by skilled health personnel; and to achieve universal access to reproductive health, including improved antenatal care. To reach anywhere near these targets may well demand the incorporation of TBAs more formally, to improve training and to have them work alongside qualified midwives and nurses. Some countries, such as Sierra Leone, have been looking at ways of repositioning TBAs and training them to work as maternal health promoters (MHPs). This can be a good strategy as TBAs are widespread and accepted, so their advice has the potential to be heeded. They could encourage women to use various health services appropriately and provide support throughout pregnancy, childbirth and new motherhood. Crucially, they can also advise on family planning services and HIV and other STD prevention.

In terms of TBAs globally, it is difficult to make an evaluation of skills because training, background and support (if any) for birth attendants are so variable. Results from impact studies are also variable. Some WHO reviews show improvements following training in Pakistan and elsewhere (MacArthur, 2009), but other studies are less optimistic. Indeed, earlier evidence from Pakistan suggested that training 60,000 TBAs had relatively little impact on maternal mortality (Midwifery Association of Pakistan, n.d.). In Malawi, TBAs were even temporarily banned between 2007 and 2010, as the Health Ministry attributed the high maternal mortality rate to a lack of skills among them. It was claimed that TBAs were unable to recognize and react quickly to obstetric emergencies and were failing to provide measures to prevent transmission of HIV from mothers to their newborn children. This ban did appear effective, and the maternal mortality rate was stated to have fallen from 800 to 510 women per 100,000 live births. However, many mothers continued to use TBAs because of a lack of alternatives. An overstretched public health system and other reasons meant the ban was controversially lifted in 2010 amid criticism from the medical establishment (Ngozo, 2011). Discussions are similar elsewhere, although there are few other, if any, examples of outright bans on TBAs in low-income countries.

Critics, especially from the formally trained midwifery sector, argue that TBAs have made relatively little impact on reducing mortality and that adding traditional midwives alone will not be sufficient to meet the MDG targets. An inter-agency report by UNFPA (2011) estimated that, for example, across fifty-eight countries, 3.6 million maternal, foetal and newborn deaths could be avoided if all women had access to a full range of reproductive, maternal and newborn care services (see Figure 8.5). It has been recognized for some time that the place of delivery is a crucial factor in maternal and baby survival rates and those giving birth in proper facilities and with trained personnel fare much better, though the strategies can vary. China, for example, has focused on strengthening hospital services rather than community midwifery and recorded a huge 62 per cent fall in newborn deaths between 1996 and 2008. In the mid-1990s, fewer than half of all births were in hospitals, whereas these were the norm by the later date. It seems the facilities were important, and provided a safer environment than home deliveries, though other factors may also have been

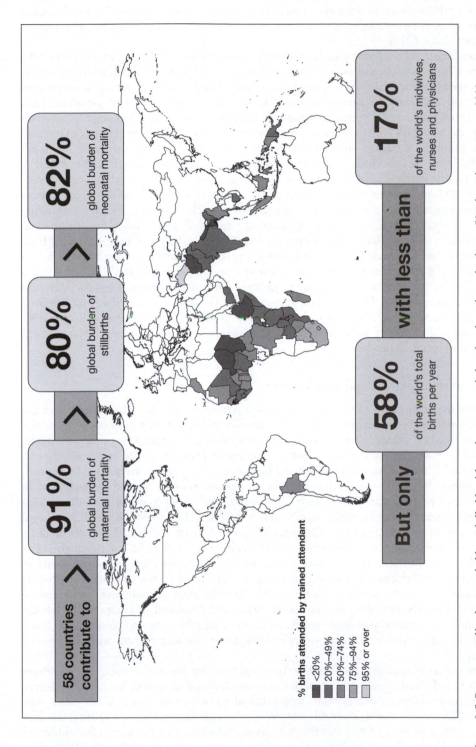

Figure 8.5 Proportion of births attended by a skilled health worker; maternal, foetal and newborn deaths, in 58 selected countries, c. 2009

Source: WHO and *The Lancet's* Stillbirths Series, as presented in UNFPA, 2011. Adapted from WHO and *The Lancet's* Stillbirths Series, as presented in UNFPA's *The State of the World s Midwifery 2011. Title:* UNFPA and partners (2011) *The State of the World's Midwifery 2011.* UNFPA, New York. Year of publication: 2011

significant (Bassani and Roth, 2011). Quality of care seems crucial but the strategy of hospital births overseen by doctors can increase sometimes unnecessary medical and surgical interventions. For example, as many as two-thirds of births in China are by Caesarian section (*Shanghai Daily*, 2011).

Others argue that deliveries under a midwife's supervision are better, even if they take place in a hospital or health centre, with doctors involved only when medically necessary. Good-quality trained midwifery services, coordinated and accessible within communities and properly supported by the health system, are obviously essential in such a strategy. They will help not only safe deliveries but antenatal and postnatal care and ongoing education on care of children, HIV, contraception and many other issues. This perspective views increasing the numbers of trained midwives as the key, part of the Global Strategy for Women's and Children's Health which emphasizes stronger health systems and sufficient numbers of skilled health workers. This is especially crucial in some poorly served Asian and sub-Saharan African countries, such as Sudan and the Democratic Republic of the Congo, where maternal mortality has remained persistently high over the past two decades. Improving competencies, coverage and access, education, regulation and quality are regarded as paramount (UNFPA, 2011). Thereafter, an effective continuum of care is needed from pregnancy, through childbirth to neonatal and then child healthcare, to reduce the toll of maternal, neonatal and child deaths and improve maternal and child health (Kerber *et al.*, 2007). In the interim, there seems to be greatest agreement that, in hard-to-reach and underserved rural areas, TBAs can be a stop-gap until more formal midwifery and maternal and child health services become widely available. In the meanwhile, research on TBAs, and many other forms of traditional health services, and their roles in health systems, will continue to be much needed.

Health systems, ethics and development

One very important aspect of health services and systems which shows considerable global variation relates to respect paid to patients, families and research, which come under the theme of 'medical ethics'. The differences are sometimes due to variations in legal systems, but they are also affected in practice by the resources and time available in different health systems and what is expected and tolerated by patients and practitioners alike. In general, many richer 'Western' systems have in place complex systems for the management of patients and professional–patient interactions, patients' rights and responsibilities, professional standards, and regulation of research in health (Mason and Laurie, 2011). Legal systems are often complex, especially regarding treatment protocols and end-of-life decisions, the application of reproductive health technology and rights of the foetus. For example, there has been much emotional debate but, in English law and increasingly in many other jurisdictions, the foetus – the potential person – does not have legal rights that can trump those of the mother (Plomer, 2005). As technology becomes ever more sophisticated and widely available, as mentioned earlier and discussed in Chapter 11, debates regarding the 'appropriate' legal involvement in acceptable use of interventions, and, importantly, the withdrawal of active care and the right to die with dignity, will undoubtedly increase.

Some poorer systems also have similar codes and legal frameworks on paper but find them difficult to enforce. Clinical and social health research is also an area of considerable debate and variation among health systems. International agencies such as the WHO have published codes relating in particular to research involving human subjects, requiring the lack of coercion, provision of full information about risks and potential benefits, informed consent and the ability to withdraw from research without penalty (CIOMS, 2002). The definitions of what are fair and reasonable standards of care are, however, by no means universally accepted and have been the subject of widespread, often critical, debate (Benetar and Singer, 2000, 2010). Given the difficulties in agreeing ethical boundaries, debate has shifted in many legal and philosophical aspects towards a human rights focus (Plomer, 2005). In recent decades, the recruitment for clinical research by multinational companies of participants from low-income countries has intensified concerns on the rights and bioethics of international research, especially regarding coercion and informed consent. Concern over recent years has focused particularly on protection and possible exploitation of vulnerable subjects in poor countries and less well-regulated health systems, potentially for the benefit of people in richer areas (Office of the Inspector General, 2000; Hawkins and Emanuel, 2008). This is clear evidence of the complex, and often ambiguous, interrelationships in global health systems between richer and poorer countries and groups.

Discussion topics

1 What do you understand by 'health sector reform', and can you provide examples of it in your own health system?
2 What are the main sources of paying for healthcare in your own system?
3 Do you think that incentivizing people to stay healthy by giving them some form of payment will work?
4 What major impacts of improved access to healthcare technologies could you see as benefiting the poorer countries of the world?

9 Global environmental change and health

Introduction

Environmental parameters are often important determinants of health, particularly with respect to infectious diseases. For example, temperature can be crucial in some instances: the minimum survival temperature for anopheline mosquitoes, the vectors of malaria, is between 8 and 10 degrees Celsius, while the actual *plasmodium* malaria pathogens have minimum temperature threshold limits for development of around 18 degrees Celsius in the case of *P. falciparum* and 15 degrees Celsius for *P. vivax*. Humidity is also an important factor, as mosquitoes generally cannot survive long enough for malaria transmission to occur if average monthly relative humidity falls below 60 per cent. Dengue fever, the other leading mosquito-vectored scourge, in turn has minimum temperature thresholds of 6–10 degrees Celsius for the *Aedes* carriers and approximately 12 degrees Celsius for the pathogen, and hence a wider geographic range. Non-arthropod vector-borne infectious diseases likewise have thresholds. The *Cercariae* larval parasites involved in schistosomiasis, for instance, on being released by the disease's freshwater snail vector, have a minimum temperature threshold of approximately 14 degrees Celsius for disease transmission (McMichael *et al.*, 2001).

Many non-communicable health conditions also have environmental factors in their aetiology, ranging from the direct injury and death toll from sudden extreme events (such as earthquakes, tsunamis, storms, heatwaves and floods) to long-term illness (such as air pollution-related respiratory disorders, various skin cancers from solar ultraviolet radiation, drought-induced undernutrition, and immune and central nervous system disorders resulting from exposure to toxic chemical residues, e.g. from pesticides, in soil and water and food supplies). Changes in environmental parameters thus inevitably have implications for human health ranging from the major to the minor.

With the massive growth of population, urbanization, industrialization and economic development over the past two centuries or so, humans have placed an ever-increasing ecological footprint on the planet and – sometimes inadvertently – set in train fundamental changes in many of the earth's vital environmental systems. Climate change is arguably the most fundamental and important of these, and the one we hear about most frequently. However, global environmental change is much wider than mere changes in, say, temperatures or precipitation. Other critical dimensions include stratospheric ozone depletion, deforestation, land degradation, air, water and soil pollution, freshwater depletion, ocean change and biodiversity loss (see Figure 9.1). While listed individually here, there are many complex and sometimes unpredictable interrelationships between these changes. Deforestation, for example, is an important contributor to global warming, and to land degradation and shrinking biological diversity. Likewise, climate change, apart from its linkage with deforestation, is associated with biodiversity loss, air pollution and other environmental processes. All have implications for health – some positive but most negative.

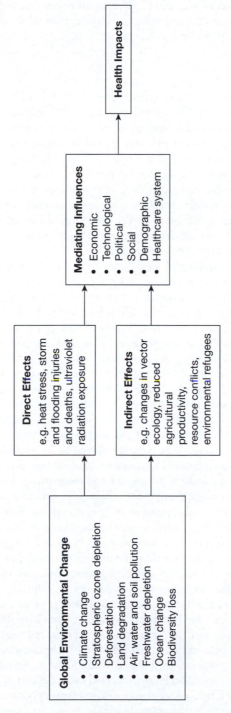

Figure 9.1 Global environmental change and health

The adaptive capacities of all societies will be challenged but people in less developed countries are likely to suffer most, having fewer economic, technological and healthcare resources to call upon (Ashdown, 2011). Within all countries, the poorest sections of the population, with the fewest choices, will generally be most adversely impacted, continuing the long-established social gradient of health.

Climate change

Climate change has been a recurrent feature of the Earth's history, and there are well-documented periods of cooling being followed by global warming rebounds. Prior to the industrial era, these perturbations were triggered by the planet's natural system dynamics. At present, the Earth is in another period of global warming, but this time human activity is most likely the main cause through the release of greenhouse gases into the atmosphere. These human-induced emissions add to the naturally occurring greenhouse gases in the atmosphere to give an 'enhanced greenhouse effect', trapping additional heat from the sun and making the Earth's surface warmer. The main greenhouse gas is carbon dioxide, principally from fossil fuel combustion and the burning of forests by farmers in developing countries. Methane and nitrous oxide, generated from a variety of activities, are other important anthropogenic greenhouse emissions.

Since the start of the Industrial Revolution, the global atmospheric carbon dioxide concentration has increased from about 280 parts per million (ppm) to 379 ppm in 2005; the methane concentration from about 715 parts per billion (ppb) to 1774 ppb; and the nitrous oxide concentration from around 270 ppb to 319 ppb (IPCC, 2007). These and any future emitted gases will have very long lifetimes and cause major warming. Significant warming has unequivocally already occurred. The IPCC (2007) reported that the linear warming trend over the last fifty years was nearly twice that for the last hundred years and that the estimated average global total temperature increase from 1850–99 to 2001–05 was 0.76 degrees Celsius, with the bulk being attributed to human activities. Alternative scenarios prepared for the fourth IPCC Assessment Report meanwhile project further warming this century of between 1.8 and 4.0 degrees Celsius. The actual temperature increase will depend on the extent and effectiveness of global mitigation efforts.

While global climate change is popularly referred to as 'global warming', the facets of climate encompassed go well beyond temperature and also involve precipitation, humidity, wind patterns, cloud cover and the frequency and magnitude of extreme weather events. From changes to these parameters will come other environmental consequences, such as sea level rise due to oceanic thermal expansion and polar melting, desertification, and land and marine ecosystem damage. Also, while climate change is a global phenomenon, there will be considerable regional variations: temperature changes will vary; some areas will get more precipitation, others less; severe weather events will become more likely in some regions, less likely in others. The impacts on different populations will thus also vary around the globe, mediated by differing local, national and regional adaptive capacities.

These climatic changes are likely to have a wide range of impacts on global population health. While there will be some beneficial impacts, the net overall impact is expected to be negative. Not all of this lies in the future, though. There are signs that climate change is already exacting a toll on human life. The World Health Organization, for example, estimates that over 150,000 deaths a year are attributable to climate change and that 5.4 million DALYs are lost (see Table 9.1). The Global Humanitarian Forum (2009), in turn, puts the death toll at twice the WHO figure. Children are the main victims and poor countries the most affected.

Projecting climate change health impacts is difficult due to the uncertainties surrounding the nature and magnitude of both future climate change and disease dynamics, plus similar

Table 9.1 Deaths and DALYs attributable to climate change, by WHO income group, 2004

	Population (,000s)	Deaths (,000s)	DALYs (,000s)
World	6,436,826	141*	5,404*
Income Group:			
High-income	977,189	0	16
Middle-income	3,044,634	11	471
Low-income	2,412,669	130	4,915

Note: * Around 12,000 additional deaths hastened by increased temperatures are not included because the years of life lost were uncertain and possibly brief.

Source: WHO, *Global Burden of Disease* website

uncertainties regarding the future mediating impact of socio-economic, demographic, political and other factors. However, the impacts already becoming evident, coupled with rigorous scientific modelling research, point to diverse health effects. Some of the increasing deaths and DALYs will be due to direct exposures to changing climatic conditions, but most will flow from indirect exposures.

Direct effects of climate change

Thermal stress

Global warming will bring mixed consequences, fewer deaths due to less exposure to cold, but more deaths due to high temperatures. These effects will vary geographically: temperate (high-latitude) countries will benefit from warmer winters and fewer cold spells. In the United Kingdom, for instance, it has been estimated that, by the 2050s, milder winters could see a fall in cold-related deaths of up to 20,000 per year, against an increase in heat-related summer deaths of 2,800 per year (Expert Group, 2001). In other places, extra heat stress deaths will outweigh any reduction in cold-related ones. Temperature variability will probably be as important in this regard as overall mean temperature increases (see Box 9.1). City populations will be particularly at risk of thermal stress in a warming world due to the urban 'heat island' effect. Many of the deaths during heatwaves are accelerated mortality (sometimes called 'harvesting') of frail/elderly persons with serious pre-existing cardiovascular and/or respiratory diseases, who probably would have died soon anyway, making it difficult to compute true heat/cold tolls.

BOX 9.1 Glimpses of the future?

Over recent years there have been a number of extreme weather-related events around the globe, all with major health impacts. Examples include extraordinary heatwaves in Western Europe in 2003 and in Eastern Europe/Russia in 2010; intense cyclones/ hurricanes, such as Cyclone Nargis, which struck Myanmar in 2008 and Hurricanes Katrina and Wilma during the 2005 Atlantic hurricane season; country-wide floods in Pakistan (2010) and Thailand (2011); and severe drought in the Horn of Africa (2011).

continued

A number of commentators have firmly attributed these events to climate change, but specific episodes such as these cannot be directly linked to climate change, even though their occurrence and magnitude fit with global warming predictions. They do, however, give us an opportunity to appreciate the potential consequences of global warming and other climate changes projected for the twenty-first century.

The 2003 and 2010 European mega-heatwaves, for example, likely broke 500-year temperature records across half of Europe. In the 2010 episode, weekly to monthly maximum temperature anomalies exceeded the 1970–99 mean by more than 10 degrees Celsius, slightly exceeding the 2003 event in amplitude (Barriopedro et al., 2011). In the 2003 episode there were an estimated 72,000 heat-related deaths and in Russia in 2010 around 56,000 (IFRC, 2011). The 2010 heatwave was so extreme that climate modelling suggests low probability of a similar episode over the next few decades. However, 2010-like extreme weekly heat spells are projected over highly populated areas of Europe between once and twice per decade by the end of the century, with 2003-like anomalies even more frequent.

Reported climatological, hydrological and meteorological disasters over the past two decades show an upward trend (see Figure 9.2), but longer-term data will be necessary before firm statements about change can be made. Also, disaster data suffer from lack of standardized collection methodologies and definitions (IFRC, 2011).

(Sources: Barriopedro et al., 2011; IFRC, 2011)

Other extreme weather events

Besides more frequent and intense heatwaves, climate change is also predicted to bring more cyclonic, storm and flooding activity with likely associated increases in deaths, disease and injury, and reduced well-being because of damage to property (homes and workplaces). The health impacts of these types of threats will almost certainly be greatest in poor countries where large and growing populations live in vulnerable locations and where household and societal capacity to adapt is weakest. Apart from the immediate injuries and loss of life from such events, longer-term health impacts (such as infectious disease outbreaks, stress disorders, food shortages, population displacement) usually follow from their initial destruction and dislocation. In the abnormally heavy and widespread monsoonal floods in Pakistan in 2010, for example, over the eight weeks after the onset of the floods, there were 832,000 cases of acute diarrhoea reported, 964,000 cases of acute respiratory infections, 256,000 cases of suspected malaria and 1,107,000 cases of skin diseases (Ministry of Health, Pakistan, and WHO, 2010). We discuss sea level rises later in this chapter, but it should be noted that in some poor countries, such as Bangladesh, even very small increases in sea level associated with climate change will render large areas of the country uninhabitable (see, e.g., BBC, 2009). In the interim, it is likely to increase the incidence of flooding with associated increase in many forms of disease and direct or indirect loss of life. Some richer countries, notably the Netherlands, are also at risk from sea level rise, but their resources to address this are greater, at least for the near future.

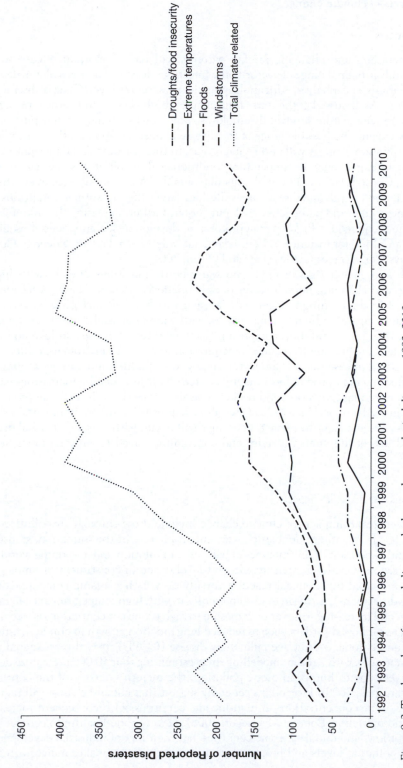

Figure 9.2 Total number of reported climato-, hydro- and meteorological disasters, 1992–2010

Source: IFRC, *World Disasters Report* (various years)

Indirect effects of climate change

Infectious diseases

Rising temperatures and changing rainfall patterns will have important effects on the geographic and altitudinal range of vector-borne infectious diseases, such as malaria, dengue, lymphatic filariasis, encephalitis, African sleeping sickness, yellow fever, Chagas' disease and schistosomiasis. As discussed at the start of the chapter, both vectors and pathogenic agents have minimum temperature survival thresholds, so any increase in mean temperatures will theoretically expand the possible range of the disease concerned and also the transmission season. Precipitation changes will also be important. In the case of malarial mosquitoes, for example, expanding favourable temperature conditions will be offset in some regions (e.g. the Amazon, Central America) by evolving unfavourable lower rainfall regimes and hence likely contraction of endemic disease areas. Besides range effects, warmer conditions will result in some vectors and pathogens developing faster, further increasing the risk of infection. The time required for *P. falciparum* protozoa to develop inside anopheles mosquitoes at 20 degrees Celsius, for instance, is 22–23 days, but only 12–13 days at 25 degrees Celsius and 9–10 days at 30 degrees Celsius (Patz and Olson, 2006).

There are also greater risks of food- and water-borne infectious diseases with higher temperatures and changing rainfall patterns. Salmonellosis, *Escherichia coli, shigellosis* and other forms of food poisoning increase with warmer weather. *Vibrio cholerae* bacteria also proliferate more rapidly at higher temperatures, with warmer coastal and inland waters in conjunction with poor sanitation comprising a serious threat. Changes in lake and river water levels and quality due to reduced precipitation also favour microbial proliferation. Further infectious disease impacts are in turn likely to come from more frequent droughts adversely affecting food production in many poorer countries, thereby increasing malnutrition and weakening protection and resilience against infections. In extreme prolonged droughts, as in the Horn of Africa in 2011 (see also Chapter 10), large environmental refugee flows to under-resourced, unhygienic relief camps will occur, with heavy diarrhoeal disease sickness and loss of life almost certain, and concomitant need for international health assistance.

Non-infectious disease health impacts

Other indirect health impacts of climate change include those through air pollution and aeroallegen levels. Weather variables play an important role in the formation, transport, dispersion and deposition of several types of harmful air pollution and a warming world will likely see these relationships intensify. Ground-level ozone (a constituent of 'smog'), for example, is produced by chemical reactions involving volatile organic compounds (e.g. unburned hydrocarbons), nitrogen oxides and sunlight, with high temperatures accelerating its formation and increasing its severity. Exposure to high ozone concentrations is associated with several respiratory disorders, such as reduced lung function growth in children, asthma, pneumonia and chronic obstructive pulmonary disease (COPD). It is also associated with premature mortality, with a recent modelling study estimating that 50,000 premature deaths occur each year due to European ozone pollution, the majority outside of the continent itself (Duncan *et al.*, 2008). Projections generally suggest that climate change will increase tropospheric ozone concentrations in high-income countries, with consequent increasing morbidity and mortality (Ebi and McGregor, 2008). Fewer ozone-health projections have been done for low- and middle-income countries, but their mix of industrial development-driven high pollution levels and projected temperature increases makes increasing ozone levels and higher morbidity and mortality likely. Particulate matter (PM) air pollution is also very bad for human health, but whether climate change will increase the days with high dangerous fine PM concentrations is uncertain (projection studies reported by Ebi and McGregor (2008) produced differing results for different regions). The IPCC (2001) notes that concentrations of fine PM depend in part on temperature and humidity, so changes in those parameters thus may affect PM concentrations and, by extension, human health. Aeroallergen concentrations (e.g. airborne pollen grains) are also associated with weather and climate factors. Increased pollen production, lengthening of the pollen season, and increased pollen allergenicity are considered likely with rising atmospheric temperatures, heightening allergic respiratory disease problems, sometimes called atopic diseases, such as allergic asthma and allergic rhinitis (Beggs and Bennett, 2011), some of which can be life-threatening as well as causes of disability.

Adverse effects on food production and nutrition are probable for many developing countries, as we discuss further in Chapter 10. Apart from the impact of droughts mentioned above, other aspects of climate change will have negative impacts on food production and nutrition which flow on to health: for example, loss of productive low-lying coastal agricultural areas through inundation by rising seas and associated coastal land and aquifer salinization; and from declining crop yields due to climatic influences exacerbating plant diseases and pests. Violent physical conflicts over water supplies and land resources are also likely in some regions. Against these negatives, modelling research suggests that under currently projected climate change cereal production would increase in high and middle latitudes.

Overall, of the numerous impacts of climate change on health discussed above, reduced access to food and safe water will likely be the most important. Food availability may be reduced and food costs considerably increased, very likely substantially caused by climate changes. (The potential increased costs and consequences are discussed in Chapter 10.)

Stratospheric ozone depletion

As we have discussed, ozone in the Earth's lower atmosphere (the troposphere) is harmful to human health. Ozone, however, is also found in the next higher layer of the atmosphere (the stratosphere) as a naturally occurring gas. In contrast with 'bad' ground-level ozone, stratospheric ozone is 'good', protecting life on Earth from harmful ultraviolet radiation (UV) from the sun which, though necessary, in excess can cause skin cancer, cataracts, immune system damage and possibly other health disorders (Lucas *et al.*, 2006). The ozone in the stratosphere forms a layer that absorbs between 97 and 99 per cent of incoming solar UV radiation. Any diminution of the stratospheric ozone shield means increased amounts of UV radiation reaching the Earth and accordingly health effects. Adverse effects are most likely, but some beneficial consequences, such as enhancing Vitamin D production, may also occur (Norval *et al.*, 2011).

As long ago as the early 1970s, researchers identified threats to the ozone layer from increasing atmospheric concentrations of man-made chlorofluorocarbons (CFCs) and other ozone-depleting industrial chemicals (e.g. halons, hydrochlorofluorocarbons, carbon tetrachloride) used as refrigerants, solvents, foaming agents, aerosol propellants and the like. A few years later, definite evidence of stratospheric ozone thinning was found, with substantial so-called 'holes' observed over the Antarctic and later the Arctic.

Alarm at the burgeoning use of CFCs and other ozone-depleting substances (ODSs) and declining ozone levels prompted the establishment in 1987 of the Montreal Protocol – an international agreement by governments to cut down and phase out CFCs. Several other agreements have subsequently been reached to accelerate the phase-out and widen the range of chemicals covered, with developing countries given longer to phase out ODSs than more developed nations.

Levels of ODSs in the stratosphere are now falling and there are signs that ozone depletion has been arrested. However, full recovery back to 1980 levels of stratospheric ozone will not be achieved until around mid-century, as ODSs take a long time to degrade. The exact health effects of the ozone depletion to date and likely future effects until ozone levels recover are difficult to assess and predict, due at least in part to the mediating effect of behavioural changes on increased exposure to UV radiation. Without governments worldwide agreeing to address the depletion problem there would, however, certainly have been significant health consequences. McKenzie *et al.* (2011) claim that, without the Montreal Protocol, peak values of sunburning solar UV radiation could have been tripled by 2065 at mid-northern latitudes, with serious consequences for human health and the environment.

Deforestation

One of the major human impacts on the biophysical environment has been the removal of forests and conversion of the land to agricultural, urban and other non-forest uses (see also Chapter 11). Deforestation has been an ongoing process since at least Neolithic times and the advent of agriculture, with the result that only a small fraction of the Earth's original forest cover now remains. At present, the Food and Agricultural Organization (FAO, 2011) estimates around 13 million hectares of forestland, mainly tropical forests, are converted to other uses or lost through natural causes each year. According to the FAO, this is down from around 16 million hectares per year during the 1990s, although some researchers dispute the FAO figures and argue there has been no reduction in the rate of destruction. Accepting FAO figures, new forest plantings make the current net annual loss approximately 5.2 million hectares, still a worryingly high figure. Also, new plantings do not replace all the ecological and human benefits of culled original forest stands. As we discuss further in Chapter 11, a variety of forces drive contemporary deforestation – population pressures, increasing demand for forest products, perceived greater economic returns from alternative land uses (e.g. mining, palm oil plantations, cattle ranches), road construction, poverty, greed, corruption, ignorance – and major reduction of remaining old-growth stocks is likely to continue.

This large-scale, ongoing deforestation has important, though not commonly appreciated, adverse consequences for human health. Deforestation is one of the leading factors behind emerging and re-emerging infectious diseases. In clearing forests and converting the land to alternative uses the microclimatic, soil, water, flora and fauna characteristics of old ecosystems are changed and new ecological conditions created. These new conditions frequently encourage the proliferation and spread of infectious disease vectors and pathogenic agents and closer contact with humans. Mosquitoes are often particularly favoured, as the removal of forest stands and shade creates suitable new temperature, humidity and stagnant-puddle breeding sites. Increased malarial transmission has been a frequent result; likewise yellow fever and dengue. Pooling of water on newly deforested agricultural developments (e.g. in dams, irrigation canals and rice paddies) has had similar effects. A variety of non-mosquito-borne diseases have also been associated with deforestation and new land uses, amongst them snail-borne schistosomiasis, onchocerciasis, loiasis, leishmaniasis, Nipah virus, Lyme disease and Rocky Mountain spotted fever.

Threats to health are also experienced by people involved in the actual deforestation process – subsistence slash-and-burn farmers, plantation and ranch owners, commercial loggers, road construction workers, mine employees. All are brought in direct contact with forest-based pathogens to which they may have little or no immunity. Where the deforestation is large scale and involves burning, another health risk can be the smoke generated, causing respiratory problems hundreds of kilometres away from the actual forest-clearing activities. The haze from forest and plantation fires in Indonesia in 1997, and several other years since, for instance, spread as far north as the Philippines and caused serious health problems across the South-east Asian region. Massive deforestation burn-offs in Amazonia have also created widespread respiratory dangers.

Unthinking destruction of rainforest areas and associated loss of biodiversity are almost certainly costing humanity valuable medicinal resources. Many vital modern pharmaceuticals come from compounds derived from forest plants. Some major examples include:

- Taxol: for treatment of breast and ovarian cancer. Derived from Pacific yew tree – *Taxus brevifolia.*
- Topotecan and Irinotecan: for treatment of breast, thyroid, small cell lung, colon and ovarian cancer, malignant melanoma, lymphomas and leukaemias, as well as AIDS. Derived from *Camptotheca acuminata* (popularly known as the 'Cancer Tree' or 'Happy Tree'), native to China.
- Vinblastine and Vincristine: for treatment of leukaemia and lymphoma and several other cancers. Derived from the rosy periwinkle (*Catharanthus roseus*), native to Madagascar.
- Prostratin: for treating HIV. Derived from the *mamala* tree (*Homolanthus nutans*), found in Samoa.

Others are presently under development, for example EBC-46, an anti-cancer chemical derived from the blushwood tree (*Hylandia dockrillii*), found in northern Queensland, Australia.

Deforestation also adversely affects health through its major contribution to climate change, rating as the second-largest source ('up to one-third'; IPCC, 2007) of anthropogenic carbon-dioxide emissions into the atmosphere, after fossil fuel combustion. Trees remove carbon dioxide from the atmosphere through photosynthesis and sequester (i.e. store) it as carbon in their bodies, thus acting as carbon 'sinks'. When trees are burned, cut down or decay, however, their stored carbon is released back into the atmosphere as carbon dioxide, contributing to the enhanced greenhouse effect. Forest clearance also makes a second contribution to global warming through the reduction in number of trees available to absorb atmospheric carbon dioxide – that is, to act as carbon sinks. The health impacts discussed in the 'Climate Change' section of this chapter thus need to be kept in mind here.

Land degradation

Land degradation, the decline in land quality, is a serious problem in all regions around the world and one of the major environmental threats to both current and future global population health. More than half of the world's land used for agriculture is now moderately to severely degraded, with around 2 billion hectares of land for crop production lost every year (UNCCD, 2011). Degradation takes many forms – loss of soil stabilizing vegetative cover, soil compaction, erosion, pollution, salinization, acidification, leaching and nutrient depletion, damaging siltation and pollution of inland waters, contamination of groundwater, desertification, etc. Natural forces can play a part, for example droughts, wildfires and coastal zone storm surges, but human factors are the main determinants. In essence, land degradation reflects a mismatch between land use and land quality. In the developing world, this mismatch is often driven by growing population pressures and widespread poverty, leading to overuse of farmlands and inappropriate expansion into ecologically fragile areas. In the more developed countries, poor land use practices are also found, but driven more by desired market returns than the food-survival imperative facing many people in poorer countries (see also 'Soil Pollution', below).

The health consequences of land degradation are generally most felt in the developing world, though they are to be seen almost universally, and work through several pathways. Most immediate is the impact on food production and nutrition. As land degrades, crop and livestock productivity falls and food insecurity intensifies. Food prices also become higher and more volatile. Already close to a billion people worldwide suffer from hunger, and the danger is that with continuing land degradation this number will increase (see Chapter 11). With malnutrition comes enhanced vulnerability to infectious diseases, particularly among children. Likewise, child cognitive development is at greater risk. In degrading drylands, declining water supplies make maintaining hygiene more difficult and water- and food-borne diseases accordingly more likely. In the case of extreme land degradation, populations may be forced to abandon areas and relocate elsewhere, potentially spreading infectious diseases. In recognition of the seriousness of the threat of land degradation to global population livelihoods and health, the United Nations has designated 2010–20 as the 'Decade for Deserts and the Fight against Desertification'. In September 2011, the General Assembly convened a special high-level meeting on desertification, land degradation and drought.

Pollution

Over the past two centuries, pollution has become one of the most pervasive and multi-faceted threats to human health. Air, water and soil resources are all severely compromised through human activities. The types and extent of pollution vary around the world, but it is safe to say that no person on the planet today is totally free from exposure to some type(s) of hazardous anthropogenic environmental pollutant.

Air pollution

Air pollution harms people both outdoors and indoors. Outdoor air pollution is mainly due to emissions from motor vehicles (e.g. carbon monoxide and dioxide, hydrocarbons, nitrogen oxides, particulates), industrial facilities and fossil fuel-based power plants (e.g. particulate matter, lead, sulphur dioxide, carbon dioxide, methane) and agriculture (e.g. through fertilizers, pesticides, burning off). These are all so-called *primary* pollutants – that is, pollutants in their own right. Some of these in turn undergo chemical reactions in the atmosphere and create further (*secondary*) pollution. Ground-level ozone, discussed earlier in this chapter, is a major secondary pollutant. Acid rain, formed through the combination of sulphur and nitrogen oxides with water, is another.

The World Health Organization estimated that in 2008 1.34 million premature deaths worldwide could be attributed to urban outdoor air pollution, 2.4 per cent of total deaths (see Figure 9.3). Fine particulate matter pollution is considered to have the greatest adverse effect on human health: it is estimated to cause about 9 per cent of lung cancer deaths and 5 per cent of all cardiopulmonary mortality (WHO, Outdoor Air Pollution website). Particulate matter pollution is a health problem worldwide, but particularly in middle-income countries where vehicular ownership and surging industrial production have not been matched by environmental pollution controls.

An important feature of outdoor air pollution is the long-distance transport of some emissions (e.g. ozone, particulates, persistent organic pollutants, mercury) by high-altitude winds. Pollution from East Asia, for example, can be carried to western North America. In turn, some North American pollution flows to Europe, while some European pollution

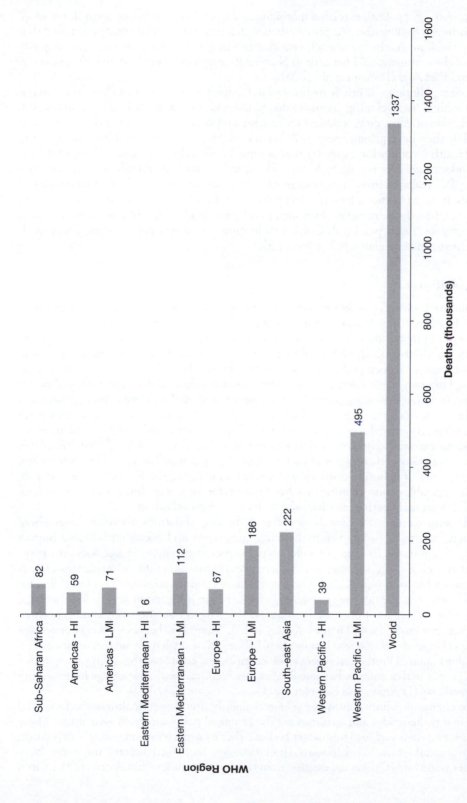

Figure 9.3 Deaths attributable to urban outdoor air pollution in 2008, by WHO region

Notes: HI = high-income; LMI = low- and middle-income.
Source: WHO, *Burden of Disease Associated with Urban Outdoor Air Pollution for 2008* website

travels to Asia. Air pollution-related morbidity and mortality, and hence control, therefore is not entirely a local matter. As previously noted, a recent modelling study estimated that 50,000 premature deaths occur each year due to European ozone pollution, the majority outside of the continent – 37 per cent in North Africa and the Near East and 19 per cent in South and East Asia (Duncan *et al.*, 2008).

Indoor air pollution was briefly mentioned in Chapter 5. As explained there, it is a major health problem in developing countries due to the widespread use of biomass fuels (wood, charcoal, animal dung, crop residues) for heating and cooking. Women and girls are most affected as they have primary responsibility for cooking and house tending. In sum, the World Health Organization estimates that around 2 million lives are lost globally each year due to indoor smoke from solid fuels, virtually all in low- and low-middle income countries (WHO, 2009a). Exposure to hazardous indoor air pollutants also occurs in more developed countries, in homes, offices, factories and public buildings (e.g. formaldehyde emitted from pressed wood products, mineral fibres such as asbestos, lead dust, pesticides, disinfectants, tobacco smoke, radon gas, etc.). Considerable illness is caused but, by comparison with developing countries, relatively low loss of life.

Water pollution

Contamination of water bodies is one of the most serious dimensions of global environmental degradation by humans, with all types of water resources being compromised – surface and groundwater, freshwater and oceans. There are three basic types of water pollutants: toxic chemicals, biological materials and thermal discharges. The capacity and will to prevent or reduce pollution vary greatly around the world. It tends to be closely monitored in many richer countries, although pollution events and accidents do still occur. However, in many developing countries, discharge of untreated industrial contaminants and their almost inevitable seepage into the water supply is often accepted as a necessary price for achieving economic development. Similarly, hygienic improved sanitation facilities are available only to around half of the developing world's population (WHO/UNICEF, 2010), the excreta of many of those without such facilities being dumped in available water bodies, running the risk of polluting drinking water supplies, entering the food chain (e.g. in fish, shellfish, vegetables), and creating breeding grounds for infectious diseases such as cholera, typhoid, infectious hepatitis, giardia, salmonella and cryptosporidium.

While sewage removal is overall far better in developed nations, there are cases where insufficient treatment occurs before discharge into rivers and ocean outfalls and human health is compromised. In many parts of Eastern Europe, for example, sewage disposal is poor. Inadequate and/or ageing sewerage infrastructure and stormwater infiltration into sewer lines also cause problems in older cities. The River Thames running through London (UK), for instance, suffers regular raw sewage overflows from the city's Victorian sewers. In an average year, 39 million tonnes of untreated sewage are discharged into the river, and up to three times that in wetter years (Thames Water, 2011). Many UK beaches also suffer sewage overflows (Ungoed-Thomas and Krause, 2010). The UK, though, is by no means alone. The US's Environmental Protection Agency, for example, has estimated that each year up to 3.5 million people in that country become ill from beach contact with raw sewage from sanitary sewer overflows (Dorfman and Rosselot, 2011).

Toxic chemical pollution of water resources mainly involves agricultural and industrial contaminants. Pesticides and fertilizers are the principal pollutants from agriculture. These chemicals find their way into freshwater bodies either by surface run-off or direct deposition by drifting aerial sprays. Many industrial pollutants are discharged directly into rivers, lakes and other waterways. Others are emitted from industrial chimneys and distributed by wind.

Both types of emissions can travel large distances from the original source. Farm fertilizers and pesticides can also be transported long distances down rivers and deposited in estuaries and coastal waters, altering estuarine and coastal marine ecosystems and frequently reducing fish stocks and the food security of fishing-based communities. Thermal pollution, such as heated water discharges from power stations or industrial plants, can have similar ecosystem altering impacts. As discussed below, extraction of oil from undersea (and on land) poses many risks of pollution from leakages and accidents.

Groundwater resources, the source of drinking water for many population groups, can also be contaminated. The nitrogen in inorganic fertilizer, for example, can leach through soil as nitrate and accumulate in groundwater. Other substances, such as pesticides, petroleum products and radioactive materials, can also infiltrate to groundwater, as can human and concentrated animal (e.g. confined feedlot) wastes. There is currently strong debate in a range of countries about the risk of groundwater contamination and dangers to health from the chemicals used in the hydraulic fracturing ('fracking') method of coal-seam gas extraction. Fears have also been expressed about the waste water brought out during the process causing pollution at the surface.

Soil pollution

The build-up of contaminants in soil through human activities has become increasingly recognized as one of the major faces of land degradation around the globe. The effects on human health occur in two main ways: through impacts on food security and nutrition due to declining agricultural productivity; and through exposure to toxic materials. The most dangerous soil pollutants are urban and industrial wastes (e.g. chemicals, liquids, plastics, gases, heavy metals) and agricultural chemical pesticides and fertilizers. Industrial wastes enter soil through both deposition of air- and water-distributed emissions and direct on-land dumping. Illegal and/or poorly managed dumping, which is widespread in many countries, is particularly dangerous. Health effects from dumped toxic materials sometimes take decades to emerge, as starkly seen in the 1970s Love Canal (Niagara Falls, NY) pollution crisis. Fertilizers and pesticides, meanwhile, clearly have benefits for farming, but can highly contaminate soils (and groundwater) if overused. Other serious, but generally fairly localized, soil pollution can be caused by mining activities. Nuclear accidents, such as those at Chernobyl (Ukraine) in 1986 and at Fukushima (Japan) in 2011, are also obvious long-term soil (and air and water) pollution health hazards. A lengthy legacy of serious soil contamination and adverse health effects was left in parts of Indo-China after the Vietnam War following US forces' use of powerful chemical defoliants. Agent Orange, the most widely used of these, contained TCDD dioxin, a highly toxic organochlorine and known human carcinogen.

Dioxins are one of the so-called POPs – persistent organic pollutants. Other well-known POPs include DDT, PCBs, chlordane, dieldrin and heptachlor. As their group name suggests, POPs last a long time in the environment, resisting natural processes of degradation, and are among the most dangerous pollutants released by human activities. POPs can be transported large distances by wind and water and migratory species, so those generated in one country can contaminate soil (and water) and affect wildlife and people in distant other parts of the world. A range of serious human health effects have been associated with POPs, among them cancers, neurological damage, reproductive disorders, developmental problems and immune system disruption. POPs accumulate in the fat tissues of living organisms and biomagnify with movement up the food chain. Human exposure to POPs is mainly through contaminated foods. In 2004, a United Nations Treaty to eliminate or restrict the production and use of POPs ('The Stockholm Convention'; United Nations, 2001) came into effect, and by early 2011 more than 170 nations had become parties to the convention.

In many countries, especially in locations which have undergone 'de-industrialization', varied forms of moderate to severe pollution can be associated with so-called 'brownfield' sites. These are sites reclaimed from previous industrial activities for residential purposes. They may retain assorted toxic traces in the soil, with some posing hazards to health and necessitating extra costs to deal with the contaminated land.

Freshwater depletion

Over 70 per cent of the Earth's surface is covered by water, but only 2.5 per cent of that is freshwater. In turn, less than half of that freshwater is accessible for human use, as nearly 70 per cent is locked up in ice caps and glaciers. With all human life on the planet personally and domestically dependent on sufficient freshwater supplies, plus agricultural, industrial and environmental water needs, the importance of freshwater resources is readily apparent. Freshwater stocks, however, are under multiple threat (Gleick *et al.*, 2001). Both surface and groundwater stocks are being compromised through pollution, while global climatic change is changing precipitation regimes and reducing water availability in some areas. Coastal freshwater aquifer loss through rising sea levels and infiltration is also a prospect. On top of these developments, in many parts of the world there are increasing demographic pressures, inexorably inflating aggregate water demand. Rising incomes are also significant, increasing per capita demand. Production of goods, crops and animals for consumption (ranging from cotton goods to beer and beef) all requires significant amounts of freshwater. The amounts used are sometimes disproportionate to the product, which has led to the calculation of 'water budgets' to show the amounts of water required to produce, say, a cotton shirt. In many parts of the developing world, small-scale, traditional-crop agriculturalists are facing increasing competition for scarce water (and land) resources from new, large-scale commercial agricultural enterprises. A substantial number of countries already face severe water scarcity and, although much can be done to improve water management and conserve water usage, more countries will almost certainly join them over coming decades, with inevitable negative health consequences – decreased food production and poorer nutrition, sanitation problems, increased risk of infectious disease, and so on.

Ocean change

Brief reference has been made in earlier parts of this chapter to changes to the world's oceans and their health impacts: for example, rising sea levels, land inundation, coastal marine pollution, seafood contamination. The magnitude and importance of anthropogenic ocean changes and the implications for human health, however, are far greater than this (National Research Council, 1999). Oceans around the world are undergoing unprecedented changes caused by a variety of human impacts. In a recent global study of seventeen anthropogenic drivers of ecological change for twenty ocean ecosystem types, it was found that no area is unaffected by human influence and that a large proportion (41 per cent) is strongly affected by multiple drivers (Halpern *et al.*, 2008). The most seriously damaged waters include the North Sea, the South and East China seas, the Caribbean Sea, the Mediterranean Sea, the Red Sea, the Persian Gulf, the Bering Sea, several parts of the Western Pacific, and the east coast of North America.

Climate change is the leading anthropogenic driver. Global warming is increasing ocean as well as land temperatures. The main oceanic impact of this – and the one that probably first comes to mind – is sea level rise through thermal oceanic expansion and melting of ice caps. Ocean warming, however, has other important consequences with links to human health. Warmer water is associated with increased harmful algal bloom (HAB) outbreaks that cause shellfish and fish poisoning. Aerosol exposures to HAB toxins are also dangerous. Climate change is additionally involved in HAB occurrence through the increasing amounts of dust in the atmosphere due to drought and desertification. This dust is iron laden and when deposited in the ocean acts like a fertilizer for the blooms. Warmer waters and the iron fertilizing also promote oceanic microbiological growth, such as *Vibrio* bacteria. Increased nitrogen and phosphorous levels (known as eutrophication) in coastal oceanic zones from agricultural fertilizer run-off also encourage the proliferation of algae. In an increasing number of areas around the world these chemical nutrients and enhanced phytoplankton activity have depleted dissolved oxygen levels in the water to the extent of producing 'dead zones' that are unable to support most marine life. The drainage of sewage and industrial wastes into coastal waters can have similar effects. Fisheries and shellfish beds are thus lost to populations in these areas. Over 400 dead zones have been identified along coastlines around the world, and the United Nations Environment Programme has categorized the phenomenon as one of the biggest environmental problems of the twenty-first Century.

Ocean chemistry is also changing through taking up a significant proportion of human-made carbon-dioxide emissions from the atmosphere. This absorption has the beneficial effect of slowing the rate of climate change, but causes ocean acidification. Direct human health effects of acidification are uncertain, but marine organisms that use carbonate to build shells or skeletons (e.g. molluscs, corals, crustaceans) will probably be adversely affected by the decreased saturating concentrations of calcium carbonate. Threats to the health and ultimate existence of such organisms could potentially have human impacts, ranging from diminishing seafood stocks to lost opportunities for marine-derived pharmaceutical products.

Oceans are also changing due to a variety of more immediately visible human activities, such as shipping traffic, oil exploration and production, and commercial fishing. While international shipping is critical to the global economy, oil leaks and spills and dumped rubbish are a more negative side of the industry. Also, the ballast water of ships can inadvertently transport human and animal pathogens (viruses, bacteria, protozoa) from one part of the world to the other. Cholera, in particular, has been suspected of 'hitch-hiking' in this manner to a number of locations. Oil spills due to accidents on exploration and production rigs have also caused serious damage to local- and regional-scale ocean areas with flow-on effects to human health ranging from loss of food sources, to chemical exposures, to mental health and stress disorders due to destroyed livelihoods (e.g. in commercial fishing and tourism) in affected populations. The largest such accident in the petroleum industry's history was the Deepwater Horizon spill in the Gulf of Mexico in 2010 (McCoy and Salerno, 2010).

Another major oceanic change has been the progressive depletion of marine fish stocks by large-scale commercial fishing operations. Many areas and fish species have been seriously overfished, with fish simply being caught faster than they can reproduce. Overcapacity is a major problem – the global fishing fleet being around two to three times larger than is needed. Much of the fishing is also indiscriminate (e.g. massive drift-netting and bottom-trawling) and wasteful. A large proportion of the fish caught are 'bycatch' (i.e. not targeted) and thrown back dead (Giuliani *et al.*, 2004). The Food and Agricultural Organization (FAO) of the United Nations estimates that the proportion of marine fish stocks over-exploited, depleted or recovering has increased from 10 per cent in 1974 to 32 per cent in 2008, and that 53 per cent of global stocks are fully exploited with no room for further expansion (FAO, Fisheries and Aquaculture Department, 2010). This overharvesting of the oceans is both a threat to the health security of the very large number of people around the world who depend on seafood as their principal source of animal protein and to the future health of oceanic ecosystems. How different fish species will react to continued ocean warming is another uncertainty.

Biodiversity loss

One of the major consequences of the various types of global environmental change we have been discussing is loss of biodiversity, mentioned briefly earlier. Whole ecosystems in forests, dry lands, the oceans and inland waters are being modified and in some cases totally destroyed by human pressure – land conversion, pollution, overuse of resources, excessive population numbers, anthropogenic climate change, and so on. With the assaults on these ecosystems, plant and animal species are becoming extinct at an unprecedented rate. In short, the world's biodiversity bank is shrinking. Ecologically and philosophically, this impoverishes the planet. All forms of life are intrinsically important and deserving of preservation. Over and above this ethical position, however, is the less recognized fact that biodiversity loss is harmful for human well-being and health. Living organisms, for example, provide essential environmental services, such as purifying air and water, maintaining soil fertility, retarding soil erosion, breaking down wastes, cycling carbon and pollinating crops. Plant and animal biodiversity also provides invaluable genetic resources for enhancing food production. Moreover, a wide array of important human drug compounds are derived from plant, fungi and animal organisms, with the very high likelihood that many more such pharmaceutical discoveries wait to be made. We touched on this in the discussion of deforestation, but the potential for medicinal discoveries lies in all ecosystems – land and water (Herndon and Butler, 2010; Chivian, 2002; Grifo and Rosenthal, 1997). Continuing human-induced biodiversity loss thus probably means unthinking squandering of novel bioactive resources.

Concluding comments

In this chapter we have attempted to show the many ways in which the Earth is experiencing major human-induced environmental change and the significance – and, crucially, the *potential* significance – of those changes for human health. We made the point at the start that climate change is the most fundamental and important dimension of global environmental change and the one that receives most publicity, but that environmental change is in fact much wider than that. We take this opportunity now to emphasize that multidimensionality of change. We also pointed to the many interrelationships between the various biophysical changes, and likewise take this opportunity to reiterate those interlinkages.

Discussion topics

1 Should the United Nations have the authority to force nations to reduce carbon-dioxide emissions to a global standard per capita level? Justify your view.
2 What do you believe are the main problems in projecting the health effects of global environmental change?

10 Geopolitics, human security and health

Introduction

In this chapter, we turn to the question of the many and often complex relationships between geopolitics, security and health. We indicated such relationships, as you will remember, in our diagrammatic model of health determinants (Figure 3.1). The linkages between health and these spheres are important and operate in both directions: geopolitics and security have effects on health; and health, in turn, has significance for geopolitics and security. Also, in the discussion we extend the notion of security beyond the traditional international and national territorial conceptualizations to encompass individual human security, too. We are aligning ourselves in this regard with the United Nations Development Programme's 1994 *Human Development Report*'s (p. 23) notions of 'safety from such chronic threats as hunger, disease and repression . . . [and] protection from sudden and hurtful disruptions in the patterns of daily life'. We begin with a consideration of one of the most important features in the globalizing world – population movements which can stem from a wide range of reasons and can have enormous implications for long- and short-term health status of individuals, communities and even nations.

Population movements, migration and health

Population movements, voluntary or involuntary, are potentially a very influential factor in global health patterns and health changes. Indeed, involuntary population movements after disasters and emergencies have been identified as a major issue in global health, sometimes with greater impacts (especially in terms of the spread of disease) than the events themselves (Watson *et al.*, 2007). The population movements may be associated with the spread of widely recognized infectious diseases, such as cholera, but, as these movements often occur in tropical areas, they may also be associated with deaths from causes such as malaria (National Research Council, 2003). Population movements can be common after certain types of disaster, such as floods, volcanic eruptions and landslides (PAHO, 2000). As well as being associated with the possible spread of infectious diseases, population movements may well give rise to the need for extra healthcare, temporary or longer term, in the receptor areas. Migration and health have long been recognized as having important and complex interrelationships (Allotey and Zwi, 2007).

Over history, people have moved for a huge variety of reasons, ranging from voluntary movements for work, leisure, retirement or family reasons, to forced movements associated with war, civil conflict, natural and humanitarian disasters and discrimination. When people move, they not only take with them their own immediate health status but introduce a new statistical and biological component into the places and populations they join. It is often assumed that disaster and wars are major causes of diseases and misery, but analysts note that it often tends to be the movement of people following, or associated with, such events that cause health impacts (see Chapter 9).

Migration is generally analysed as internal (within a country) or international (crossing a national boundary). Distances can be large or small in either case, although the geopolitical and administrative restrictions tend to differ between the two forms. An example of long-distance internal migration can be seen in China, where as many as 200 million people within a large country have migrated hundreds, even thousands, of kilometres over the past thirty years to work in the rapidly developing eastern seaboard provinces. But these people are often not accurately recorded as they are moving within a country and may not acquire residential rights in their destinations. By contrast, many people may travel far smaller distances from Hong Kong to China for residence, work or leisure. While technically moving within the same country, because they cross a formal immigration frontier their data will be recorded. International migration, on the whole, is better recorded and more rigidly controlled than internal migration within countries, and of course it can have profound health consequences. Arrivals to new countries may not have access to or be eligible for public healthcare, if it exists. They may have knowledge, language and social difficulties in accessing needed services and they may be disoriented in a new setting, with possible psychological health consequences as well as physical health needs. This is especially likely to be the case when the migrants are refugees or displaced people who have, willingly or unwillingly, ended up somewhere new.

Migration and migration policies have become major socio-political and security issues in many developed and developing countries over the past few decades, as migration flows have grown rapidly. The immigrant population in the OECD countries, for example, has more than tripled since the 1960s, but it is highly subject to fluctuations due to economic conditions, especially downturns (OECD, 2011b). There are many crucial migratory links between richer and poorer countries and, for some lower-income countries (such as the Philippines, Indonesia, India and several countries in Central America), remittances – legal or illegal – from their citizens working abroad comprise substantial and crucial parts of national income, and support millions of people and families 'at home'. In terms of 'who migrates', migration has long been recognized as being age, gender and qualification dependent (UNDP, 2009). There is, for example, considerable concern over loss of well-educated, young personnel (especially, ironically, in the health sector) from poorer countries to cluster in richer countries. For instance, almost half of foreign-born doctors or nurses working in OECD countries were in the USA, about 40 per cent in Europe, and the balance in Australia and Canada (OECD, 2007). Almost invariably, the people who can move most easily are the active, best qualified and most talented – the people many countries can ill-afford to lose.

As a result, emigration rates for better-educated people are almost always much higher than total emigration rates. This difference is especially large for African and Asian countries. The emigration rate of highly skilled persons born in Africa is 10.6 per cent (and, for Latin America, 8.8 per cent), well above the world average of 5.4 per cent. Moreover, the highest rates of highly skilled migration are often from small and/or poor countries, among which several stand out, having highly skilled emigration rates above 50 per cent. Barbados, Guyana, Haiti, Trinidad and Tobago, Belize, Mauritius and Tonga have more tertiary-educated people born within them but living abroad than at home. By contrast, many richer or populous countries have low emigration rates of highly skilled persons, such as the United States, Japan, Saudi Arabia and China (Dumont et al., 2010). It is often lamented that outflows denude poor donor countries of skills. However, when local education systems are good but domestic employment opportunities limited, and migration a possibility, human nature tends to seek out greener pastures.

Table 10.1 Number of refugees and internally displaced persons (millions), 2000–10

	2000	2005	2010
Refugees	15.9	13.0	15.4
Internally displaced persons	21.2	23.7	27.5
Total	37.1	36.7	42.9

Source: Based on data in UNDESA, 2011

Some migrants may be classed as refugees, because they have been forced to flee their home countries as a result of wars, ethnic conflicts or other security reasons. In such cases, the United Nations High Commissioner for Refugees and other humanitarian governmental organizations and NGOs may be involved as these people have crossed an international border. Others may be internally displaced persons who have had to move within their own country, perhaps due to similar conflict reasons, but they will often not be eligible for the same levels of international protection and assistance (Jacobsen, 2008). Their psychological and physical health status may be harmed just as much as that of international refugees, but their needs may not be as well identified or met. The numbers fluctuate quite considerably but, as Table 10.1 indicates, there was an increase, especially in internally displaced persons (IDP), over the first decade of this century. Of the data listed by UNHCR (2011), in 2010, the nations with the largest numbers of 'refugees and people in refugee-like situations' were Iran, Pakistan and the Syrian Arab Republic, each with over a million people. In terms of IDPs protected or assisted by UNHCR and 'people in IDP-like situations', Colombia had 3.67 million, the Democratic Republic of the Congo 1.72 million, Sudan 1.62 million, Somalia 1.46 million and Iraq 1.34 million.

Health needs of people in emergency and conflict situations

'Emergency situations' are many and varied, arising from natural and human-induced circumstances, and combinations of the two. They range from unexpected natural shocks, such as earthquakes, tsunamis and sudden flooding, through to longer-term, sometimes more anticipated, effects of, for example, conflicts or climate change, resulting in population exodus and resultant health needs. Effects can be very extensive, affecting huge numbers and extensive areas of countries and regions. An example is the Asian tsunami of 2004, which touched three continents and heavily impacted many countries in South-east and South Asia and even as far as Somalia. Alternatively, effects can be more localized with, say, impacts on specific cities and sub-regions. The health impacts of emergencies that grab headline attention are generally those in the immediate aftermath of the event. However, the more important health and humanitarian effects can often be associated with the long-term needs for rebuilding and regaining infrastructure for life and health, long after international attention has drifted elsewhere.

The health and welfare needs of people following disasters and conflicts are naturally very varied. At the immediate time of the event or conflict, many people may be injured and killed, with the wounded needing urgent care and dead bodies requiring hygienic disposal. There is often also immediate disruption to food, water, welfare and other human needs, including supplies of medication for the sick and those needing long-term care, and separation of families. In some situations, especially in conflict zones, there can be the danger of reprisals, rape and other violence. Longer-term, post-disaster and post-conflict situations frequently need the rebuilding and reprovisioning of health services (see Chapter 8), welfare and psychiatric services, and the replacing of lost infrastructure. In addition, specific risks, such as the clearance of unexploded bombs, mines and improvised explosive devices, can be very important. In Cambodia, Mozambique and elsewhere, for example, landmines and unexploded ordnance have gone on killing and maiming humans – especially children – and animals for decades after the conflict concluded.

Armed conflict as a global health problem

Conflict situations cause considerable mortality and disability. In its 2004 global burden of disease estimates, the WHO rated war and civil conflict as causing 184,000 deaths and 7.4 million DALYs annually. Sequels, such as morbidity and mortality from malnutrition, famine, infectious disease and the like, can add hugely to the long-term toll. Perhaps rather belatedly, armed conflicts are now being recognized as a major, often growing, public health issue (Murray *et al.*, 2002). The UK government, for example, has included reduction of the humanitarian and health impacts of conflicts as one of its 'top twelve' global health targets for 2015 (HM Government, 2011). Deaths in conflicts form just the 'tip of the iceberg', and many more health consequences occur during and subsequently, though they are often not well documented due to lack of witnesses. They include disability, economic and social decline, associated endemic poverty and malnutrition and, very importantly, longer-term psycho-social illnesses (Murthy and Lakshminarayana, 2006). However, in spite of the magnitude of the direct and indirect health consequences, military (and severe civil) conflict has not received the same public health research and policy attention as have many other causes of illness and death. Sadly, as Murray *et al.* (2002, p. 346) note, 'political scientists have long studied the causes of war but have primarily been interested in the decision of elite groups to go to war, not in human death and misery'. This lacuna should be an increasingly important area of attention for global health, although it is often subsumed under research on accidents and injuries. Rapid reporting, the internet and other sources can now help us to know about new areas of conflict almost immediately. However, if those conflicts become prolonged, public interest tends to wane. Moreover, reliable data on almost all aspects of most conflicts are often absent, which makes an accurate assessment of the health impacts and ways to reduce the consequences very difficult. In addition to battlefield deaths, the health consequences from the displacement of populations, disruption of many health and social services, and the heightened risk of disease transmission may be the major collateral effects, as follow from many natural disasters (see Chapter 11).

The *World Report on Disability* (WHO, 2011c) emphasizes that injuries and outcomes are often exacerbated in conflict situations by delays in obtaining emergency healthcare and lack of longer-term rehabilitation. A 2009 assessment of the consequences of conflict in Gaza found that problems included long-term disability from traumatic injuries, because of lack of appropriate follow-up; and complications and premature mortality in people with chronic diseases, because of disrupted treatment and access to healthcare. Many people suffered from permanent hearing loss from explosions, and long-term mental health problems from the continuing insecurity and lack of protection.

Wars and other conflicts may be short and relatively contained within a country or district, or they may be long lasting, involving many nations and protagonists. Often, conflicts drag on for years without satisfactory resolution, especially civil wars. For example, while there have been no world wars since 1945, in the twenty-two countries of the WHO's Eastern Mediterranean region alone, since 1980, over 80 per cent of the population have either experienced or remain in conflict situations (Murthy and Lakshminarayana, 2006). In extreme cases, such as in the conflict between North and South Korea, which has never had a formal end, wars can lead to isolation and oppression. In the case of North Korea this has led to untold human suffering in lack of development, nutrition and health terms for its population. In many situations, especially those of internal political or inter-ethnic strife and civil war, problems may never be properly or permanently solved.

A first non-military casualty of most conflicts is the provision and maintenance of regular health and welfare services. External international assistance may also be discontinued. Another immediate effect can be disruption of supplies, food and agriculture that often accompanies both intense and drawn-out conflicts. Economies are disrupted, people flee or are driven away, they may abandon their homes and farms in an attempt to seek safety and often become medium- or long-term aid-dependent as a result. It can also be very difficult to draw a line that ends the conflict to permit aid workers and others to re-enter a former conflict area.

Psychiatric and psychological impacts of armed conflict

Both immediate and subsequent, longer-term, psychiatric and psychological disorders are prominent among the health consequences of most conflicts, among both children and adults (Pedersen, 2002; López-Ibor *et al.*, 2005; Murthy and Lakshminarayana, 2006; Neria *et al.*, 2009; Wang *et al.*, 2010). The WHO (2001) attributes great importance to dealing with psychological traumas of war. It has estimated that, in situations of armed conflict globally, 10 per cent of those who experience traumatic events would have serious mental health problems and a further 10 per cent would develop behaviour that would affect their ability to function effectively. Anxiety disorders, post-traumatic stress disorder (PTSD), substance abuse and misuse, depression and prolonged grief, other psychological, psychosomatic problems such as insomnia, back and stomach aches, and behavioural problems may be widespread after violence and also other disasters. The capacity of humans to cope with adversity and recover from armed conflicts and their aftermath is becoming a major area of interest in psychology and psychiatry (WHO, 2001; Neria *et al.*, 2009). Prevalence rates of problems are associated with the level of trauma and the availability of physical, social and emotional support, and also post-conflict support. High post-conflict emergence of mental problems has been seen in many countries and regions, including Afghanistan, the Balkans, Cambodia, Chechnya, Iraq, Israel, Lebanon, Palestine, Rwanda, Sri Lanka, Somalia and Uganda – all places with histories of long-term, violent and very troublesome conflict, either within communities or between countries (Murthy and Lakshminarayana, 2006).

Gender and age risks in conflicts

In terms of risk factors and risk associations, women tend to have an increased vulnerability to the psychological consequences of war, and there is high correlation between mothers' and children's distress in war situations. Maternal depression can be common but, in spite of their vulnerability, women are often resilient under stress. Higher rates of trauma-related psychological problems are also noted in children, especially adolescents. Child soldiers forcibly recruited and taught to fight and kill face particularly difficult problems of recovery from exposure to and participation in violence (Coalition to Stop the Use of Child Soldiers website).

While not an issue of wholly global reach, involvement of children in conflicts is so widespread in some areas as to be a major health problem, and it is particularly but not exclusively associated with developing countries (Gates and Reich, 2009). The problem is at its most critical in Africa, with children as young as 9 involved in armed conflicts, but children are also used as soldiers in a number of Asian countries, and parts of Latin America, Europe and the Middle East. Most child soldiers are aged between 14 and 18, and while some may enlist on a 'voluntary' basis, many are coerced or see few survival alternatives. In Africa, many child soldiers are AIDS orphans. The Coalition to Stop the Use of Child Soldiers' *Child Soldiers Global Report 2008* documents nineteen countries where child soldiers were recruited or used in hostilities between 2004 and 2007, mainly in non-state armed groups – Afghanistan, Burundi, Central African Republic, Chad, Colombia, Cote d'Ivoire, the Democratic Republic of the Congo, India, Indonesia, Israel and the Occupied Palestine Territory, Iraq, Myanmar, Nepal, the Philippines, Somalia, Sri Lanka, Sudan, Thailand and Uganda. It is recognized the numbers and locations fluctuate considerably as conflicts wax and wane, but tens of thousands of minors are probably involved every year. Moreover, over sixty countries, including many in the West, still permit the recruitment of under-18s into their armed forces (Coalition to Stop the Use of Child Soldiers, 2008).

Somalia: two decades of conflict

The prolonged conflict in Somalia in the Horn of Africa sadly exemplifies many of the health and welfare problems in prolonged conflict zones. Conflict broke out in 1991 and, twenty years later, the various sides appear as far apart as ever. Many people are fleeing the countryside and moving to the capital city, Mogadishu, where all services are under great strain and there is minimal safety. It is estimated that a million people have lost their lives directly from violence or from the famine or disease associated with the prolonged conflict and drought. Many more have been injured, the bulk of them civilians. The ICRC (2011), present in Somalia permanently since 1992, notes the impact is very hard on civilians, particularly women and children caught in the crossfire. Warring factions often fail to distinguish between civilians and fighters and use indiscriminate tactics; they do not respect and protect medical staff, hospitals or clinics. The ICRC has nevertheless been attempting to provide emergency aid to people affected by armed conflict and natural disasters, especially the prolonged drought driving people from their farms. They have also striven to restore and improve the livelihoods of those made vulnerable by the continuing humanitarian crisis. The worst regional drought in sixty years has impacted geographically more broadly than Somalia, affecting more than 12 million people by 2011 (Oxfam, 2011a), including parts of Ethiopia, Kenya, Uganda and Djibouti, with resulting famine and substantial migration.

In Somalia itself, the number of war-wounded treated at the two main referral hospitals, Medina and Keysaney, both in Mogadishu, increased sharply to 6,000 patients in 2010, compared to 5,000 in 2009 and around 2,800 in 2008. Over a third of the wounded were women and children, caught in fierce fighting between the Transitional Federal Government forces (supported by some 8,000 African Union troops) and various armed factions. Both hospitals are supported by the ICRC, and Medina, a community-based hospital, has been working around the clock because of the almost continuous fighting. In 2010, the hospital treated over 3,000 war-wounded, of whom over 1,100 were women and children. People caught in mortar or artillery fire, or in landmine explosions, made up three-quarters of the hospital's patients. The staff themselves – doctors, nurses and others – work at great personal risk; armed guards patrol the grounds and staff have been targeted with death threats and assassination attempts in a bid to destabilize services. Nevertheless, the hospital maintains a policy of treating war-wounded and the sick regardless of clan, armed faction or political camp (ICRC, 2011). Yet more sadly, however, there seems to be little prospect of an early return to normality and bomb attacks are regularly reported (War Victims Monitor, 2011).

The situation in Somalia, and elsewhere in the region, is exacerbated by the numbers fleeing from the drought in the countryside. Some Somali men have turned to piracy, one of the few remunerative occupations, but one fraught with risk and violence. As well as the million unnecessary deaths from the conflict and ensuing disruption, there are many other health side-effects of war and civil disturbance in this region and elsewhere, such as parts of South and West Asia (e.g. Afghanistan, Pakistan, Sri Lanka, Gaza, Iraq). These include the people who have been injured and handicapped, who can be identified and perhaps assisted. However, there are millions more hidden casualties, including people with psychological injuries, and children without parents who lose family life, education and upbringing, and others suffering in the extensive social disruption. Murthy and Lakshminarayana (2006) note ex-combatants have high psychiatric morbidity and use of drugs such as khat. For many children, the prolonged conflict has brought deep psychological scarring.

Sadly, in the face of such need, mental health services have been almost totally disrupted in Somalia, as they so often are in such circumstances. Moreover, the continuing, endemic violence and a tolerance of lawlessness, including piracy, prevent anything resembling good governance, making the provision of community health, education, welfare and other infra-structural and housing provision practically impossible. As a result, the well-being of almost all Somali citizens is very much reduced.

The remnants of war: landmines and unexploded ordnance injuries and risks

Many countries with histories of conflict have in the past been very heavily mined or blan-keted with a wide variety of different explosive weapons. While considerable progress has been made in international restrictions on and clearance of such military ordnance, they can still pose an immediate risk to military personnel but, yet more problematic, an ongoing huge risk for local residents for years and even decades after the conflict has ended. Unexploded weaponry (e.g. bombs, shells, grenades, mines) poses especial dangers to children and people involved in agriculture or living in former conflict zones. Such weapons are still doing damage, for example, in parts of South-east Asia, such as Vietnam, Cambodia and Laos, more than three decades after conflict ended there. Precise data are very hard to gather but several institutions and NGOs are involved in mine clearance and are estimating the extent of danger. In the 1990s, the most heavily mined countries were identified as Angola, Cambodia, Afghanistan, Iraq, Vietnam, Mozambique, Sudan, Somalia and Ethiopia, as well as Bosnia and Croatia. The numbers of amputees in the worst-affected countries ranged as high as 30 per 10,000, whereas the average in a landmine-free country, such as the USA, was about 1 per 22,000. In some countries, such as Egypt, very large numbers of mines have been laid but in remote or border areas, thereby causing less human injury than those in more populated areas. In the densely populated areas of South-east Asia, the majority of casual-ties are generally civilians, especially children, who are also at higher risk of being killed. Civilians often account for over 30 per cent of casualties, and as many as 90 per cent in some places. This was seen in Namibia in the 1980s, Mozambique in the 1990s and Afghanistan in 2002–03, where 81 per cent of victims were civilians and 46 per cent were under 16. In Erbil, Iraq, between 1998 and 2007, the figure was 97 per cent (New Internationalist, 1999; Bilukha *et al.*, 2003; Shabila *et al.*, 2010).

Not only do landmines and unexploded ordnance ('uxo') kill, but their wider effects can be very serious for individuals and communities. For every two people killed by mines, approximately three are injured (de Smet *et al.*, 1998). Therefore, the acute trauma, surgery, pain management and rehabilitation (physical and psychological) needs in many areas with landmines and unexploded war ordnance are enormous. Many of these weapons that cause indiscriminate injury have been outlawed by international agreements, such as the 1980–83 annex to the Geneva Convention and the 1997 Ottawa Treaty. The former restricted cer-tain types of conventional weapons, such as landmines and non-detectable fragments. The latter stopped the production and distribution of anti-personnel mines after 1999 and gave signatories four years to destroy their stockpiles and ten years to clear all mined areas. Some countries have subsequently announced complete clearance. However, others, including several permanent members of the UN Security Council, have not even signed the treaty, and, indeed, not all types of 'uxo' are covered by it. About forty states are still estimated to have stockpiles of anti-personnel mines, and the ICRC (2010) notes that compliance with stockpile destruction is one of the major challenges facing the treaty. Mines are still in use in some countries and, more importantly, as noted above, will continue to cause casualties for decades. Considerable unexploded ordnance also exists from historic conflicts in many parts of the world, and this still causes injury and death, too.

An important factor complicating treatment and rehabilitation is that many of those injured in this manner are poor and live in remote areas, so access to acute surgery and long-term rehabilitation is very difficult. Many suffer from chronic conditions, such as phantom limb pain, which is often hard to treat. Moreover, the effects of explosions can have huge social and economic impacts on individual victims and their families and wider communities. The injuries lead to loss of productivity and seriously reduce people's ability to care for themselves and relatives. Clearance to make areas free from landmines and other 'uxo' is very lengthy, risky and expensive: estimates suggest it costs over 300 times more to clear a mine than to lay one. Development agencies spend some $400 million annually on land-mine clearance and some cost–benefit analyses even argue against its cost-effectiveness, except in humanitarian terms (Cameron *et al.*, 2010). In some places, the fear of landmines can cause people to abandon farming areas, even if the actual number of mines is relatively few. Until clearance can be completed, whatever the distribution, preventive strategies have to focus on education and changing behaviour, especially among high-risk groups, such as children, who may pick up and play with explosive devices (Surrency *et al.*, 2007). The other two action foci are victim assistance and stockpile destruction and clearance. As increasing numbers of countries join the landmine ban convention, and its success grows, this helps focus attention on post-conflict consequences of other weapons, and especially cluster munitions and unexploded ordnance (ICRC, 2010).

Terrorism

A particularly dark side of violent conflict and global health is the loss of life and injuries sustained in terrorist attacks. Terrorism has a lengthy history but, in recent decades, it has become an area of increasing concern due to the greater killing power now available to perpetrators. The 11 September 2001 attacks in the United States are a good example, showing how simple commercial airplanes could be easily converted by non-specialists into lethal missiles capable of killing thousands of people very quickly. Other readily accessible and commonly employed terrorist weapons include suicide vests, AK-47s, rocket-propelled grenades, missiles, landmines, improvised explosive devices and fertilizer truck bombs. Potential killing devices on a larger scale include biological, chemical and radioactive 'dirty bombs' or other delivery mechanisms.

Quantifying the exact magnitude of terrorism's health toll is impossible due to lack of consensus as to what counts as a terrorist act. Each year, the US State Department compiles a report on attacks for Congress. Figures from the 2010 report are presented in Table 10.2. The 11,604 reported attacks in that year occurred across 72 countries. South Asia and the Near East had the most attacks and victims, led by Afghanistan (3,307 attacks) and Iraq (2,688 attacks). The State Department figures, however, fall short of a true global accounting. On the basis of the aphorism that 'one man's terrorist is another man's freedom fighter', many other deaths around the world could be seen as terrorism casualties: for

Table 10.2 Incidents of terrorism worldwide, 2006–10

	2006	2007	2008	2009	2010
Attacks worldwide	14,371	14,414	11,662	10,969	11,604
People killed as a result of terrorism worldwide	20,487	22,719	15,708	15,310	13,186
People injured as a result of terrorism worldwide	38,413	44,095	33,885	32,651	30,665

Note: Terrorism is defined as 'premeditated, politically motivated violence perpetrated against noncombatant targets by subnational groups or clandestine agents'.

Source: United States Department of State, 2010

example, civilian fatalities in Afghanistan and Pakistan from unmanned, drone-delivered missile strikes and similar deaths during Israel's bombing and invasion of the Gaza Strip in 2008–09.

Health threats to national and international security

Over the past fifteen–twenty years disease has increasingly come to be seen as a security issue, posing potential threats to peace and stability both within countries and internationally. The emergence and worldwide spread of the HIV/AIDS pandemic has been the main factor behind this thinking, reinforced by the huge array of other new and re-emerging infections. A landmark point in this evolving view of health was the UN Security Council's discussion of HIV/AIDS as a security issue at its 10 January 2000 meeting, the first time it highlighted disease as a threat to security. In the same month the US National Intelligence Council released a major report warning that new and re-emerging infectious diseases 'will complicate US and global security' (NIC, 2000).

Not surprisingly, most attention has focused on the HIV/AIDS security issue, although other debilitating infectious diseases, such as malaria and tuberculosis, also have security ramifications. The HIV/AIDS threat to national and international security is seen as having two main dimensions: weakening of military forces (particularly of developing nations); and undermining the economic foundations of affected nations. HIV/AIDS and other serious infections weaken armed forces in a number of ways: for example, by eroding the available recruitment pool; by the loss through premature illness and death of experienced personnel; by reducing effectiveness; and by weakening operational capacity (including participation in international peacekeeping missions). These have been particular problems for many African armed forces as a result of the high HIV/AIDS prevalence rates found across much of the continent. HIV/AIDS, though, is not only an issue for African armed forces (UNAIDS, 2005). The recruitment implications of the disease, for example, have received attention in both the United States and Russia. It is argued that nations and militaries weakened by heavy infectious disease burdens are less able to defend themselves and thus more vulnerable to external political threats, but as yet there has been no obvious real-world case of any such threat transpiring. Alongside the threats to their armed forces, high HIV/AIDS prevalence has caused enormous damage to the economies and social fabric of many African nations and in cases contributed (with other factors) to internal political unrest and instability. The above all relates to 'naturally' emerging infectious disease threats to security. Additional potential threats are posed by 'deliberate' infection through bioterrorism and biowarfare (Peterson, 2002–03; Curson and McRandle, 2005).

In concluding this section, we should briefly note that infectious diseases are not the only health conditions that shrink military recruitment pools. For example, obesity, asthma, mental health disorders and drug abuse are important rejection factors in many Western countries. Over a quarter of young Americans, for instance, are too overweight to join the military, and when other health problems are added, over half of young adults cannot join because of health issues (Mission Readiness, 2009). We will leave it to our readers to decide whether smaller armed forces are a good or a bad thing!

Health of people after natural disasters

We discussed the health impact sequences to natural disasters in Chapter 9 when looking into climate change and natural disasters, and we consider certain other aspects in Chapter 11, when looking to the future. This is a complex topic, in which health effects are precipitated by and interact with not only the disaster situations but local social, health and other conditions. Availability of healthcare, technical support, engineering back-up and general quality of infrastructure can all mean the same types of occurrence have very different impacts in different situations. The recovery time, particularly, demarcates the better-equipped richer countries from the poorer countries when such events happen, though this is not always a clear equation. While some rich countries recently have recovered relatively well from severe natural events (for example, earthquakes in Japan and New Zealand; tsunamis in Japan; and Hurricane Katrina in the southern USA, especially New Orleans), there were nevertheless many deaths and injuries, considerable social and economic effects, and potentially long-term psycho-social health effects.

Similar natural disasters affecting poorer countries tend to cause much greater and often much longer-lasting health and other problems. Examples in the first decade of this century include earthquakes in China and Haiti; flooding in Bangladesh and Pakistan; the massive 2004 Asian tsunami; and major cyclonic devastation in Myanmar (Cyclone Nargis) and Central America (Hurricane Wilma). Safety, health, food and shelter are generally the immediate concerns of both affected and displaced people. Infectious disease outbreaks and spread usually go hand in hand with these disasters in poorer nations due to water and sanitation problems, loss of local health services, and especially, as noted, the temporary or permanent migration of people affected by the events.

Older people in emergency situations

Older and disabled people have been identified as a particular population group often at heightened risk during and after natural disasters, conflicts and related situations. Sometimes older groups may be better able to report the damage from disasters or the pain of conflict situations than younger persons (Wang *et al.*, 2010). Unfortunately, though, their sometimes special needs are often overlooked or ignored (WHO, 2008d). Many have less chance of being able to quit the scenes of conflict or emergencies and their conditions, and age may make it more difficult to gain acceptance in new areas even if they are able to relocate (WHO, 2008d; Global Action on Aging, 2010b).

As the WHO notes, conflicts are only one of many disaster types impinging on older people. Given the global ageing trends noted earlier, and especially the growth of older populations in low- and middle-income countries which are often subject to natural disasters and emergency situations, emergency planners must consider their needs. Hutton (2008) notes that poor health and reduced mobility all too often increase their risk of serious injury and illness in disasters. Data indicate that older people have often sustained more injuries in disasters than other groups (see Box 10.1).

BOX 10.1 Older people can be disproportionately affected in disasters and emergencies

Older people may have greater vulnerability than other groups because of health, mobility and economic status, as well as potential neglect within some communities and even families. Evidence suggests they have often suffered disproportionately in emergencies and disasters, with recent examples:

- France, 2003, heatwave: 70 per cent of 14,800 deaths were of people aged over 75.
- Aceh, Indonesia, 2004, tsunami: highest age-specific death rates were for adults aged 60–69 (22.6 per cent) and 70-plus (28.1 per cent).
- Louisiana, 2005, Hurricane Katrina: most of the estimated 1,330 people who died from effects were older persons: 71 per cent were older than 60 and 47 per cent of this group were over 77. Detailed studies of almost 1,000 deaths found 49 per cent were of people aged over 75, with drowning the most common reason.
- UNHCR worldwide: estimates that older persons make up 8.5 per cent of the overall refugee population, and in some cases comprise more than 30 per cent.
- In 2005, approximately 2.7 million people aged over 60 were living as refugees or internally displaced persons.
- China, 2008, Sichuan earthquake: of the estimated 69,000 deaths, many were older people, and post-traumatic symptoms and psychiatric morbidity were greater in the 60-plus group.
- Japan, 2011, tsunami: as almost one in four people were aged over 65, older people were very heavily involved in the estimated 20,000 deaths and also suffered from loss of care, medicines and facilities. People aged over 60 were estimated to comprise 65 per cent of deaths, with 24 per cent in their seventies.

(Sources: Based on Hutton, 2008; WHO, 2008d; Brunkard *et al.*, 2008; Jia *et al.*, 2010)

Social health of women and girls: unacceptable levels of gender-biased social violence?

As we have noted previously (Chapters 4, 5 and 6), in the vast majority of countries, women on average outlive men, sometimes by a substantial number of years. However, social equality for females is still lacking in many poorer countries, especially among low-income groups, and health suffers accordingly. In many such countries, religious and cultural practices subordinate and disadvantage women and female children (both born and unborn). In most more developed nations, equality is entrenched legally and socially, even if it sometimes does not always work fully in practice. Elsewhere, and in certain cultural settings in particular, women struggle daily for the most basic human rights. Many girls are denied education and their welfare, education and nutrition are often regarded as much less important than those of boys. To counter this, female education, and especially maternal education, has long been identified as a key to raising women's and girls' health and general well-being. But there are many aspects of (lack of) rights and access to education and other societal goods that severely hamper the achievement of global health equality for women and girls. A selection of examples will help us consider whether future progress in some areas of global health can be achieved.

For many years, the United Nations has identified that a wide range of violence affects millions of women worldwide, from all socio-economic and educational backgrounds. It notes violence often transcends cultural and religious barriers, hindering any entitlement of women to participate fully in society and violating fundamental human rights. Sadly, gender-based violence (GBV) often occurs with the explicit or tacit agreement of states and laws. UNFPA (2009) stresses that violence against women and girls is both a human rights violation and a public health priority. Unless it is stopped, we cannot prevent the spread of HIV, many other STDs, and numerous other forms of ill-health associated with or directly resulting from such violence and discrimination.

The United Nations Department of Public Information (1996, p. 1) noted that violence against women 'takes a dismaying variety of forms, from domestic abuse and rape to child marriages and female circumcision'. A decade and a half later, the situation is not much better. Many forms of violence are elevated in poorer countries, but some types, especially domestic abuse, are widespread, ignored or condoned even in the richest countries (see Box 10.2). Following the UN definition (UNFPA, 2009, p. 6), GBV encompasses but is not limited to acts of physical, sexual and psychological violence, wherever or by whomever it is perpetrated, or whether condoned by the state:

> The acts include spousal battery; sexual abuse, including of female children; dowry-related violence; rape, including marital rape; female genital mutilation/cutting and other practices harmful to women; non-spousal violence; sexual violence related to exploitation; sexual harassment and intimidation at work, in school and elsewhere; trafficking in women; and forced prostitution.

Sex ratio imbalances: culture versus biology

In a number of countries and among some groups within certain countries, there is evidence of gender imbalances, sometimes severe, in which primarily more boys are being born than girls (see also Chapter 5, Box 5.2). This phenomenon has indirect health implications and also important social and care consequences for the countries and localities where such imbalances are developing. Imbalances have come about for many reasons, some with a political element, but they are generally socially and culturally influenced. The reasons may

---

BOX 10.2 Violence against women: a universal phenomenon

- Women are subjected to various forms of violence – physical, sexual, psychological and economic – both within and outside their homes.
- Rates of women experiencing physical violence at least once in their lifetime vary from several per cent to over 59 per cent, depending on where they live.
- Current statistical measurements of violence against women provide only limited information. Statistical definitions and classifications require more work and coordination internationally.
- Female genital mutilation is the most harmful mass perpetuation of violence against women and shows only a slight decline.
- In many regions of the world, longstanding customs place pressure on women to accept abuse.

(Source: UNDESA, 2010, p. 127)

be underpinned by factors such as cultural son preference, tied in with feelings that sons will contribute more to the family and be less costly (for example, in terms of dowries) than girl children. Gender selection has ironically been made easier by the increasing availability of medical technology (especially cheap ultrasound tests) and other tests that indicate a foetus's gender. Even when such gender-identification tests are outlawed, they are often used and abortion of female foetuses can occur. When gender determination is not available, female infanticide sometimes happens. China and India (see Box 5.2), the two most populous nations in the world, are showing quite alarming gender imbalances nationally and especially in specific places. China has developed an increasingly imbalanced birth gender ratio, now standing at about 120 males per 100 girls (as opposed to the 'normal' ratio of around 105:100). Other Asian countries, such as Vietnam and Pakistan, are developing similar imbalances (Chatterjee, 2009; United Nations in Vietnam, 2011; WHO, 2011l). Vietnam now has a ratio of around 112:100, notably among wealthier families. While this is a smaller imbalance than China's, it has grown relatively rapidly between 2000 and 2010, and is forecast to rise further.

In China, the government is particularly concerned that a large number of men will not be able to find wives, in a country where marriage has previously been almost universal. Such a situation is unprecedented, so the social and family consequences (such as care for older persons in the absence of daughters, and family continuity) are unpredictable. Some commentators suggest that the end result will be social and even political unrest. There is also likely to be rising demand for sex workers and trafficking of women. The demographic and sex structure of the population of Asia will certainly be seriously affected. As the UN (2011, p. 1) has noted, 'There is huge pressure on women to produce sons, which not only directly affects women's sexual and reproductive lives with implications for their health and survival, but also puts women in a position where they must perpetuate the lower status of girls through son preference.' It also undermines the attainment of MDG 3 on gender equality.

So, what can be done now and in the future to avoid disastrous socio-economic situations developing? This is an example of real and potential abuse of medical technology and procedures. Ultrasound and abortion services are often legal and easily and cheaply accessible, even when foetal sex determination *per se* is illegal. Many governments in Asia have tried to ban antenatal foetal sex diagnosis and sex selection, and to punish medical professionals involved. However, knowledge and access have spread so widely that it is very difficult to control. In India, medically assisted sex selection is illegal but the law is widely ignored and prosecutions are rare. In 2010, China considered relaxing its one-child policy, which has probably exacerbated the sex imbalance, and proposed extending this to the major cities as well as some rural areas. This is to counter population ageing as much as the birth gender imbalance.

Optimistically, perhaps social change will also be effective, as some studies have found that young couples in major Chinese cities are now happy with a girl or a boy child, provided the baby is healthy. In India and elsewhere, it is hoped that education will gradually counter the deeply imbued preference for sons. However, the UNFPA (2011b) and WHO (WHO, 2011l) note the only known successful campaign against sex selection was in Korea, which targeted healthcare providers and religious leaders using ethics arguments. The sex ratio at birth fell from 116 boys to 100 girls in 1991 to nearly normal by around 2010.

Rape and abuse of girls and women are common in many countries

Rape has been used over the centuries as a weapon of war, to subjugate, humiliate, terrify, punish and oppress opponents, and especially civilian populations. Unfortunately, the practice continues to this day, occurring in recent and current conflicts in several African nations and elsewhere (e.g. Sri Lanka and the Balkans). In extreme and unstable conditions, violence against women is often even systematized. The long-conflict-ridden Democratic Republic of the Congo (DRC) is a prominent example. A 2011 report on the country estimated that over 400,000 females had been assaulted between 2006 and 2007 (significantly higher than official UN reports of 16,000 per year) – meaning forty-eight women were raped every hour over those two years. As many as 1.8 million women reported being raped in their lifetime (Peterman *et al.*, 2011; Gettleman, 2011). The DRC study attributed the much higher figures to the fact that women were feeling more able to report sexual violence. Sadly, many of the women had also been forced into sex by partners, so the violence was not restricted to enemy forces. Moreover, sexual violence was widespread outside the conflict zones of eastern DRC, supporting earlier reports that found sexual violence was spreading outside of war zones and becoming more endemic in DRC's civil society. The study suggests that even its much higher figures are conservative estimates of the true prevalence of sexual violence. Chronic under-reporting still exists, because of stigma, shame, perceived impunity, and exclusion of younger and older age groups as well as data on male attacks, and the inaccessibility of many parts of the DRC. Human Rights Watch reported that sexual violence in 2009 was twice that of 2008, which, if accurate, suggests the current prevalence of sexual violence is likely to be even higher than the study suggests (Peterman *et al.*, 2011).

In some, mainly less developed, countries, gang rape, 'honour killings' and mutilations of females for alleged misconduct, adultery or even social sins of their families have been common. Some of these abuses have become so prevalent in some situations that they form personal and public health issues of tragic proportions. Within individual communities, even in some Western counties, so-called 'honour rape' is tolerated and even condoned. A notable, controversial case in Pakistan achieved global coverage. This involved Muktaharan Mai, who won worldwide acclaim when she went public after she was gang raped in 2002. In Pakistan, rape conviction rates are extremely low. Her rape had been ordered by village elders in response to the alleged adultery of her younger brother (perhaps meaning as little as walking with a girl from a rival clan). Human rights groups supported her in her complaint to the authorities and six rapists were convicted, only to see the High Court overturn all but one conviction in April 2011. Muktaharan Mai, like other women in similar situations, was then faced with her rapists returning to live in her home area, and the acquittal has been seen as a huge setback for women's rights in Pakistan (BBC, 2011a).

That such an internationally high-profile case could be overturned by the nation's highest courts, and the police's evidence and investigation found so faulty, sends a very negative signal to other women in such circumstances seeking redress for sexual abuse. This example seems a clear case of cultural factors and incompetent and insensitive legal systems overriding human rights, and national law even being used to undermine human rights. Hopefully, future governments and police forces worldwide will stand up to such alleged religious 'laws' and cultural practices, and strengthen good governance and justice. Most importantly, the international community must lend support to those who wish to do so and severely reprimand national governments that do not protect their female citizens.

However, at the moment, there are many areas of weakness. Even in established democracies, such as India, widespread rape of women, especially in rural areas and some states, is acknowledged. Many women fear going out alone after dark, and even educated women feel they must dress in a discreet manner and take care in case their behaviour is interpreted as inviting sexual assault. After years of ignoring this phenomenon, it is finally becoming a political issue (Krishnan, 2011). However, almost everywhere, improvement is taking an unacceptably long time and much pressure, as well as attitudinal change.

Food security and the global community

Most people in the richer countries take the availability of food – basic and luxurious – for granted, even if there are poor groups who cannot afford to eat adequately and others who eat improper diets. However, for many people in poorer countries, food is a great source of stress and food insecurity a major cause of ill-health and starvation. The *World Disasters Report 2011* has a focus on hunger and malnutrition and states bluntly that almost a billion people are hungry or malnourished, and that the global food system is failing (IFRC, 2011). There is little chance of hitting the MDG 1 target of halving the number suffering from hunger by 2015, and the current food crisis has, to some extent, taken the world by surprise in terms of preparedness. Numbers reported suffering from hunger had been increasing over the decade to about 2009, although they fell slightly in 2010 (FAO, 2010).

Why, with modern technology and distribution methods, international linkages and awareness, is this the case, with hunger afflicting close to 15 per cent of the world's population? A lack of priority in development policies on agriculture and the effects of aid on local food production are important factors, but global agribusiness and distribution systems, as well as local and regional security crises, have been held as much to blame. It is also important to consider the other side of the nutrition coin, the more than a billion people globally who are suffering overnutrition and the effects of poor diet and associated risks of many NCDs. 'Hunger and malnutrition (both under and overnutrition) are as much a threat to the world's health as any disease' (IFRC, 2011, p. 9).

Looking forward from a global population of around 7 billion in 2011 to projected populations (medium series) of between 9 and 9.5 billion by 2050 (UNDESA-PD, 2011), food availability must become an ever more pressing health, social, economic, geopolitical, security and human rights issue. Many international and local governmental, NGO and charitable groups are focusing on this topic, but several key problems are emerging involving the interactions between growing demand for food, faltering production, waste and increasing prices (Oxfam, 2011b). Food prices are an important immediate and leading indicator of the intersections between population, climate, ecology and supply and demand. Oxfam (2011b, p. 21) feels that conditions are deteriorating, noting, 'demography, scarcity and climate change: a perfect storm scenario for more hunger'. A predictable but probably largely avoidable reversal of human development is anticipated over the next few decades due to huge, unprecedented increases in prices of basic food staples, which disproportionately hit the increasingly poor sub-populations in times of economic depression. Hunger, malnutrition and associated ill-health will unfortunately likely increase again, especially in poor households where already half or more of spending goes on food, leaving very little for other necessities, let alone luxuries. The potential for political conflict and violence both within and between nations from deteriorating food security is clearly high.

In *Growing a Better Future*, Oxfam (2011b) predicts that prices of staple foods such as maize may well more than double by 2030 unless world leaders (and agribusiness) take action to reform the global food production and distribution systems. So, we may well expect to see average cost of key crops increase by between 120 and 180 per cent. The reasons are complex, and include bad management, lack of investment in agriculture (including research, development and production methods), diversion of land and subsidies to biofuels, in some cases 'land grabs' by international companies, and speculation in commodities. However, as seen in Chapter 9, overwhelmingly, climate change is likely to be the key underlying factor, threatening production in many countries and fanning financial speculation.

As much as half the increase in price will probably be caused by climate change, which clearly demands coordinated international action, but increased volatility in prices will also be related to availability and distributional factors. In particular, Oxfam identifies shortages and costs of land, water and energy. Four 'food insecurity hotspots' illustrate the potential increasing risks in areas already having problems feeding their people, summarized by the BBC (2011b) as:

- In Guatemala, with 865,000 people at risk of food insecurity because of lack of state investment in smallholder farmers, and high dependence on imported food.
- In India, people already spend more than twice the proportion of their income on food than people in Britain, especially for basics.
- In Azerbaijan, wheat production fell 33 per cent in 2010 due to poor weather, forcing the country to import grain from Russia and Kazakhstan. Food prices were 20 per cent higher in December 2010 than they had been in 2009.
- In East Africa, as noted earlier, 12 million people in 2011 faced chronic food shortages due to drought. Women and children, as always, tended to be worst affected.

Rising food prices help push people into extreme poverty, with dire consequences for well-being all round. Although the World Bank did report that prices declined somewhat during the last quarter of 2011, the annual food price index was still 24 per cent above 2010. However, prices may stabilize as supplies improve (World Bank, *Food Crisis* website). Because of high food prices, many people cannot afford to invest in education, health and basic important domestic facilities (shelter, water, electricity), which can cause an upward spiral of infant and child mortality and a reluctance to reduce fertility rates if parents fear the loss of their children. Many also try coping strategies, substituting different or cheaper foods, and also eating less or going hungry, perhaps leading to undernutrition or malnutrition.

Specific geopolitical and natural events can cause food prices to spike beyond the effects of 'regular' inflation. For example, food prices in April 2011 were 36 per cent above levels a year previously, driven by problems in the Middle East and North Africa. Overall, it is estimated that almost a billion people, or almost 15 per cent of the world's population, are undernourished (Oxfam, 2011b) and that, in 2011, the lives of an additional 400,000 children might have been at risk because of high food prices (World Bank, *Food Crisis* website). The World Bank established a Global Food Crisis Response Program (GFRP) in May 2008 in response to the severity of the crisis. However, its research suggests that the subsequent 2010–11 surge in food prices hit poor people globally above the peak of the 2008 crisis level. Precise effects varied very considerably between countries because of wide variations in transmission of global prices locally and differences in households' patterns of production and consumption. The effects globally were to push a further 44 million people into extreme poverty (below \$1.25 per day; Ivanic *et al.*, 2011), with inevitable dire consequences for nutrition.

Oxfam, the International Federation of Red Cross and Red Crescent Societies and others emphasize the need for greater transparency in commodities markets, fairer regulation of futures markets and scaling up of food reserves. There needs to be discouragement or reduction of biofuels policies which divert production from food crops and consume food-producing land. There also needs to be increased investment in small farmers and women in agriculture. Food and other aid programmes that inadvertently undermine local food producers also need careful administration. Production systems must be enhanced and water supplies improved and planned for, especially in places of marginal environmental production where climate change will almost certainly have the greatest impact. Fundamental and interrelated issues, such as poverty and inequality, are of course very high on the agenda. Despite the clear need for these developments, progress is slow and food security for all the world's peoples remains an elusive goal. Unfortunately, there is scant evidence that world leaders can deal effectively even with clear current global crises in many sectors. Based on their performance to date, effective global political action to address a largely 'hidden' future crisis, such as potential food shortages and price increases, and many other impending problems in global health, seems highly unlikely.

Discussion topics

1   What are the major impacts of politically caused population movements in terms of health?
2   Discuss the major risks experienced by populations before and after armed conflict.
3   What is the likelihood of effective elimination of landmines in the near future?
4   How and why is violence, including gender-based violence, a major public health issue?
5   'Food is often consumed excessively in rich countries and insufficiently in poor countries.' How far do you agree with this statement?

11 Global health futures?

Introduction

Who knows what the future holds in terms of global health? All our futures are likely to be influenced by similar trends, but just how far we are impacted will depend on where we live, who we are and how well our environments are managed. We *exist* in a global world but we *live* locally. So, we are all affected by a complex interactive web of our national and local circumstances and environment, influenced more or less by pervasive global effects.

In this chapter, we speculate, based largely on evidence but also on some imagination, on possible health futures and risks. A confounding feature is that some potential developments – for example, urbanization – may have both positive and negative health implications. In this final chapter, we speculate selectively on how some of the issues discussed earlier may develop in terms of global health in the coming decades.

As we have emphasized throughout, global health futures will be influenced by a combination of political, technological, demographic, economic and social factors, plus natural environmental changes and incidents (speculative examples are given in Box 11.1). Some of these factors are reasonably predictable (for example, global demographic ageing, increasing urbanization), others less so (such as natural hazards, global political cooperation). It is also hard to say definitively whether some of the issues will be positive or negative. An example is global ageing, which can be a hallmark of success in health and population terms yet leads to great challenges if not properly catered for. Moreover, many of these forces will affect various areas of the globe differently, and the impacts on different socio-economic groups are also likely to be variable. Periodic global economic shocks will almost certainly continue to occur in the future and will affect the ability of governments, employers and individuals to care for their health. Healthcare inflation may put new technical, clinical and pharmacological developments beyond the reach of even moderately well-off people and governments and force explicit or *de facto* healthcare rationing. Because as much as a quarter of the world's population is likely to continue to struggle to meet day-to-day necessities and health costs, investment in education or environmental improvements may be unaffordable, of low priority, or in the luxury category.

In Chapter 10, we discussed the issue of food insecurity, for which problems are particularly focused in some countries and parts of the globe. Many predict that this is likely to continue and that food prices and availability will become even more volatile, which will likely have huge implications for health. This operates in several ways: the direct health impacts of malnutrition on everyone, especially on females and children; possible population effects, as parents may opt for larger families when infant and child mortality is high; and a lack of money to spend on health, education and domestic improvements as poor households are pushed into extreme poverty by high food prices.

So, is a longer-term future of cycles of economic downturn and poverty inevitable? Are many countries or groups likely to become increasingly aid-dependent, and small farmers in

BOX 11.1 Scenarios in global health futures?

Mainly positive:

- Population growth levels off.
- Technological improvements improve diagnosis and life-sustaining techniques.
- Better training of health and support personnel.
- New classes of drugs found.
- New and effective antibiotics and antivirals developed.
- Cure or effective treatments for dementias.
- NCDs become more controllable.
- Treatments that make many cancers liveable conditions.
- International networkings lead to improved health knowledge.
- Improvements in food security (production, GM sources, etc.) boost health.
- Health and education policies encourage lifestyle improvements (increased exercise, better nutrition, declining prevalence of cigarette smoking), leading to longer, healthier lives.
- Narrowing of socio-economic inequalities between and within countries.
- Greater gender equality.
- Genetic engineering and anti-ageing research.

Potentially mainly negative:

- Population and ageing pressures grow, numbers render services non-providable/non-affordable.
- Technology costs run above rates of inflation, increase costs and decrease access.
- Drug resistance renders most or all classes of antibiotics useless.
- Super-bugs and new viruses and other new forms of disease emerge.
- Periodic global pandemics increase.
- Urbanization exposes millions very quickly to infections, environmental pollutants and potential effects of industrial accidents.
- NCDs run out of control, reducing life expectancy.
- Increasing global criminal activity (people trafficking, drug smuggling).
- 'Lifestyle' education fails: increasing alcohol and drug abuse; growing obesity epidemic.
- Natural disasters impact more people (earthquakes, tsunamis, floods, fires).
- Climate change shifts disease vector boundaries and pathogen dynamics.
- International rivalries raise risks of conflicts; religious intolerance and conflicts.
- Food production disrupted by climate change and other factors.
- Food distribution disrupted by conflicts; starvation increases.
- Conventional war increases; nuclear war; biological and other terrorism threats increase.
- Violence against women and children continues unabated.
- Adverse technological effects; biological, chemical, nuclear accidents.
- Global financial crises impact well-being, health and healthcare.

many countries forced to quit agriculture because they cannot compete globally or because local climate change ruins their cropping capabilities?

There is increasing awareness of the very complex interaction between education, especially of mothers, and the long-term health of children and adults. Any unforeseen circumstances that disrupt such social developments may have huge impacts on health. Therefore, war, conflict situations, refugees, marginalization of some social or religious groups, and effects of long-term natural disasters, such as floods and droughts, are all likely to affect people's ability to improve their lot. Food security, and its associated circumstances, is one of the foremost items impacted by such events.

In global health terms, many feel the major issues will almost certainly involve the changing balances between non-communicable diseases (NCDs) and infectious conditions, all of which are heavily influenced by demographic factors, social conditions, individual behaviours and technological advances. Many have heralded NCDs as 'the future' but, as we have noted throughout this book, infectious conditions are by no means on the retreat or likely to be vanquished in the foreseeable future. Furthermore, humanity is very likely to lose some of its main medical weapons for treating infections, with many antimicrobial drugs losing their effectiveness and in some cases becoming wholly ineffective. So, individuals and communities who have become accustomed to easy access to antibiotics and even antiviral medicines will be thrown back onto behavioural and environmental means to achieve infection prevention and control after outbreaks. A bleak picture of a future with few new drugs for even common infectious conditions is not wholly implausible.

The demographic and epidemiological crystal ball

We will first consider likely broad trends in global population health over the coming century or so – specifically, developments in life expectancy, infant and child mortality, and disease patterns. With that demographic and epidemiological canvas painted, we will then look in more detail at selected prospective health determinants and developments.

Life expectancy

Most population health specialists project significant human life expectancy gains over the twenty-first century, although a few are less optimistic on the basis of concerns regarding the growing obesity epidemic and consequent implications for non-communicable disorders (Olshansky, 2004). The general optimism, however, is not surprising for several reasons. First, there is obvious scope for further increases in most countries. While many places and some groups currently have woefully short life expectancy, there are already several population groups that have attained life expectancy at birth levels of 90 years or more (such as Asian Americans in New Jersey – 90.9 years; Pennsylvania – 90.7 years; Connecticut – 90.1 years; and Arizona – 90.0 years; (Lewis and Burd-Sharps, 2010). So, average lifetimes of at least that length are clearly biologically attainable at the population level. Second, the knowledge and medico-technical capacity to achieve such levels exist: much mortality in both the developing and developed world is clearly preventable ('avoidable') through primary, secondary and tertiary prevention actions, even if the scope for huge gains is perhaps shrinking in developed countries. Third, this knowledge and technical capacity will inevitably expand greatly over the course of the century. Fourth, many achievable life expectancy gains do not involve high costs. That said, economic capacity, political will and other determinants of health, both national and international, will inevitably vary, and 2100 will still be far short of seeing a globally equitable healthscape.

Regular projections of life expectancy for countries and world regions are produced by the

United Nations and the US Census Bureau and made available online (e.g. UNDESA-PD, 2011 and US Census Bureau, *International Database* website). All such calculations are by definition underlain by assumptions about future mortality trends and thus will vary according to the particular assumptions adopted and the data and methodology employed. Differences in these areas will lead to different results, as the comparison of United Nations and US Census Bureau projections for selected countries for 2050 in Table 11.1 shows. As indicated, eleven of the twelve largest differences listed relate to African countries. This is perhaps not unexpected, given the demographic uncertainties surrounding those nations, though the magnitude of some of the differences is arresting. But as the listing of Singapore shows, quite substantial differences sometimes occur in projections even for more demographically advanced nations. For the *broad* development level groupings of countries, however, the figures for the two agencies are very similar.

Always in the background when considering future life expectancy is, of course, the possibility of major 'demographic shocks'. For example, projections of global mortality made before 1980 had no inkling of the HIV/AIDS epidemic that was to emerge over the last two decades of the century and put a whole new face on life expectancy futures for many populations around the globe until the introduction of highly active antiretroviral therapy (HAART) ultimately made the disease no longer an automatic death sentence. Also, as with all projections, greater confidence can be placed in shorter-term as opposed to longer-term figures.

Table 11.2 and Figure 11.1 plot the latest United Nations life expectancy at birth projections for the world and major groupings of countries from 2010 through to the end of this century. At the global level, an additional 12.6 years of life are anticipated; for the more developed regions a gain of 10.9 years; for the less developed regions 13.5 years; and for the least developed countries in the less developed bloc an additional 19.8 years. US Census Bureau projections go through to only 2050, but show similar trajectories up to that point for the three country groupings (see Table 11.2). If achieved, these gains will clearly be significant improvements in longevity, globally and regionally, but will still mean a world of marked health inequality, with inhabitants of the least developed countries and the less developed regions on average bearing life expectancy disadvantages of 10.7 and 8.1 years,

Table 11.1 Differing life expectancy at birth (years), projections for 2050

Country	United Nations	United States Census Bureau	Absolute difference
	Years	Years	Years
Lesotho	58.7	72.3	13.6
Namibia	70.0	57.8	12.2
Equatorial Guinea	64.3	74.5	10.2
Gabon	72.2	62.1	10.1
Kenya	68.6	76.4	7.8
Democratic Republic of the Congo	62.4	70.2	7.8
Sierra Leone	62.6	70.2	7.6
Zambia	63.0	70.6	7.6
Mozambique	63.9	70.8	6.9
Burundi	65.3	72.2	6.9
Togo	69.8	76.2	6.4
Singapore	85.4	91.6	6.2

Sources: UNDESA-PD, 2011; United States Census Bureau, *International Database*

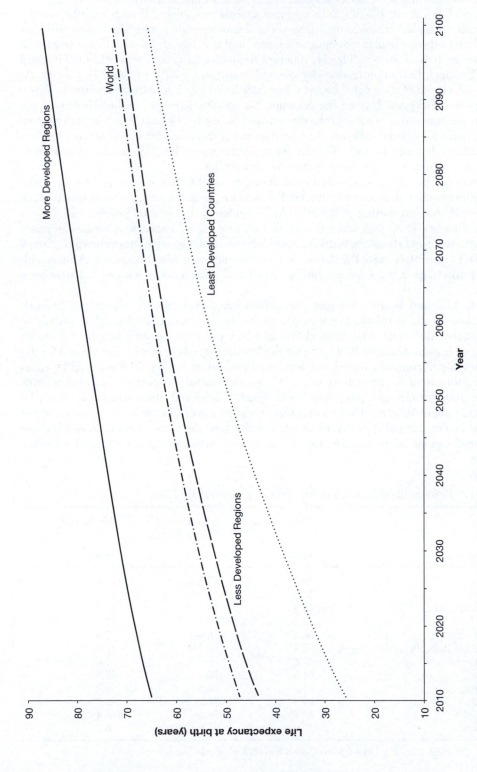

Figure 11.1 Projected life expectancy at birth, World and UN major regions, 2010–99

Source: UNDESA-PD, 2011

Table 11.2 Projected life expectancy at birth (years), World and UN major regions, 2010–99

Year	World	More developed regions	Less developed regions	Least developed countries
2010	68.6	77.5	66.7	57.9
2050	75.9 (75.7)	83.0 (83.0)	74.7 (74.9)	69.7 (70.4)
2099	81.2	88.3	80.2	77.7
% increase 2010–99	18.4	14.0	20.3	34.1

Note: 2050 figures in parentheses are US Census Bureau projections.

Sources: UNDESA-PD, 2011; United States Census Bureau, *International Database*

respectively, relative to people in the more developed regions. At the country level the life expectancy gap will be even wider (see Figure 11.2).

It is worth reminding readers of the notion of cohort life expectancy (explained in Chapter 2) here. All the above graphed, tabular and text data are period figures. Realistically, health levels will continue to improve through newborns' lifetimes and so cohort figures will be higher than these period ones. An indication of what the difference may turn out to be is given in Table 11.3, which details period and cohort projections recently released in the United Kingdom and the United States. (Note, the projections for the two countries are not comparable, however, as, in addition to the different reference dates, they are based on different assumptions of future mortality decline.)

Infant and child mortality

As has been spelled out in earlier chapters, a major feature of the global healthscape, despite substantial improvements over recent decades, relates to the marked disparities around the world in infant and child mortality. There is realistic reason, however, to anticipate that these inequalities will have narrowed markedly by the end of this century. The knowledge and technical capacity to prevent the bulk of such premature death is available. With an economically fairer world and increased global political will, this unnecessary loss of life could be drastically reduced. Table 11.4 presents the latest United Nations child (under-5) mortality projections. Achieving these gains will be one of the major health challenges of the century for the global community.

Table 11.3 Projected period and cohort life expectancy at birth (years): United Kingdom, 2058 and United States, 2086

Projected level of life expectancy (years)						
United Kingdom, 2058	*Low*		*Principal*		*High*	
	Males	*Females*	*Males*	*Females*	*Males*	*Females*
Period	81.2	85.7	86.0	89.4	90.7	93.2
Cohort	81.3	85.7	94.8	97.8	110.9	112.2
United States, 2086	*Low*		*Intermediate*		*High*	
	Males	*Females*	*Males*	*Females*	*Males*	*Females*
Period	79.4	83.2	83.4	86.8	87.7	90.4
Cohort	81.6	85.2	87.6	90.6	94.5	96.7

Sources: United Kingdom Office for National Statistics, 2010; US Social Security Administration, 2011

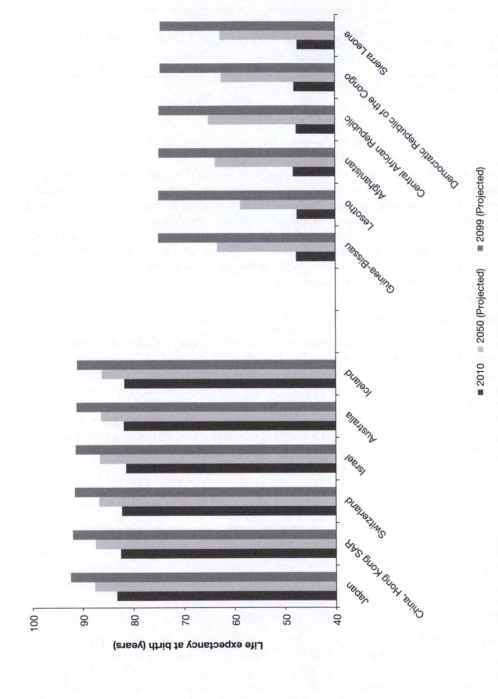

Figure 11.2 Actual and projected life expectancy at birth, selected countries, 2010–99

Source: UNDESA-PD, 2011

Table 11.4 Under-5 mortality rates,* World and UN major regions, 2010–99

Year	World	More developed regions	Less developed regions	Least developed countries
2010	62.6	7.9	69.0	118.3
2050*	30.0	5.5	33.1	45.3
2099*	14.3	3.7	15.8	19.2
Percentage decline 2010–99	−77.2	−52.5	−77.1	−83.8

Notes: * Deaths under age 5 per 1,000 live births; * projections.

Source: UNDESA-PD, 2011

Causes of death and DALYs

Outside the (hopefully unlikely) catastrophic emergence and global spread of some new ultra-virulent infectious disease, cause of death patterns over this century should see a continuation of the broad epidemiological transition of the last century to ever more deaths being due to non-communicable conditions (NCDs). However, we are unlikely to get to the stage at any time this century where, to reuse United States Surgeon General William Stewarts's oft-quoted supposed words in 1967, 'we can close the book on infectious diseases'. Indeed, that day will probably never come. As we shall see, new pathogenic microbes will continue to emerge, and old ones will go on adapting to new hosts, environments and preventive measures. With the already high interconnection and rapid transportation between countries certain to intensify, infectious disease in any part of the world is potentially a problem for all other peoples around the globe.

As part of the Global Burden of Disease project, the World Health Organization has produced projected cause-specific death and DALY figures for the year 2030 for the world as a whole and various groupings of countries. Table 11.5 summarizes the projected global pattern and those for World Bank income groups of countries. These projections can be compared with the 2008 figures in Table 4.9. The cautionary comments in the preceding section about understanding and interpreting projections are equally pertinent here.

In this projection series, the WHO foreshadows more than three-quarters (76.1 per cent) of global deaths in 2030 being due to non-communicable disease, up from 63.2 per cent in 2008 (see Table 4.9). The proportion is projected to be considerably higher in high- and middle-income countries, but lower in low-income nations, where communicable, maternal, perinatal and nutritional causes are expected still to be taking sizeable tolls. As we discussed in Chapter 7, the projection of increasing NCD deaths is the standard expectation of global health specialists, but the exact magnitude of the rise will have to await 2030 due to the uncertainties around future mortality calculations. For example, in projections released just two years before the Table 11.5 series, the baseline scenario NCD proportion for 2030 was 69 per cent (Mathers and Loncar, 2006). In that earlier projection series, HIV/AIDS deaths were projected to total 6.5 million in 2030, but in the subsequent series two years later that figure had been revised down to 1.2 million.

The specific mix of NCD deaths will vary somewhat between countries due to differing age structures, development levels, dietary and lifestyle patterns, and other health determining factors. The age structure factor will most overtly underlie the evolving pattern of dementia mortality. In low- and middle-income countries chronic obstructive pulmonary disease (COPD) is highlighted by the WHO to be a significantly larger proportional contributor to NCD deaths than in the richer developed nations, in line with (but intensifying) the current pattern. Cerebrovascular disease is similarly projected to be a proportionately

Table 11.5 Major causes of death and DALYs, World and WHO income groups, projections for 2030

Cause	World %	High-income countries %	Middle-income countries %	Low-income countries %
Deaths				
Communicable, maternal, perinatal and nutritional conditions:	13.8	5.2	7.0	24.4
Infectious and parasitic diseases	6.2	1.7	3.0	11.3
Respiratory infections	4.2	3.2	2.6	6.4
Perinatal conditions	2.8	0.2	1.1	5.6
Non-communicable diseases:	76.1	88.7	84.1	62.9
Malignant neoplasms	17.6	24.3	20.0	12.6
Neuropsychiatric disorders	2.6	6.5	1.7	2.1
Cardiovascular diseases	34.8	38.1	38.3	29.8
Respiratory diseases	10.9	5.8	13.9	9.4
Injuries	10.0	6.0	9.0	12.7
DALYs				
Communicable, maternal, perinatal and nutritional conditions:	19.9	3.8	10.0	29.9
Infectious and parasitic diseases	8.9	1.7	4.5	13.2
Respiratory infections	3.3	0.9	1.5	5.1
Perinatal conditions	5.6	0.6	2.7	8.6
Non-communicable diseases:	66.0	87.7	76.2	54.9
Malignant neoplasms	8.1	13.9	10.5	5.3
Neuropsychiatric disorders	17.1	27.6	18.7	14.2
Cardiovascular diseases	13.1	14.7	15.2	11.3
Respiratory diseases	6.3	5.3	7.6	5.4
Injuries	14.0	8.5	13.7	15.2

Note: These projections for 2030 are part of the same projection series as the 2008 figures presented in Table 4.9.

Source: WHO, *Global Burden of Disease* website

more important NCD cause of death in low- and middle-income countries, to essentially the same degrees as at present. Cancer deaths, on the other hand, are projected to be more important percentage-wise in richer nations than in low- and middle-income countries, albeit by a narrowing margin.

The burden of disease (DALYs) panel in Table 11.5 similarly shows an NCD-dominated world by 2030, but not to the same degree as deaths alone. In low-income countries, communicable, maternal, perinatal and nutritional conditions are projected to be responsible for 30 per cent of total DALYs – the *double burden* (see Chapter 4) persisting. With respect to NCDs, the most ominous projected trend is a dramatic increase in neuropsychiatric disorders we have noted before and discuss below (e.g. unipolar depressive disorders, alcohol use disorders, Alzheimer's and other dementias, schizophrenia). In rich nations, these conditions are projected to account for over one-quarter of total DALYs by 2030. The proportion will be somewhat lower in middle- and low-income countries, but still significant and likely to

BOX 11.2   Extracts from Political Declaration of the High-Level Meeting of the General Assembly on the Prevention and Control of Non-communicable Diseases

We, Heads of State and Government and representatives of States and Governments . . .

1   Acknowledge that the global burden and threat of non-communicable diseases constitutes one of the major challenges for development in the twenty-first century . . .

2   Recognize that non-communicable diseases are a threat to the economies of many Member States, and may lead to increasing inequalities between countries and populations.

3   Recognize the primary role and responsibility of Governments in responding to the challenge of non-communicable diseases and the essential need for the efforts and engagement of all sectors of society to generate effective responses for the prevention and control of non-communicable diseases . . .

15   Note also with profound concern that non-communicable diseases are among the leading causes of preventable morbidity and of related disability . . .

22   Note with grave concern the vicious cycle whereby non-communicable diseases and their risk factors worsen poverty, while poverty contributes to rising rates of non-communicable diseases, posing a threat to public health and economic and social development . . .

33   Recognize that the rising prevalence, morbidity and mortality of non-communicable diseases worldwide can be largely prevented and controlled through collective and multisectoral action by all Member States and other relevant stakeholders at local, national, regional, and global levels, and by raising the priority accorded to non-communicable diseases in development cooperation by enhancing such cooperation in this regard.

(Source: United Nations General Assembly, 2011)

swell in later decades of the century. In recognition of the great and growing health and socio-economic harm caused by NCDs, the UN General Assembly held a special high-level meeting on the prevention and control of such diseases in September 2011, deeming them a development challenge of 'epidemic proportions' (UN General Assembly, 2011; Box 11.2).

Statements about likely causes of death and DALY patterns beyond 2030 obviously become ever more conjectural. The relative importance of different health disorders, however, can be confidently expected to continue to evolve as their determinants and the capacities to prevent, treat and cure them likewise evolve. Table 11.6 presents scenarios for 2050 and 2100 that were recently published by the US Social Security Administration (Bell and Miller, 2005): cancer replacing heart disease as the dominant cause of death; respiratory disease assuming more importance; heart disease declining in proportionate importance by more than half; and vascular disease falling away to almost nothing. Only time will tell how accurate these predictions are, though.

Table 11.6 Cause of death patterns, United States, 2000–2100

Cause of death	2000 %#	2050* %#	2100* %#
Heart disease	30	19	12
Cancer	23	27	30
Vascular disease	10	5	2
Violence	6	5	5
Respiratory disease	10	14	18
Diabetes mellitus	3	4	4
Other	19	25	29

Notes: # Average of male and female percentages; * projections.

Source: Bell and Miller, 2005

Non-communicable diseases (NCDs) – the way of the future?

As seen above, NCDs have widely been predicted as humanity's future: 'epidemics' of cancers, dementias, cardiovascular conditions, diabetes, and underlying conditions such as increasing obesity, risky behaviours, poor nutrition, smoking; the list is extensive. So, prevention being far more important than cure in many NCDs, lifecourse behaviour modifications, education and environmental management all become crucial. Preventing the development for as long as possible of chronic, non-communicable conditions, especially in the context of global demographic ageing, has been a major focus for some time. The WHO (2010b) already has distinct strategies that will and must continue, usually in combination, though often with different emphases in different places and groups:

- promoting physical activity;
- reducing overweight and obesity;
- reducing sodium (salt) intake;
- promoting fruit and vegetable consumption;
- reducing alcohol-related harm; and
- tobacco control.

The 'causal pathways' for NCDs introduced in Chapters 3, 4 and 7 are also important avenues for action: underlying determinants, common risk factors, and the ultimate development of NCDs. The specific foci of these strategies may well shift within the NCD group globally over the coming decades. Very few conditions are likely to become more important than the expected huge increases in dementias.

Dementias and the future

Within the varied NCD group, psychological conditions form a huge component, and increasingly prominent are conditions associated with ageing. Looking to the future, with greater life expectancy and increased numbers of older people in almost every country worldwide, dementias are likely to increase as they are principally disorders of older years. As we noted earlier, prevalence basically increases exponentially with age, with the rate doubling every five years (Jorm *et al.*, 1987; Alzheimer's Disease International, 2009), from below 1 per cent among people in their early sixties to close to 25 per cent in the 85-plus age group. The nature and growing incidence of dementias were discussed in Chapter 7 but, looking to the future, estimates suggest that, from 35 million people with dementia worldwide in 2009–10, numbers are likely to double every twenty years. In reality, the actual rates of increase may be much higher (Dementia Research Group website). Unless significant developments occur in the treatment of dementias, which seems unlikely at the moment, the numbers affected in both rich and poor countries will increase considerably (see Figures 11.3 and 11.4). This epidemiological feature is very concerning and many feel its already major prevalence in the USA (see Box 11.3) and other demographically advanced Western nations is likely to be repeated globally within the first half of this century. This is especially worrying for low- and middle-income countries:

- Most poorer countries lack residential and daycare facilities for such conditions.
- Environments at home and in neighbourhoods are rarely 'elderly friendly', especially for people with cognitive impairments.
- In many countries, regardless of development status, carers are themselves growing older and strains on family and community resources will be enormous.
- Internal migration in many countries means younger family members are frequently geographically separated from their older relatives and are therefore not in a position to provide care.

Alzheimer's Disease International (2009, 2010) estimates that over 115 million people globally will have dementia by 2050, at least 10 per cent more than previous estimates (published in 2005). In turn, applying the average age-specific prevalence rates calculated by Jorm *et al.* (1987) to the latest United Nations population projections (UNDESA-PD, 2011) produces a total of close to 200 million sufferers by the end of the century. Large increases will occur in the developed nations, but by far the greatest, by dint of demographic weight, will be in the developing world. (Readers can refer to Chapter 7 and specficially Box 7.12 for a discussion about causes of mortality from dementias.)

Research and services are particularly needed in poorer countries. The 10/66 Dementia Research Group, part of Alzheimer's Disease International, works on dementia, non-communicable diseases and ageing in low- and middle-income countries. They suggest that

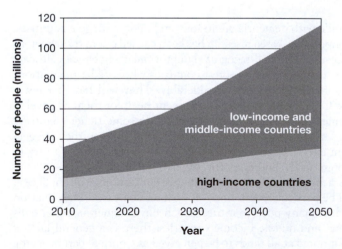

Figure 11.3 The growth in numbers of people with dementia in high-income countries compared with low- and middle-income countries, 2010–50

Source: Alzheimer's Disease International, 2010, Fig. 3, p. 16

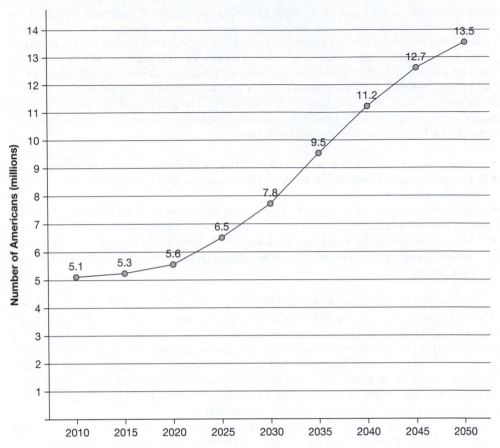

Figure 11.4 Americans aged 65-plus with Alzheimer's disease, 2010–50 (projected numbers)

Source: Alzheimer's Association, 2011, p.3

two-thirds (66 per cent) of people with dementia are in low- and middle-income countries, but only 10 per cent or less of population-based research has been carried out in those regions (Dementia Research Group website). The well-recognized improvements in basic healthcare and longevity will impact most on the current poorest countries whose older populations (and, accordingly, dementia sufferers) will grow considerably. They will have far fewer formal resources available (see Chapter 8), so there is an urgent need for them to develop practical dementia care strategies. This is now being attempted in some richer countries, such as Australia, France, the United Kingdom and elsewhere, though even they struggle and, without current long-term effective treatments, the most important thing is to try to improve care management, coordination and support.

Richer countries will have a huge amount to do, but this epidemiological challenge, alongside so many others, will be particularly enormous for poorer countries. The situation is yet to be widely recognized in many poor countries which have numerous other calls on their services. In many low- and middle-income countries, there is a general lack of awareness of dementia, which if noted at all tends to be perceived as a normal part of ageing (Alzheimer's Disease International, 2010). Many governments still unrealistically rely on family and/or well-intentioned but unresourced and largely untrained community care. This will clearly have to change globally.

BOX 11.3 A bleak picture: baby boomers and Alzheimer's in the USA

Unless we find a treatment or a cure, Alzheimer's will become the defining disease of the Baby Boom Generation. They will be 'Generation Alzheimer's'.

In 2010, 5.3 million Americans had Alzheimer's, which will increase, fast. 'Early' baby boomers are turning 65; by 2030, the US population aged over 65 will have doubled, with many more people with Alzheimer's:

[P]ossibly 16 million by mid-century, when there will be nearly a million new cases every year . . . One in eight baby boomers will likely get the disease after they turn 65. At age 85, that risk increases to nearly one in two . . . [Crucially,] if they don't have it, they will very likely be caring for someone who does. Alzheimer's was a disease boomers saw in their parents or grandparents. [Today,] Alzheimer's is their disease, their crisis, their epidemic.

Right now, we are unnecessarily losing the battle against Alzheimer's disease. Death rates for other major diseases – HIV, stroke, heart disease, prostate cancer, breast cancer – are declining. Our country's significant commitment to combat these conditions has saved lives. But for Alzheimer's disease, the federal government's efforts have been meager, and deaths are skyrocketing.

About 80,000 Americans die each year of Alzheimer's,

but only after a very long good-bye, and years of suffering endured by individuals, family and friends. Today, there are no Alzheimer survivors – none . . . Alzheimer's is not just a little memory loss. It eventually kills, but not before it takes everything away.

(Source: Alzheimer's Association, 2011, pp. 1, 2, 6, 6)

The global picture on dementia is currently gloomy, although there have been considerable recent advances in the understanding of all dementias, and Alzheimer's in particular. Looking to the future, parallel paths of seeking treatments or cures and developing practical, and affordable, care-management strategies are essential. Scientists are increasingly working towards treatment and, of course, ultimately a cure (Alzheimer's Association, 2011, 2012). However, in this respect, the immediate future is not optimistic and, as noted in Chapter 8, costs associated with dementias are likely to become enormous. Even in the USA, one of the wealthiest countries, the future is very worrying:

- Alzheimer's disease is the sixth leading cause of death in the USA, causing 78,889 deaths in 2009 (preliminary data).
- The number of Americans dying each year from Alzheimer's disease rose by about 60 per cent between 2000 and 2009.
- Alzheimer's kills more Americans every year than breast and prostate cancer combined.
- Alzheimer's is the only disease in the 'top ten' causes of death in America without a way to prevent it, cure it or even slow its progression.
- Death rates for most other major diseases, including heart disease (the number-one

cause of death), have declined, mainly due to research, policies, behavioural change and treatment.

Childhood cancers: a possible future success area?

Adult cancers may still be at very high rates in many countries, but several types now have reasonable treatments and prognoses. Moreover, the situation is even better for many childhood cancers, which can now have cure rates of 80 per cent or even higher (see Chapter 7). However, these success rates are largely confined to rich countries and rich groups in poorer countries. Elsewhere, cure rates are as low as 10–30 per cent. Misdiagnosis, lack of trained staff, lack of technical resources, cost and availability of drugs, abandonment of treatment, toxic deaths, accessibility and co-morbidities with other ailments mean that survival rates are still very low in most developing countries. So, why is this an area of potential optimism?

Several promising interconnected initiatives are emerging, which will hopefully improve survival rates: global health partnerships involving twinning between doctors in rich and poor countries; increasing access to care centres and use of satellite centres in poorer countries; lowering the costs and availability of drugs; and, increasingly, using remote technology to diagnose and discuss treatments. The Global Task Force on Expanded Access to Cancer Care and Control focuses on these issues and feels that there are possibilities for significant advances in childhood and women's cancers, as well as palliative care. It also states that 50–60 per cent of cancer mortality in low- and middle-income countries is avoidable by using country-specific strategies for prevention and treatment (Knaul et al., 2011).

We see an example of these issues and potential in the Queen Elizabeth Central Hospital in Blantyre, Malawi, one of just two hospitals in the country that treat child cancer. It is twinned through World Child Cancer with hospitals in the Netherlands and Britain which assist in specialist medical training visits to transfer knowledge and skills to medical staff in Malawi. Currently, because of a lack of diagnostic equipment in most rural areas and access, by the time many children reach the Queen Elizabeth, it is too late for them (Hammond, 2011). Many have aggressive forms of cancer, such as Burkitt's lymphoma, which are treatable if caught early. It is hoped such twinning arrangements, one of many examples internationally, will improve survival rates and local initiatives to increase awareness and accessibility to the centres.

But even greater potential for future improvement may be through local initiatives involving the use of satellite centres and technology to improve communications, as in parts of the Philippines. Here, geography separates the population between many islands, and even on the larger islands, such as Mindanao, distances and travel times are enormous. Therefore, satellite clinics can be linked with the only specialist centre and staff, often via video conferencing for initial diagnoses, sharing x-rays and pictures. These give access to the sole paediatric oncology specialist, who cannot travel frequently to see distant young patients. Follow-ups via email and texts help to bridge the distances.

A major factor in cures will be in the maintenance of treatment regimes, which are often abandoned in poor countries because of the costs and difficulties of continuation. Potentially, local staff can also gain access to advice from the largest and most advanced treatment centres anywhere in the world. This use of technology and satellites to increase access to specialist support is a reason for optimism, as cure rates of many common childhood cancers, such as leukaemias, may be brought to levels nearer to those currently seen in the developed world.

Will acute and infectious conditions continue and may they become much worse?

A *future without effective antimicrobial drugs?*

Humans almost everywhere have become used to medicine supplying treatments for commonplace and rarer conditions, both infectious and non-infectious. A huge global pharmaceutical industry exists which functions in part to find new and more effective medicines or therapies as we live in a 'microbial world' (Hofkin, 2010). Conditions that were considered life threatening even a generation ago are now routinely treated with drug interventions, such as high blood pressure, several cancers, most non-resistant tuberculosis cases, severe systemic infections and many others. Almost all antibiotics, drugs effective against bacteria, have been discovered and become widely available within the last seventy years or so (see Chapter 4). Most adults alive today and children born in all but the very poorest countries or living in the worst circumstances have been raised during a period in which drugs have been able to defeat many bacterial infections. Indeed, some drugs have also been developed to combat certain viruses (e.g. HIV, hepatitis B and C, influenza A and B), although to date viruses have proved much more recalcitrant to treatment than bacteria.

BOX 11.4 'Combat drug resistance! No action today, no cure tomorrow'

On World Health Day, 7 April 2011, the WHO warned of a possible return to the days before antibiotics were developed unless urgent global action is taken to combat the growing problem of drug resistance.

> The misuse and irrational use of drugs are weakening the fight against diseases, such as tuberculosis and malaria, that should have been contained decades ago. At the same time, other age-old diseases are on the rise, with the possibility of no cure.

Antimicrobial drug resistance is a complex problem and a global concern. It kills but also increases health costs and threatens patient care:

- An estimated 440,000 new multidrug-resistant TB cases globally annually, with extensively drug-resistant TB (XDR-TB) identified in fifty-eight countries so far.
- The fight against malaria is hampered by the emergence of resistance to the frontline drug, artemisinin.
- Treatment for gonorrhoea is threatened by growing resistance to the last-line treatment for this sexually transmitted infection.
- Emergence of hospital-acquired 'superbugs', resistant to major antibiotics, is becoming increasingly frequent.

The WHO targets health policy-makers and providers, the public, patients and civil society, the pharmaceutical industry, health institutions, prescribers and dispensers. The media will be an important influence.

(Sources: WHO, 2011d, 2011k)

However, what happens if this rapid evolution and development of medicines slows or the medicines themselves become less effective? The WHO issued a grim warning in 2011 about the future if drug resistance is permitted to continue (see Box 11.4). It is already widely recognized that many drugs used to treat diseases such as cancers can become less effective as cells become less responsive to them. Similarly, *antibiotic resistance* is increasingly common. This is the tendency for certain bacteria to develop a resistance to one or more antibiotics (see Box 11.4). It often occurs when antibiotics are used repetitively or at sub-lethal initial doses when most but not all targeted bacteria are killed by a dose of antibiotics. Inappropriate prescribing (for example, antibiotics for viral conditions), non-prescription use of antibiotics (in India and China, for example) and failure to complete drug treatment regimes are other contributory factors. The use of antibiotics as growth promoters in food animal production also plays a role in the build up of resistance. Frequent or over-exposure to an antibiotic provides conditions that allow the evolution of germs resistant to that particular antibiotic. One of the latest reinforcements of Zinsser's (1935) classic statement that 'Nothing in the world of living things is permanently fixed' is the NDM-1 enzyme, first detected in 2008 and found in many rich and poorer countries since. This enzyme makes bacteria resistant to a broad range of 'last-ditch' drugs used in antibiotic-resistant cases. Kumarasamy *et al.* (2010) see bacteria with resistance to carbapenem conferred by NDM-1 as a potentially major global health problem.

In many countries, and for some conditions in almost all countries, several antibiotic types have become either less effective or wholly ineffective. This necessitates the use of new and/or stronger antibiotics, which almost inevitably are also more expensive. Eventually, resistance can develop to all types. This has already become so serious that the New Zealand Ministry of Health (2011), for example, has warned that 'antibiotic resistance is a global threat to the treatment of bacterial infectious diseases'.

The threat of resistance is not confined to antibiotics. For example, many forms of malarial parasites in certain locations are immune to the commoner and safer, or cheaper, prophylactic drugs. *Plasmodium falciparum*, for instance, has developed resistance to most current antimalarials (e.g. chloroquine, mefloquine, sulfadoxine-pyrimethamine), although the geographical distribution of resistance to individual drugs varies (Boland, 2001; WHO, 2011d). Antiviral resistance also occurs and is potentially a major future global health risk, particularly in relation to influenza. Flu viruses can genetically mutate significantly from year to year and even change during the course of a single influenza season, making them resistant to previously effective drugs. For example, widespread resistance among influenza A (H1N1) viruses to oseltamivir (trade name Tamiflu), one of the most prescribed anti-flu drugs, has been detected in recent years. In the event of a genetically dramatically new flu virus emerging, existing drugs could prove totally ineffective and massive loss of life could occur in the time required to develop an effective new drug.

Major resistant pathogens have been called the 'ESKAPE' microbes: *Enterococcus faecium*, *Staphylococcus aureus*, *Klebsiella pneumoniae*, *Acinetobacter baumannii*, *Pseudomonas aeruginosa* and *Enterobacter* species (Boucher *et al.*, 2009). Some types of resistance, such as MRSA, are relatively new, evident only since the 1990s (see Box 11.4). Others, such as resistance to commoner penicillins, have evolved gradually over decades (see below). To date, many of the resistant bacteria or strains have been encountered either in special settings (such as hospitals) or among certain groups and individuals (such as people co-infected with HIV and tuberculosis; drug users; or people with very chronic conditions). However, there is already growing evidence in many parts of the world – especially in Asia and Latin America – of, for example, MRSA becoming acquired in the wider community, not only in institutions.

A very serious concern is that some bacteria have become resistant to almost all of the easily available, and especially the cheaper, antibiotics. They are therefore becoming more dangerous and increasingly a major public health problem. In addition to MRSA and VRE, multidrug-resistant *Mycobacterium tuberculosis* (MDR-TB) can be a major problem. Individuals in some countries with MDR-TB may be a walking health hazard and are forced to undergo prolonged treatment regimes under controlled conditions. Large numbers have been reported in poorer countries where control and health services are less able to treat them. Kerala State, India, for example, reported 200 cases and a shortage of basic and second-line drugs in 2010. In some major cities in the USA, prisons, homeless shelters and hospitals have been prime sites for transmission, especially among HIV-infected people who are particularly vulnerable to TB. Health specialists fear the spread of resistant strains widely into the community. This is a particularly dangerous threat as TB can be spread by relatively little contact. China is reported to have the second-highest numbers of MDR-TB globally and around one-quarter of the world's cases. Worryingly, a detailed study in Shandong Province found almost half of new TB cases were MDR, and mainly of the Beijing genotype strain, possibly more virulent and easier to transmit, and common throughout Asia. This suggested transmission, previously slower, may be becoming easier. As the condition is difficult to treat, it threatens TB control overall. MDR-TB in China tends to be found in the lower socio-economic groups, so it is likely to be related to poverty and lack of education, emphasizing the need to target these groups (He *et al.*, 2011).

Earlier, in the USA, increased prevalence of resistant strains spread throughout the country in the 1980s. This was assumed to be caused by a lack of compliance with drug regimes, since such medicines typically need to be taken for many months while the person may feel better after only a few weeks and stop treatment. Resistance therefore develops. The migration of people from affected areas, especially internationally, can exacerbate the spread of resistant strains.

Progress can nevertheless be achieved. New York had more cases of MDR-TB in the 1990s than other American cities but, by sustained public health measures, the problem has been reduced. Almost a quarter of TB cases were drug resistant in 1992 but sustained DOT (directly observed therapy) for people who might not take their medicines regularly, involving concerted tracing and daily follow-up of such individuals, was introduced and in the following few years new cases were reduced by 30 per cent (Schneider, 2011). Similar problems are to be seen today in parts of the former Soviet Union, China and India, but control mechanisms are unfortunately much weaker.

Yet more worrying for the future is the emergence of extensively drug-resistant tuberculosis (XDR-TB). In MDR-TB, the strains are resistant to the more common anti-tuberculosis drugs; XDR-TB, however, is resistant to virtually all, giving a 50 per cent death rate or more. The worst scenario is a return to an age when tuberculosis was not treatable. If this is replicated for some other diseases, widespread problems could emerge, even restricting international travel and leading to extreme cases of fear and isolation when persons display symptoms. 'In the struggle between microbes' ability to evolve new variations and human ingenuity in devising new defenses against them, the microbes are gaining' (Schneider, 2011, p. 168).

Unfortunately, some microbe strains which were formerly fairly innocuous are now apparently becoming more deadly, making the 'superbug' threat a real potential epidemiological future. Humans, as a species, may once again be forced to rely on old-fashioned ways of avoiding diseases, with emphasis on sanitation, isolation, avoidance, surveillance and infection control. Almost everywhere, health departments and healthcare units are emphasizing 'good practices', such as rigorous personal hygiene, hand washing, avoidance of coughing, and the like. Most importantly, health professionals and the public are being urged to minimize the use of antibiotics and, when necessarily prescribed, to complete the course. Patients need to be told to 'expect to leave your doctor empty handed' and not to demand antibiotics for conditions such as colds, caused by viruses against which antibiotics are ineffective.

Changed behaviours are especially important for many 'social' diseases, particularly sexually transmitted infections, for which prevention is much better than cure; indeed, cure may be much more difficult in the future as resistant strains emerge. In the United Kingdom in 2010, for example, annual new cases of STDs numbered almost 500,000, about two-thirds of them in women aged under 25. These diseases can have serious long-term implications for individuals' physical and reproductive health, so education and behaviour modification, and public health campaigns to promote these, are essential strategies.

Can research and industry come to the rescue?

Is the pharmaceutical industry responding to the need for new drugs? Unfortunately, as Bartlett (2011) notes, with the huge investment required to develop and test any new drug, estimated at nearly a billion dollars, and limited patent periods, the potential return on investment for any antibiotics is generally small. European health agencies remark that the last new class of drugs active against gram-negative bacteria was developed nearly forty years ago. More worrisome, around 2010, no new drug classes for gram-negative bacteria were under development. As it has historically taken about eight years from drug discovery to FDA approval, there is no new class on the horizon at the moment (Bartlett, 2011). A similar lack of research and investment has generally been seen with respect to research into drugs to fight many common 'poor country' diseases, such as malaria, over the years. However, for malaria at least, as noted below, there was some renewed hope in 2011.

Realistically, it is highly unlikely that future new drug developments will be sufficiently rapid. Demands for, and access to, drugs are growing hugely and resistance may well accelerate as more people use antibiotics and the commoner cheaper types become more accessible. Moreover, modern transportation allows people, animals, plants and pathogens to meet and mix very easily, in a short time frame. Many more people are travelling for tourism, work and migration, and they connect once-remote or isolated areas with one another, eliminating many of the geographic and cultural barriers that once limited the spread of disease. Almost nowhere is isolated these days and global interconnectedness allows infectious diseases to emerge more frequently and spread over greater distances. Some types pass more easily between humans and animals and evolve into new and more virulent strains (Relman *et al.*, 2010) and, of course, spread resistant strains, too.

Efforts are under way, such as the WHO's attempts to deter the emergence of antibiotic and other drug resistance. The Global Antibiotic Resistance Partnership (GARP) focuses on selected developing countries, where the need to maintain (cheap) antibiotic effectiveness is often paramount. In most high-income countries, antibiotic resistance has been widely recognized and is already prioritized, but this is not the case in much of the developing world, where antibiotic resistance may not even be mentioned. This is particularly a problem in low- and middle-income countries. Their burden of infectious diseases is greatest, as is their propensity to use cheaper established drugs. Poor patients with resistant infections are far less likely to have access to, or be able to afford, expensive alternatives.

Consequently, many experts are pessimistic. The Institute of Medicine (IOM, 2010, p. 1) notes, 'Infectious diseases remain among the leading causes of morbidity and mortality on our planet. The development of resistance in microbes – bacterial, viral, or parasites – to therapeutics is neither surprising nor new.' The IOM notes that evolution of resistance to antimicrobial drugs has been known but either underestimated or ignored 'since the dawn of the antibiotic era over seven decades ago' (p. 3). Indeed, evidence of resistance started to emerge almost as soon as the 'miracle drug' penicillin was introduced in 1943, and significant resistant strains had been identified by 1946. 'However, the scope and scale of this phenomenon is an ever-increasing multinational public health crisis as drug resistance accumulates and accelerates over space and time. Today some strains of bacteria and viruses are resistant to all but a single drug, and some may soon have no effective treatments left in the "medicine chest'" (p. 1). For future global health, many people feel we seriously need to address the question: what if most antibiotics become useless by, say, 2022? This could happen even sooner, as there is growing evidence in parts of Asia and in some European and North American hospitals that, for example, *Clostridium difficile* and MRSA are now effectively drug resistant, along with the HIV-related pneumonias and TB mentioned above. For antivirals, already of limited effectiveness, what if wholly untreatable strains of 'spreadable' infections, such as avian flu, become the norm? Scientists increasingly agree that multidrug-resistant gram-negative bacteria pose the greatest risk to public health, with rapid growth, and there are few new antibiotics, or ones under development, active against such bacteria. Indeed, 'drug development programmes seem insufficient to provide therapeutic cover in 10–20 years' (Kumarasamy *et al.*, 2010, p. 597).

There have been some success stories: for example, the announcement of the first new drug in twenty years that is effective against hepatitis C, a major underlying cause of liver cirrhosis and cancer; and, unusually, there may be others in the pipeline (Enserink, 2011). However, on the whole, new antimicrobials for major infections are few and far between and new ones are badly needed (*The Lancet*, 2009).

Research and clinical trials for some drugs to fight infrequent and 'orphan' drug diseases are sometimes sponsored by governments, industry and donors. Organizations such as the Bill and Melinda Gates Foundation have recently attempted to redress neglect of poor country conditions by subsidizing both research into new drugs and the distribution of existing medicines, especially those for conditions that affect children and their long-term physical and cognitive development. They hope for a future in which, for instance, polio is eradicated (Gates Foundation website). They also view education, poverty eradication and resultant better nutrition often as important as pharmaceutical developments.

There are also some other positive infectious disease fronts. Hopes, for example, are held for vaccine development with some diseases. In 2006 a vaccine preventing certain types of human papillomavirus (HPV) was approved and introduced. Over the years, much research has been devoted to malaria and HIV/AIDS vaccines and some limited successes have appeared. Malaria vaccine research and trialling has taken two basic approaches – trying to make people immune to the disease; and preventing malarial mosquitoes from spreading it (i.e. transmission blocking) – with promising results from both approaches. A vaccine conferring almost 50 per cent cover was announced in 2011, although its long-term effectiveness for all age groups is still to be ascertained. Encouraging progress towards an HIV vaccine has also been made in recent years. As of July 2010, there were two Phase II, three Phase I/II and seventeen Phase I clinical trials of preventive HIV vaccine candidates in progress, although researchers know that we have 'been here before' and success has slipped away.

Another issue related to medicines that deserves mention, and which may well increase in the future, is counterfeit or fake drugs: 'Spurious/falsely-labelled/falsified/counterfeit (SFFC) medicines', as WHO (2010c) calls them. They are deliberately and illegally mislabelled with respect to identity and/or source. This is recognized as an important problem, very widespread globally, but very difficult to quantify. It has been noted as particularly prevalent in some regions, often poorer countries where there is a strong demand for cheap, over-the-counter drugs from pharmacies, such as certain countries in West Africa and China. Counterfeit drugs may contain inert ingredients or excess amounts of effective drugs; they may even be poisonous. Drugs such as anti-malarials, anti-cholesterol, anti-diabetics, antibiotics and even anti-cancer medicines can be affected, and those for problems such as obesity and erectile dysfunction (e.g. Viagra) are especially commonly counterfeited. Generic or brand-name drugs may be involved. Depending on the type of drug, effects can range from merely ineffectual to lethal. All such drugs are unreliable, and dealing with SFFC medicines is now a considerable public health challenge that is being pursued by the WHO and Interpol, among others.

Will the world be overwhelmed by infectious diseases?

While antimicrobial resistance is a huge and increasing concern, most health Doomsday scenarios involve global infections from new or mutant viruses, for which there is little or no natural immunity and no effective antiviral drugs. How likely is this? In the 1980s, for example, in the face of a newly identified virus, HIV, it was widely predicted that this was a death sentence. It was claimed that HIV and its variants, which cause immune failure (AIDS, in this case), would kill millions and perhaps billions of people. As we now understand better, this proved to be overly pessimistic. HIV infection did not spread very easily; behavioural changes and care could avoid transmission and, today, basic antiretroviral therapy (such as Stocrin) is effective and can be subsidized to be available even in poor countries.

However, the most extreme scenarios today are predicted to involve droplet spread or easy contact-transmitted variants, especially involving influenza viruses that are spread or mutated via birds and pigs (such as avian and swine flu). Drawing fairly extensively on the potentially dangerous SARS outbreaks of 2003, there have been increased 'interdisciplinary' warnings of new or re-emerging infectious diseases in the 'global networked city', interlinked by global travel (Ali and Keil, 2008). As Frenk (2010, p. 20) notes, infectious diseases have a long record of cosmopolitan presence but 'what is new is the scale of what has been called "microbial traffic", which has expanded as a result of an explosive increase of trade and travel'. Prior to several flu-variant outbreaks, Osterholm (2007) was warning that the world was 'unprepared for a pandemic'.

Infectious disease outbreak information is available from, for example, the WHO's Global Outbreak Alert and Response Network (GOARN). This is a technical collaboration of existing institutions and networks which pool human and technical resources for the rapid identification, confirmation and response to outbreaks of international importance. Networks of networks for infectious disease surveillance can provide confirmed reports of communicable diseases through various government and university research institutes in communicable diseases such as the US Centers for Disease Control and Prevention, the UK Public Health Laboratory Service, the French Pasteur Institutes, plus global networks of schools of public health and the Training Programs in Epidemiology and Public Health Intervention Network (see, for example, the TEPHINET website). There are gaps, however, which are sometimes filled locally, regionally or globally via the internet by health professionals, local authorities, media and the general public (Box 2.5 outlined some of these, such as ProMed-mail). What most have in common is a desire to provide informed, accurate and timely views of infectious disease status locally.

The WHO's epidemic preparedness and response

Once a communicable disease outbreak has been confirmed, relevant information can be accessed by all interested parties (e.g. via http://www.who.int/csr/don/en/). An international technical and humanitarian response is then mounted if required. The WHO states that its team arrives within twenty-four hours of confirmation of an outbreak, makes an initial assessment and begins immediate control measures. Preparations are then made for a more extensive response if necessary. The WHO (2011j) states that, by linking the international response to systematic global surveillance, the worldwide 'network of networks' provides support and advice, so no one country, technical or humanitarian partner is left to shoulder the entire burden. The WHO also has a specific pandemic influenza preparedness framework for the sharing of influenza viruses and access to vaccines and technology transfer, and an international network of influenza surveillance and research laboratories. A wider sharing network for flu samples was under negotiation in 2011, which will hopefully increase vaccine and anti-viral drugs production, reduce costs and make them more affordable, especially for developing countries (WHO, 2011f).

What sorts of risks are covered and what new threats are feared? These are the major questions to which surveillance has to be alert, and examples of known current diseases of concern are given in Table 11.1. Another area is the possibility of terrorism and what the WHO calls 'deliberate epidemics'. These can include threats from known diseases such as anthrax and brucellosis (perhaps accidentally spread), as well as terrorist or military strikes with chemical or biological agents (which may be of unknown origin). Of course, this is always a speculative Doomsday scenario. More generally, the WHO's Global Alert and Response programme aims to strengthen biosafety, biosecurity and readiness for outbreaks of dangerous and emerging pathogens (the WHO mentions as examples SARS and viral haemorrhagic fevers; see Table 11.7).

Table 11.7 Various categorizations of emerging and re-emerging infections

NIAID emerging and re-emerging diseases	*Diseases covered by the WHO's Global Alert and Response (GAR)*
Group I: Pathogens newly recognized in the past two decades	
Acanthamebiasis	Anthrax
Australian bat lyssavirus	Avian influenza
Babesia, atypical	Crimean-Congo haemorrhagic fever (CCHF)
Bartonella henselae	Dengue/dengue haemorrhagic fever
Ehrlichiosis	Ebola haemorrhagic fever
Encephalitozoon cuniculi	Hendra Virus (HeV) Infection
Encephalitozoon hellem	Hepatitis
Enterocytozoon bieneusi	Influenza
Helicobacter pylori	Lassa fever
Hendra or equine morbilli virus	Marburg haemorrhagic fever
Hepatitis C	Meningococcal disease
Hepatitis E	Human Monkeypox (MPX)
Human herpesvirus 8	Nipah Virus (NiV) Infection
Human herpesvirus 6	Pandemic (H1N1) 2009
Lyme borreliosis	Plague
Parvovirus B19	Rift Valley fever
	Severe Acute Respiratory Syndrome (SARS)
Group II: Re-emerging pathogens:	Smallpox
	Tularaemia
Enterovirus 71	Yellow fever
Clostridium difficile	
Mumps virus	
Streptococcus, Group A	
Staphylococcus aureus	
Group III: Agents with bioterrorism potential	

Sources: National Institute of Allergy and Infectious Diseases and WHO, *Global Alert and Response* websites

There is also a WHO Emerging and Dangerous Pathogens Laboratory Network (EDPLN), comprising global and regional EDPLN networks of high-security human and veterinary diagnostic laboratories (in recognition of potential disease crossover from animals, and of known zoonoses). The labs can collaborate to share their knowledge, biological materials and experimental research results, to support diagnosis in international responses, and rapidly detect and contain global epidemic threats due to novel, emerging and dangerous pathogens. Longer term, they facilitate knowledge transfer about safe and appropriate diagnostic technologies, practices and training to regional networks. A major aim is to improve earlier diagnosis and management of outbreaks and infections of emerging and acute endemic disease threats. Clearly, future risks are considerable, as exemplified by the risk had avian flu (H5N1) not been contained in outbreaks up to 2011.

Predicting future outbreaks

There is a great amount of information on past and current epidemics and pandemics, but the major question is: what will happen in the future? This is naturally speculative, as it is dependent on many interlinked factors: mutations of the disease-causing organisms, interactions with human (and sometimes animal) hosts, population movements, and pharmaceutical research and developments, including drug resistance, among many other things. While many emerging diseases appear new to humanity, others are re-emerging. An important factor in the emergence of new infections can be increasing numbers of immunocompromised people who can develop severe or life-threatening conditions from infections previously thought to be non-pathogenic or not serious (Beltz, 2011).

Many feel that we can learn from past epidemics and some sophisticated historical research and modelling has been conducted. In particular, Cliff *et al.* (2009) have produced a major synthesis from a historical–geographical perspective of the factors underlying how, when and where infectious diseases emerge and re-emerge. This excellent work combines statistical and spatial methods to illustrate these processes at different scales. This follows the same research team's *World Atlas of Epidemic Diseases* (Cliff *et al.*, 2004), and builds on many other important publications by these authors on the historical evolution and geographical spread of diseases. In terms of the future of infectious diseases, Cliff *et al.* (2009) identify some key needs:

- spatial detection of (re-)emerging diseases;
- emergence detection and surveillance;
- controlling re-emerging and newly emerging diseases;
- spatial barriers: quarantine strategies; and
- aspatial barriers: vaccination strategies.

In particular, they draw on past experiences to analyse the interruption of chains of infection based on *spatial strategies* – blocking links by isolation and quarantine between susceptibles and sources of infection – and *non-spatial vaccination strategy*. Clearly, the issue of barrier control will be extremely important in the case of (re-)emergence of new forms of infectious diseases against which effective vaccinations are unlikely to be immediately available. Vaccines may be developed but these take time. If a new deadly disease, or one that disables or kills a substantial portion of those who contract it, rapidly emerges, there will be little or no time to develop a vaccine. Therefore, traditional and modern forms of barriers will be needed in both dealing with infected persons (e.g. barrier nursing) and infection-control measures in hospitals and the community in the prevention of both local and global spread. In SARS outbreaks in 2003–04, for example, extensive public health campaigns were conducted on hand washing, control of droplet infections, use of masks, and temperature checks for international travellers at many airports. Hong Kong, for instance, introduced compulsory quarantines for some infected hotels, closed schools and universities, and curtailed some non-essential services. Hospitals employed infection control and barrier nursing. In the future, more extreme measures, including widespread compulsory quarantines, bans on travel and other public health and security measures, may have to be considered. The essence will be deciding in time when to implement such measures, which is often a politically highly charged decision, with many social and economic consequences. In serious outbreaks, the necessities of public health will likely need to take precedence over the principles of individual rights.

Can we predict future outbreaks? Detailed studies suggest we can learn in principle but not always predict in detail from past infectious disease outbreaks. Research on variants of influenza viruses, some of which have turned deadly and are likely to do so again in the future, shows the situation is very complex. The Wellcome Trust (2009) provides useful summary scientific background to flu pandemics. Starting with the 1918–19 global Spanish influenza outbreak that killed an estimated 40–50 million people worldwide, Taubenberger and Morens (2010) discuss what has been learned about this 'once and future pandemic'. They note that the German physician Most asked very pertinent questions of influenza almost 200 years ago. What is influenza? Where does it come from? 'How did influenza behave in the past? In what ways can we predict future occurrences, and how will future outbreaks behave?' And, most pertinent, 'through what means can its spread be halted?' (Taubenberger and Morens, 2010, p. 17). A great deal of scientific and epidemiological knowledge exists on the first two questions, but we are not a lot closer to answering the last three with certainty.

Starting with an analysis of the 1918–19 pandemic, 'the most lethal influenza pandemic on record', Taubenberger and Morens consider the detailed nature of spread and evolution of the virus. Most communities experienced morbidity of 25 to 40 per cent, with children younger than 15 years of age experiencing the highest rates of infection. The case mortality rate in the United States averaged 2.5 per cent, and mortality was concentrated in an unusually young age group – 'those younger than age 65 accounted for more than 99% of excess influenza-related deaths', a contrast with some later pandemics (Taubenberger and Morens, 2010, p. 20).

Modern criteria to identify disease suggest that there may have been at least fourteen influenza pandemics over the past 500 years (1509 to 2009), approximately one every thirty-six years. These pandemics may not have occurred randomly and some have been followed by lengthy periods of high respiratory disease activity. This suggests there may be not only pandemic events but pandemic *eras*. As Cliff *et al.* (2009) and others point out, understanding historic outbreaks – and maybe in particular the times when these are likely to occur – will help predict what may happen and how to control it.

The next pandemic

Influenza is widely thought of as the most likely pandemic threat facing humanity. Influenza A viruses infect large numbers of warm-blooded animals and can switch hosts to form new lineages in new hosts. 'The most significant of these events is the emergence of antigenically novel influenza A viruses in humans, leading to pandemics' (Taubenberger and Morens, 2010, p. 16). However, no one exactly predicted the emergence of the 2009 H1N1 swine-origin pandemic virus, and Taubenberger and Morens are pessimistic whether, given current knowledge, anyone will be able to predict future pandemics *accurately*. This includes the timing and location of the next pandemic, what sub-type it will be, and its likely impact in terms of morbidity and mortality. Indeed, Morens and Taubenberger (2011) state that although we have learned much about pandemic influenza and epidemics, there is yet more that we do not know. Puzzles surrounding the evolution and combination of viruses, transmission between other hosts and humans, and many other factors have meant pandemic influenza has produced surprises and highlighted numerous gaps in scientific knowledge. 'Understanding and predicting pandemic influenza emergence' is something we are currently far from being able to achieve (Taubenberger and Morens, 2010, p. 24).

The majority of the world's younger (under 40) population has no protective immunity to the influenza virus sub-types circulating between 1957 and 1968. So, the human susceptibility factor is one complex risk, as well as many other potential viral combinations that could underlie future pandemics. Yet, ironically, in the case of influenza, for example, improved understanding of the viruses has made for even less certainty about the determinants of, and possibilities for, future pandemic emergence. The unpredictability of sources and the potential ranges of pandemic morbidity and mortality also have to be acknowledged. Therefore, planning will have to include the range of approaches noted above.

Must we be pessimistic? In the case of influenza, a good example, until a reasonably universal influenza vaccine or better drug treatments can be developed, and made available and affordable, especially in poorer countries, humanity will have to rely on robust basic public health approaches to outbreaks and pandemic controls. For influenza in particular, these must be supported surveillance, data sharing and cooperation, to include humans, domestic animals and wild birds. The United Nations warnings that H5N1 (avian flu) might kill millions in 2006 and the WHO's declaration of an A/H1N1 (swine flu) pandemic in 2009 may have been somewhat premature, but international caution, monitoring and preparedness need to remain high (CDC, 2011b). Effective intervention strategies must be put in place to reduce transmission and disease, with the implementation of effective non-pharmaceutical interventions. As noted above, a proposed WHO network would attempt greater sharing of flu samples and hopefully lead to better and cheaper antivirals and possible vaccines, with the pricing element being especially important for poorer counties.

Scientific research is, of course, crucial to develop treatments and vaccines, with an ultimate aim of a universal vaccine against all sub-types, although difficult as many are constantly evolving. Scientific input can be in the form of vaccines, antivirals, genome sequencing and modelling. Surveillance, and research on genetic features which cause strains to become more virulent and perhaps easier to transmit between humans, is crucial for both development of prevention and treatments. Health policy may focus on initial containment and hygiene measures and, later, mitigation to minimize the impacts of an epidemic (Wellcome Trust, 2009). As Taubenberger and Morens (2010) discuss, new vaccine methodologies are almost within reach, and international agreements on production, distribution, intellectual property, costings and administration must be achieved. Once infections occur, however, antiviral drug stockpiles have generally been limited in size (although this is improving) and effectiveness. So, in terms of prevention, containment and control of outbreaks of influenza and many similar infectious diseases, strong, unified political effort and collaboration are essential, in parallel with advances in basic science. Taubenberger and Morens further note that, until scientific breakthroughs occur in understanding, prevention and treatments, humanity's ability to anticipate pandemic events will remain poor and the currently available anti-pandemic weapons weak. Therefore, much will depend on carefully planned, strong responses. But even now we may not be much more advanced than we were in 2006–07, when Osterholm (2007) noted that the world was unprepared for a pandemic.

Concern about the emergence of swine flu or an H5N1 bird flu pandemic is clearly warranted, given their possible high case fatality rate and potential for spread and mutation.

However, many other possibilities for future pandemics must also be anticipated and planned for. HIV/AIDS was a salutary reminder of the possibility of devastating epidemiological 'shocks'. It is almost certain there are unknown animal pathogens in remote areas of the world that will at some time jump species and become virulent zoonotic infections of global significance. In the past, a reactive ('wait and respond') approach has often been taken to infectious disease emergence and lives accordingly have needlessly been lost because of no early-warning system. For instance, the HIV/AIDS epidemic came slowly to world attention when cases were detected in California in 1981. However, examination of preserved plasma and lymph node samples taken in the then Belgian Congo (now the Democratic Republic of the Congo) in 1959 and 1960 has revealed HIV infection. Subsequent studies have in turn pointed to the virus circulating in Africa many years before that. With earlier detection, the disease might have been contained and millions of deaths and much ill-health avoided. This lesson from HIV/AIDS has led to more proactive approaches to disease detection now being pursued, as noted above, through such initiatives as Global Viral Forecasting (see GVF website). Wild and domestic animals and sentinel human populations living in remote geographical regions in Africa and Asia are being monitored by GVF to detect new and potential zoonotic infections before they take hold and expand into global pandemics. This surveillance work is essentially a 'one health' approach, recognizing actual and potential disease linkages between humans, animals and the environment, combining human and veterinary medicine, viral and bacterial genetics and wildlife ecology (American Veterinary Medical Association, 2008; Kahn, 2006).

Will urbanization and globalization increasingly pose disease and other health risks?

Population growth, concentration and movement of people into new areas, perhaps associated with climate boundary changes, are generally considered to be major potential reasons for the likely continuing emergence and re-emergence of many infectious diseases. Social and demographic changes, associated with urbanization and the interdependence of globalization, have facilitated and perhaps accelerated the spread of pathogens. Wilcox and Gubler (2011) note that environment and landscape changes stemming from human activities have interfered with many natural ecosystems (see Chapter 9). Especially important are the spread of settlements and agriculture into peri-urban habitats, along with deforestation, and the spread of intensive farming. Irrigated agriculture, often with inadequate drainage and sewerage systems, can lead to the spread of water-borne or water-vectored diseases (such as diarrhoeas, cholera, leptospirosis, malaria and dengue). A variety of known and new tick-borne diseases can afflict humans when they enter animal habitats for work, residence or, increasingly, recreation (see, e.g., McNeil, 2011) and there are also certainly many types yet to be identified.

Demographic changes are almost inevitably the major direct and indirect factors in the increase in infectious disease, although rather different underlying mechanisms can be at work in urban and rural environments. The huge growth of cities over the past half century is likely to continue and even accelerate in coming decades as people, perhaps optimistically, see city dwelling as the way to a better life. Even with the relatively minor counter-urbanization trends, enabled as some people choose to work from home in more congenial rural or suburban locations, the growth of cities and conurbations seems unstoppable. Two hundred years ago only about 3 per cent of the world's population lived in cities, while today 50 per cent do; and, by 2050, the United Nations estimates the figure will be close to 70 per cent. Simple demographics mean the urban surge will inevitably be strongest in the less developed world, with urban dwellers in those regions anticipated to swell by

2.7 billion between now and mid-century (UNDESA-PD, 2011). There were fewer than eighty cities of over a million people in 1950, but such places will probably exceed 1,600 by 2015. Depending on definition of city areas, in 2011 there were over twenty urban agglomerations ('mega-cities') of over 10 million people, and at least four of more than 20 million, figures unbelievable only a few decades earlier (UNDESA-PD, 2010). The city will increasingly be a unit for health analysis, in terms of risk, health policy and services (Gusmano *et al.*, 2010).

The massive scale of the urban health challenge lying ahead is starkly illustrated by the following selected figures of projected city population growth for just the fifteen-year period 2010–25: Delhi 6.4 million; Dhaka and Kinshasa 6.3 million; Mumbai 5.8 million; Karachi 5.6 million; Lagos 5.2 million; Kolkata 4.6 million; Shanghai 3.4; Luanda and Manila 3.3 million; and Lahore and Kabul 3.2 million (UNDESA-PD, 2010). Many others are facing increases of 2 million or more over this period. Massive further growth in turn lies beyond and, in many cases, it will almost certainly be impossible for urban housing, water, sanitation, employment and health service infrastructure to keep pace.

Indeed, already, urban infrastructure provision has often failed to match population growth. Wilcox and Gubler (2011) note that massive urban population increase has been matched by a similar increase in global infectious disease vulnerability from just this one factor. Cities may offer some, though by no means all, inhabitants better access to health-care, but this may be outweighed by exposure to other emerging health risks because of the conjunction and connection of so many humans.

Millions of people crowded in close proximity, often living in different socio-economic circumstances yet sharing facilities such as public transport, offices and services, gives ample opportunities for spread of both simple and serious infectious diseases. Commuting brings people together in common spaces for work, shopping and recreation from over great distances, exposing enormous numbers in multiple daily interactions. Urban living, with its many new and often changing environmental facets, provides abundant opportunities for food-, water-, air-, rodent- and vector-borne pathogens to establish and multiply in human populations (recall the epidemiological triad shown in Box 3.1). In general, each pathogen has its own transmission and adaptive characteristics, giving a minimum threshold population for survival (e.g. about 250,000 people for measles). But, whatever the threshold, the emergence of very large and mega-cities easily provides such numbers (Wilcox and Gubler, 2011). 'The triumph of public health is largely responsible for making cities more habitable' (Gusmano *et al.*, 2010, p. 4). The reverse may conceivably occur: the potential breakdown of public health in the face of an unstoppable new or resurgent disease, or, more likely, the combination of several lesser but cumulative infectious waves, also has the potential effectively to make cities death traps. The emergency medical services of many major cities are already working at close to capacity. Even a mild pandemic could overwhelm the USA's stretched healthcare system (Osterholm, 2007).

Urban growth will inevitably lead to social and environmental consequences that favour spread of infectious diseases, given population movement and concentration bringing together and exposing larger and new populations. Resistance to possible treatments may also emerge. Poverty and associated poor living conditions, particularly lack of sanitation and infrastructure for waste-water disposal and solid waste management, increase opportunities for vector-borne diseases and illnesses that may pass from animals to humans. Mosquitoes such as *Aedes albopictus* (the vector of viral infections such as dengue fever, yellow fever, West Nile virus) are well adapted for breeding in small amounts of water in discarded receptacles, and this potential vector of viral diseases has readily taken advantage of environmental change. Malaria is also increasingly transmitted within developing world cities, the parasite-carrying *Anopheline* mosquitoes finding suitable habitats associated with the watering of crops in urban farming and small amounts of water readily found in warm, wet climates. Industrial-scale intensive animal production globally may favour proliferation and spread of water- and food-borne pathogens and can encourage antibiotic resistance when these are used in the animal production food chain. Non-vectored diseases of poverty, poor housing and overcrowding (such as tuberculosis and sexually transmitted infections) will also be a growing threat.

In most rural areas, population growth may be less significant in disease emergence, especially in areas of outmigration, but the demands of urban areas for food encourage agricultural extension, as well as lumber trade and mining to supply resources. These factors often mean new, perhaps non-immune, populations move into new environments. Extractive activities, deforestation and changes in land use transform rural landscapes and make the spread of diseases easier (Wilcox and Gubler, 2011). It would be almost impossible, even if anyone wished to try, to halt or reverse the global trend of urbanization and con-comitant urban demand for accommodation, manufactured products and food. Therefore, future growth in numbers exposed to many new and old pathogens in urban areas and former rural areas is likely to continue unabated. The potential for new and unpredictable epidemi-ological futures is enormous. Health and other public policies will have to recognize this and plan accordingly; and, in particular, urban and regional planning must take careful account of health consequences of population expansion.

Alongside these health threats to urbanites will likely be continuing (perhaps worsening) threats of non-pathogenic origin. Two particularly 'urban' threats are: respiratory and cardio-vascular problems caused by air pollution emitted by industry and vehicular traffic; and road traffic-related injuries and deaths (as noted in Chapter 8). Industrial air pollution (e.g. particulate matter, sulphur oxides, carbon dioxide) is already a major health problem in many developing world cities and its health consequences are increasingly acknowledged (see Chapter 9). The danger is, however, that health concerns will be sacrificed in the pursuit of economic growth, and heavy polluters will be allowed to continue essentially unchecked. In turn, with economic growth and increasing affluence, personal vehicle ownership levels will inevitably rise among city populations, as will the total volume of emitted particulates and other pollutants (such as carbon monoxide and dioxide, oxides of nitrogen, hydrocarbons, and lead) unless rigorous air-quality policies are implemented – which is especially unlikely in cities in poorer nations. Increased road traffic in congested cities will likewise see rising numbers of accidents and casualties. Rising urbanization will almost certainly also see adverse shifts in diet and activity and rising prevalence of over-weight/obesity (with implications for NCDs such as cardiovascular disease, diabetes and certain cancers), through more sedentary lives and wider consumption of processed low-fibre, high-fat foods. Mental disorders (especially depression and anxiety) are also likely to burgeon. Additionally, numerous major cities have coastal locations and are thus particularly vulnerable to the health consequences that would follow from any significant sea level rise due to climate change (see Chapter 9).

At the basis of much concern, implicitly or explicitly, has been population growth and fear of Malthusian checks, perhaps in the form of food shortage and/or disease. On this front, projections of global population totals for the mid-twenty-first century are unpredictable, to say the least. From around 7 billion in 2011, predicted totals range from 8.1 to 10.6 billion by 2050 (UNDESA-PD, 2011). Some projections then suggest levelling off or even decrease, while others show population growth continuing unabated to 2100. The only certainty is that what actually happens will be extremely dependent on social, economic, political, environmental and, certainly, health conditions. If China, for example, totally relaxes the one-child policy, will there be a population boom in the most populous country? Social research indicates not, but equally there are many poorer countries which still have high fertility rates and, in these countries, poverty and urbanization often conjoin to provide huge problems for all classes of diseases, both infectious and NCDs.

An increasing role of natural disasters in the spread of diseases?

The first years of this century have seen a large number of natural disasters, and the internet age has helped bring reports to our attention very rapidly. As discussed in Chapter 9, with continuing global climate change, climate-related disasters (such as extreme storms, floods, heatwaves, fires and droughts) can be expected to increase, with potentially profound health effects. The future regarding other geophysical disasters, such as earthquakes, tsunamis and volcanic eruptions, is less predictable, but it will need to be a central consideration in health planning in vulnerable regions.

Natural disasters have immediate effects in terms of death and serious injury, while subsequent disrupted conditions can lead to even more death and morbidity if epidemic diseases take hold. However, the relationship between natural disasters and communicable diseases can be misunderstood. It is often assumed risks of spread of infection are high because of the chaos that often follows natural disasters, perhaps because of risks from dead bodies. But the risk factors for outbreaks after disasters often stem from population displacement (see Chapter 10). This goes on top of the loss or disruption of safe water supply, sanitation, shelter, health services and disruption of supply chains for medicines and food. People may be crowded together and be at extra risk, especially if the pre-existing health status of the population is not good. The nature of the local environment and the disease ecology all interact, as Watson *et al.* (2007) discuss in terms of risk factors for outbreaks after a disaster, likely communicable diseases and establishment of priorities.

There will be inevitable short- and long-term effects of natural disasters on, for example, the provision of health and other services, including shelter, sanitation and education. A lot depends on the efficiency of local recovery. The health disruption and social aftermath of the Haiti earthquake, for example, were still evident well over a year later, as few services had been restored and many buildings and infrastructure were still damaged. This contrasts with the relatively rapid rebuilding after the 1995 Kobe earthquake. However, in the same country but in a different context, the Japanese post-earthquake tsunami of March 2011, which killed almost 20,000 people, created ongoing disruption to healthcare services, in part because of the associated damage to nuclear power stations which rendered large areas uninhabitable.

Will technology come to the rescue?

We speculated elsewhere in the book and earlier in this chapter whether technology – perhaps in the form of pharmacological inventions such as new antimicrobial drugs or pharmacological treatments for non-communicable conditions such as dementias and obesity – might come to humanity's rescue in disease prevention and treatment. Like most other researchers, we are somewhat pessimistic. However, technology – of course, a hugely broad concept – may well have a boom-time in the next two or three decades. This will be likely in both new technology for treatment and diagnosis, and in the extension and application of existing technologies (particularly the internet and expanding mobile phone networks) to knowledge, diagnosis and treatment options. This is an enormous area, but we can speculate that technology will impact on global health in almost every respect. It could be especially important in:

- Diagnostic capabilities: blood tests for many diseases, including cancer tests and predictions; safer, faster and more accessible scanning techniques in the field of magnetic resonance imaging (MRI), computerized tomography (CT) and positron emission tomography (PET) may well emerge.

- Access to information for healthcare professionals and the public: this is most likely to be the major technological advance in the coming decade. Internationally, almost all places can already access similar data sets, information, diagnostic criteria and treatment protocols for almost all types of disease and condition. However, rising information availability via the internet is being matched by rising expectations in many countries.

- Treatment diagnosis and sharing, meaning access to specialist advice can be extended to remoter areas. This is also likely to make great strides in both richer and poorer countries in the coming decades. In particular, mobile phone technology is enabling many remote areas, especially in poorer countries, to leapfrog communications barriers and access advice and treatments.

- 'Magic bullet' research is progressing for treatments in many diseases. But, as noted earlier, there are many gaps and the future 'pharmaceutical armoury' against many common infections is not well stocked, nor are there numerous new drugs in the pipeline for many key conditions.

- Better shelf-life of medicines and, for example, vaccines that can be transported without the need for keeping them cold.

- Better, cheaper treatments for many NCDs and conditions, including the most common, such as hypertension, high cholesterol and diabetes, with fewer side-effects; research into major current and increasing conditions, such as dementias; better control for some mental disorders.

- Nanotechnology developments could revolutionize medicine across a range of areas: gene therapy, drug delivery, biomedical imaging, cell repair, diagnostic tools, disease prevention.

- Better understanding may well be achieved of the heritability and hence the prevention or anticipation of some conditions in families, especially for, say, cancers and dementias.

- Genetic engineering/stem-cell technology, both in disease prevention and treatment, and in some control of vectors, continues to advance. Already better prediction and targeted or personalized treatments are possible for some cancers, such as those sub-types of ovarian and breast cancers that are associated with defective genes. For others, diagnosis of people with certain specific defective genes can help identify those at greater risk of developing some types of cancer. At present, most of this is still research in progress or available only in specialized centres. Nevertheless, many health services, at least in richer countries, are realizing what services and treatments they may be called on to provide in the future. Research in gene therapy is a fast-moving area.

- Refinements in existing reproductive health technologies and development of new technologies are likely to provide even greater ability to extend the reproductive years of some women, but may bring unpredictable financial and social costs.

- Biological research in vector control is already yielding some results, for example in genetically modified mosquitoes in the fight against dengue and malaria. This type of high-technology research may become more widespread and yield opportunities to control the vectors of a number of diseases affecting humans and animals, although some groups are concerned about possible unexpected environmental side-effects of biological control.

- Telecare for home delivery of many simple tests, results and ultimately some treatments.

- Technology for home care: this has been researched extensively in the context of long-term care for people with disabilities and especially ageing populations. The area of *gerontechnology* is increasingly researching how technology, from communications to robotics, can assist older people to live in their own homes or support carers. While many aspects are experimental and futuristic, their applications are being extended and attempts are being made for many types to be practical and affordable.

• Technology for health care education: this too will be one of the major developments in the coming decades, as health sciences, nursing, medical and paramedical students and professionals have their depth and range of education and examples greatly extended.

Unfortunately, while the technical capacity for all the above is in the realm of the likely, it is almost certain that not all of humanity will benefit from them equally in the foreseeable future. Economic and political power will inevitably see the inequalities and gradients in health and healthcare continue, and perhaps even increase, in relation to technological advances. In short, the wealthiest 10 per cent of people in any country will have a better chance of gaining access to them than the poorest 10 per cent. Likewise, citizens of developed nations will generally obtain the benefits ahead of those in poor countries.

Longer life and better or worse health?

In concluding this chapter and the book, it is important to return to a theme raised several times in previous chapters. Health and health status are changing almost everywhere, usually but not always for the better. Globally, people are living longer and, with a few exceptions, most countries have a longer life expectancy in 2011 than they had in 2000 and certainly a few decades before. But what are the limits to longevity and, as the WHO's maxim reminds us, we need to ask if we are 'adding life to years' or simply adding years to life?

Are we perhaps approaching the limits, or are substantial further gains still likely? That question of future human longevity has attracted the attention of a wide range of disciplines – demography, gerontology, biology, medicine, economics, philosophy, etc. – and unsurprisingly has produced diverse conclusions on the topic. The following references convey a good representation of that diversity: Harper and Howse (2008); Oeppen and Vaupel (2002); Carnes *et al.* (2003); Miller (2002); Olshansky (2004); Richel (2003); Sonnega (2006); and Wilmoth (1998).

While the 'human machine' must ultimately wear out, we feel there is good reason to believe that an average life expectancy at birth of close to 100 years is achievable within some countries by the end of this century. Since 1840, best-performance life expectancy has steadily increased by three months per year (Oeppen and Vaupel, 2002) and, catastrophic global pandemic, nuclear war or environmental change shocks aside (see Box 11.5), further significant increases can be confidently anticipated, even if at diminishing rates to those of the past. As we have shown in earlier chapters, much current mortality is preventable, especially in poorer countries. That, parcelled with the likely technological advances in medicine and public health (such as disease prevention and cure, and regenerative medicine) listed in the preceding section, plus likely developments in age-retardation biology, underlies our assessment. As noted earlier in the chapter, some population groups have already attained average life expectancies at birth of 90 years or more. Offsetting this optimism in the eyes of some, however, is the potential future effect of the growing obesity and associated NCDs epidemic in both the developed and developing world (Olshansky, 2004; Swinburn *et al.*, 2011).

Assuming that longevity expansion still has some way to go, what quality of health might then be expected? Global health researchers are not uniform in their assessment of what happens as populations grow older. Are people better off in terms of health – and welfare?

Or do people have longer life and possibly poorer health, as Verbrugge asked in 1984? To many, having a good life and a good death is more important than adding some extra but possibly unrewarding years of poor health. So, global health research is increasingly having to face more difficult ethical issues and qualitative concerns about what welfare and quality of life are like for survivors.

BOX 11.5 Disaster scenarios

Nuclear conflict

For most of the second half of the twentieth century (the 'Cold War' years, 1946–91), the world lived under the threat of global nuclear war and consequent 'nuclear winter' (atmospheric smoke-induced global cooling). Approximately a billion people were seen as likely to die directly from blast, heat and immediate radiation effects in a major 'Superpowers' nuclear war, and hundreds of millions more left severely injured. Many millions more would have died in subsequent years from radioactive contamination and nuclear winter conditions (*Ambio*, 1982).

Post-Cold War, the threat of global nuclear warfare has somewhat receded, but regional-scale conflicts remain a serious possibility. Nuclear exchanges between India and Pakistan, Israel and Iran, and North Korea and South Korea/Japan, for instance, are possible. While casualties in such attacks would probably be smaller than from a global conflict, they would nonetheless be large. Estimates suggest an exchange between India and Pakistan involving 100 nuclear weapons of 15 kilotons each could produce about 21 million fatalities. A similar-sized exchange between Israel and Iran could cause around 10 million deaths (Toon *et al.*, 2007). In addition, substantial global-scale climate anomalies (e.g. surface temperatures, precipitation rates, growing seasons) from light-absorbing smoke emissions from the blasts into the atmosphere would occur, likely severely degrading agricultural productivity for many years.

On a smaller geographic and demographic scale, there is also the possibility of nuclear attacks by terrorist organizations. Nuclear weapons can be made compact and lightweight and attacks could potentially be delivered by simple land, sea or air transport.

Large abrupt climate change

The majority of climate scientists believe the world is in a period of climate warming and associated environmental change and that this is likely to continue for a long time, with significant impacts on human health around the globe (see Chapter 9). Projected changes this century, while alarming, are envisaged as relatively gradual, making adaptation to the changes easier than would be the case with larger and more abrupt change. However, palaeoclimatic records show that large, abrupt changes to the global climate system have occurred frequently. Temperature changes of up to 16 degrees Celsius and precipitation doublings, for example, have occurred in periods as short as decades or less (Committee on Abrupt Climate Change, National Research Council, 2002) and might therefore presumably happen again. Such changes occur when a threshold in the climate system is crossed. 'Triggers' external to the climate system, such as changes in the Earth's orbit or a brightening or dimming of the sun, could bring this about; so could internal triggers, such as emissions of climate-altering

continued

gases into the atmosphere. This raises the question of whether human-induced greenhouse gas emissions might ultimately trigger abrupt, larger climate change than is currently projected. This would clearly have enormous impacts on global health futures.

Major infectious disease pandemics

Catastrophic infectious disease pandemics could drastically revise the likely twenty-first-century global health future of steadily rising life expectancy that we have charted. There is the constant possibility of a deadly, completely new pathogen emerging or an existing one mutating into a new hyper-virulent form and exacting a massive global toll. Sequential visitations by different such pathogens, perhaps becoming more potent, would be the worst scenario. Highly contagious killer infections would be the most likely candidates. With a novel, swiftly spreading deadly infection, enormous numbers of deaths could occur before any effective medical treatment could be produced. Any such treatment would likely be costly, so poorer countries could probably afford only limited coverage.

As noted in several chapters, there is some, although not unambiguous, evidence of a compression of morbidity, in that many older populations have a longer life with a compression of serious or disabling illness into a shortening period at the end of life. But will this continue? We started this chapter with a rather gloomy prediction of existing and probably increasing 'pandemics' of non-communicable diseases. Several authorities paint dire pictures of the future of ageing populations with high rates of dementias and decreasing funds and personnel to provide care for them. For many, such epidemiological futures will present major challenges – to individuals, families, nations and the global community.

Faced with ageing populations and workforces and a future of population decline, some large-population countries in Europe and Asia, such as Germany, Spain, Italy, Japan and, especially, China, will have to consider seriously pushing 'population revitalizing' pro-natalist policies in the coming decades. Some, such as Russia are already attempting this. Policies to stimulate people to have more children, if successful (and past experience is not positive), will have enormous implications for health, social welfare and education systems. They will have to provide good maternal and health care, ever better education, and support systems for both younger and older age cohorts. Immigration expansion may also become a necessary demographic path for some countries, and this would also have major implications for health systems, demands for health personnel and social integration. There will also be a need to reconsider age, longevity and work. The notion of 'retiring' from formal employment in one's early or middle sixties might make sense when life expectancy is only a few years greater; but when longevity has grown well beyond that, can a retirement and pension age of an earlier demographic era be sustained? With this in mind, several developed nations (including Japan, France, Germany, the United Kingdom and Australia) have raised or signalled their intention to raise their pensionable ages, and some have effectively made formal retirement ages illegal. But, so far, there is not great evidence that many countries have fully considered the combined implications of the changing demographic dividend. This, then, may be one of the greatest future global health challenges.

Discussion topics

1 The current existence of an 'epidemic' of non-communicable diseases (NCDs) is widely reported. How do you see this developing in the coming few decades in different parts of the globe and what can be done to avert it?

2 What can be done to help avoid the emergence of ever greater antimicrobial drug resistance?

3 What forms and features of technology are likely to have the greatest impact on health and well-being in (a) low-income developing nations (b) high-income developed countries?

4 What health-related population policies do you think are likely to be needed in ageing populations over the next fifty years?

5 Discuss the cases *for* and *against* rationing of healthcare for older people in the more developed world in light of the rapid ageing of populations and rising costs of healthcare. (Read: Evans, 1997; Williams, 1997; Moody, 2010.) What is your view on the idea of age-based healthcare rationing?

Glossary

Acute disease A disease of rapid onset and usually of brief duration. The term carries no connotations about the severity of a disease. (Compare with *Chronic disease.*)

Anthropogenic Caused by humans.

Antibiotics Drugs used to treat infections caused by bacteria and certain other micro-organisms. There are various classes that target different bacteria. Common antibiotics include penicillins and streptomycin. Antibiotics cannot cure viral infections.

Arboviral disease A viral disease transmitted by arthropods (i.e. arthropod-borne). There are over 100 arboviruses that affect humans, mosquitoes being the most common vector. Dengue and yellow fever are the most serious and widespread arboviral diseases.

Bacteria Single-celled microorganisms that sometimes cause illness to humans and animals. Examples include *Vibrio cholerae, Mycobacterium tuberculosis, Yersinia pestis* and *Escherichia coli (E.coli)*. Some bacteria are beneficial and indeed essential to life.

Burden of disease A measure of disease combining years of life lost due to premature mortality and years of life lost due to time lived in states of less than full health – DALYs (disability-adjusted life years).

Cancer A group of diseases involving body cells multiplying out of control to form masses of tissue (tumours) that damage the area around them. Cancer cells frequently metastasize: that is, spread to and invade and damage other parts of the body. Cancers are termed malignant neoplasms (tumours) and comprise ICD-9 Codes 140–208 and ICD-10 Codes C00–C97.

Cardiovascular disease Any disease of the heart or blood vessels (e.g. stroke, ischaemic heart disease, peripheral vascular disease). The major cause of death in developed countries. Also referred to as circulatory disease. ICD-9 Codes 390–459, ICD-10 Codes I00–I99.

Cause of death Deaths are categorized according to the World Health Organization's International Statistical Classification of Diseases and Related Health Problems. The cause of death in this classification is defined as the underlying cause: that is, the disease or injury which initiated the train of morbid events leading directly to death. The underlying cause may be different from the immediate cause. For example, the underlying cause of death of a person who fell and broke a hip and then went on to develop and die of pneumonia in hospital would be the fall. The immediate cause would be pneumonia. The current version of the International Classification is the 10th Revision (ICD-10).

Cerebrovascular disease Abnormal condition of the blood vessels of the brain resulting in impairment of blood and oxygen flow to the brain. Interference to the circulation due to bleeding from a weakened artery (cerebral haemorrhage) or blockage of an artery (cerebral thrombosis and cerebral embolism) is known as a stroke. ICD-9 Codes 430–438, ICD-10 Codes I60–I69.

Chronic disease A disease that persists for a long time. The term carries no connotations about the severity of a disease. (Compare with *Acute disease.*)

Cohort A group of persons who experience a certain event (e.g. birth, marriage) during a defined time period.

Co-morbidity When a person has two or more health problems at the same time.

Compression of morbidity The proposition that, as mortality declines, ill-health and disability will be compressed into the later years of life (due to improving living standards and medical and public health advances).

Crude death rate The number of deaths in a specified period (usually one year) divided by the average total population in that period (usually taken as the mid-year population). The rate is normally expressed per 1,000 population.

Degenerative disease A disease that involves the biological deterioration of the body (e.g. heart disease, some cancers, rheumatoid arthritis, etc.), usually but not always associated with ageing. Sometimes referred to as non-communicable diseases (compare with *Infectious disease*).

Demographic transition The long-term shift of birth and death rates from high to low levels in a population. The decline in mortality normally occurs first, leading to a period of rapid population growth before fertility starts to fall. Some writers prefer to term this process the vital transition, using demographic transition as more of an umbrella concept covering transitions on a variety of demographic dimensions besides fertility and mortality (e.g. in age structure, causes of death, mobility, population distribution).

Determinant of disease A factor (e.g. characteristic, behaviour, event) that influences the occurrence of a disease.

Differential mortality The differences in mortality between various sub-groups of the population (e.g. age, ethnic, occupational, place of residence groups) at a particular time or within or between different cohorts.

Disability-adjusted life years (DALYs) The years of life lost to premature mortality and years lived with a disability, adjusted for the severity of the disability. One DALY is one lost year of healthy life. The DALY thus gives a wider picture of health problems (disease burden) than mortality statistics portray through incorporating the non-fatal consequences of ill-health and injuries. (See *Burden of disease*.)

Endemic disease The normal level of disease which is permanently present in a population group or geographic area.

Epidemic A mass outbreak of a disease in a particular geographic area which spreads and then disappears relatively quickly.

Epidemiological polarization The coexistence of 'old' (pre-transition) and 'new' (post-transition) diseases in a country. Sometimes termed the 'double burden' of disease.

Epidemiological transition The shift in the major causes of death from infectious diseases (e.g. tuberculosis, diarrhoea and enteritis, pneumonias) as well as famine, to chronic and degenerative ailments (e.g. heart disease, stroke, cancers) associated with the long-term decline in mortality from high to low levels.

Epidemiological triad (triangle) A model of disease causation, with disease being seen as the result of interaction between three factors: agent, host and environment.

Epidemiology The study of the patterns and determinants of health and disease in populations.

Ethnicity Refers to the classification of people into groups on the basis of a common attribute, such as national origin, ancestry, language, religion, or race. While all members of a population can be classified on these attributes the term 'ethnic group' is most often used with respect to minority groups.

Foetal death (stillbirth) The death of a foetus that occurs after twenty weeks' gestation or 500 grams.

Food insecurity When people do not have adequate physical, economic or social access to food.

Food security When people at all times have physical, economic and social access to sufficient, safe and nutritious food that meets their dietary needs and food preferences.

Globalization The increasing interconnectedness and interdependence of peoples and countries, involving global flows of goods, services, finance, people and ideas (and sometimes diseases) and the development of institutions and policies facilitating those flows.

Health A state of complete physical, mental and social well-being, and not merely the absence of disease or infirmity (WHO).

Health indicator A measure that indicates the level of health of a population or subpopulation – e.g. life expectancy at birth.

Health inequalities The differences (disparities, variations) in the health of individuals and groups between and within countries.

Health inequities Inequalities in health which are unnecessary and avoidable and involve some form of injustice.

Health transition The changes over time in a society's health. The term has a wider meaning than mortality transition, covering the positive condition of health as well as death and illness. It also refers to the cultural, social and behavioural determinants of health.

Hunger See *Undernourishment*.

Immunization (vaccination, inoculation) The production of immunity to infectious disease artificially by introducing specific antigens (dead or weakened micro-organisms) into the body. The body produces antibodies in response to the antigens, giving protection from that disease.

Incidence rate The number of new cases of a disease (or injury or other health-related condition) over a given period in a defined population, divided by the population at risk of contracting the disease. The population at risk is usually taken as the mid-period population. Theoretically, persons who have already got the disease should be excluded from the at risk population, but that is often not possible. Incidence data are valuable in investigations of disease aetiology (causes).

Infant mortality The death of a child before its first birthday. The infant mortality rate is expressed as the number of infant deaths per 1,000 live births over a specified period.

Infectious (communicable) disease Those diseases caused by pathogens (e.g. bacteria, viruses, protozoa, endoparasites, fungi). Infectious diseases which are spread by direct contact with infected persons are often termed contagious (e.g. sexually transmitted diseases, ebola), although some writers use 'contagious' more loosely as a synonym for all infectious diseases.

International Classification of Diseases (ICD) The World Health Organization's International Statistical Classification of Diseases and Related Health Problems. The current version is ICD-10, the 10th Revision. (See *Cause of death*.)

Ischaemic heart disease Heart disease resulting from reduced blood supply to the heart due to thickening and hardening (atherosclerosis) of the coronary arteries. Causes chest pain (angina) and heart attack. Also known as coronary heart disease. ICD-9 Codes 410–414, ICD-10 Codes I20–I25.

Life expectancy The average number of additional years a person of a given age and sex would live if current mortality trends were to continue.

Life table A table detailing the life expectancy and probability of dying at each age for a given population. There are *period* and *cohort* life tables. (See Chapter 2.)

Malnutrition A broad term often used as an alternative to undernutrition. Technically, however, it also refers to overnutrition. In the first sense, people are malnourished if their diet has insufficient calories and protein for growth or is micronutrient deficient. In the second sense, people are malnourished if they consume too many calories.

Maternal mortality Deaths of women from pregnancy- or childbirth-related complications.

Morbidity The levels of disease, illness, injuries and disabilities in a population. Measured by such things as health surveys, doctor visits, hospital admissions, disease registers.

Mortality The occurrence of deaths in a population. One of the three basic demographic processes (along with fertility and migration).

Mortality crisis A sudden large increase in the death rate.

Multiple causes of death statistics In many cases deaths involve several causes and conditions. Until recently causes of death statistics were tabulated on the basis of each death being assigned to a single underlying cause, all other information provided on the death certificate being 'lost'. Processing all causes and conditions reported on each death certificate gives a far more accurate summary of the mortality pattern of a population.

Neonatal death The death of a live-born infant within twenty-eight days of birth. Deaths in the first seven days of life are termed 'early neonatal'. Deaths between twenty-eight days and one year are called 'post-neonatal'.

Pandemic An epidemic that spreads over a very wide area, which can be continent-wide or world-wide (e.g. the 1918–19 Spanish flu and the mid-fourteenth-century bubonic plague outbreak across Europe).

Parasites Living things that live in or on another organism and can cause disease. Human parasites include protozoa, amoeba, worms and flukes. Examples of human parasitic diseases are malaria, schistosomiasis, sleeping sickness, tapeworm and giardia. Some sources adopt a wider definition of parasite, also including viruses, bacteria and fungi as parasites.

Perinatal mortality rate The number of stillbirths and deaths in the first week of life per 1,000 live births.

Population ageing An increase in the proportion of elderly persons in a population, usually resulting in a rise in the median age.

Potential years of life lost (PYLL) A measure of premature mortality. For example, at current average life expectancy levels in developed countries all deaths before age 75 might be considered untimely and to involve a loss of potential years of life. Thus, from this perspective, a person dying on his/her fortieth birthday loses thirty-five potential years of life.

Premature mortality Deaths that can be considered to have occurred before their due time. This concept underlies the PYLL measure of mortality.

Prevalence rate The number of people in a defined population with a disease (or injury or other health-related condition) at a given point in time (point prevalence) or during a specified period (period prevalence), divided by the average population. Prevalence data hence show the magnitude of a given health problem and are important in planning services and allocating resources. As they include persons who may have contracted the disease many years ago, however, they are not useful in aetiological (causal) studies.

Relative risk A measure of the proportionate increase in disease rates among people exposed to a particular health risk factor compared with those not exposed to the factor: for example, the relative risk smokers have of developing lung cancer compared with non-smokers. Relative risk is expressed as the ratio of the incidence rate of those exposed to a factor to the incidence rate of those not exposed.

Sex ratio The ratio of the number of males to the number of females in a population. Usually expressed as the number of males per 100 females.

Social gradient of health The tendency whereby the lower an individual's or group's socio-economic position, the worse their health.

Specific rates Any rate that is computed for specific sub-groups (e.g. age, sex, race) of a population: for example, age-specific death rates. Rates can be made specific for multiple attributes (e.g. age and sex; age, sex and race). By using specific rates the possible confounding effects of age, sex, race, etc. masked in crude rates are eliminated.

Standardized (adjusted) rates Overall summary rates which (unlike crude rates) are unaffected by compositional differences between the populations being compared. Age is the most common factor standardized for in population research, although it is frequently also necessary to adjust for sex and race, singly or in combination. In comparing mortality variations between areas, for instance, other things being equal, areas with younger populations will have lower crude death rates than areas with older populations. Standardization procedures allow this age structure effect to be controlled.

Survival curve A line graph plotting the percentage of a population surviving to different ages under a given level of mortality. (See Figures 4.1 and 4.5.)

Underlying cause of death This is the precipitating cause of death and is defined by the World Health Organization as 'the disease or injury which initiated the train of morbid events leading directly to death, or the circumstances of the accident or violence which produced the fatal injury'.

Undernourishment (undernutrition, hunger) When caloric intake is less than the minimum dietary energy requirement needed for light activity and to maintain a minimum acceptable weight for attained height.

Urbanization An increase in the proportion of a population living in urban areas. The term is also used with reference to the percentage urban at a particular point in time: that is, the level of urbanization.

Vectors Organisms (e.g. insects, snails, arachnids) which carry pathogens between humans, or from infected animals to humans: for example, mosquitoes are the vector of the malarial protozoan, *Plasmodium*; fleas are the vector of the plague bacterium, *Yersinia pestis*; freshwater snails are the vector (and intermediate host) of the schistosomiasis parasite, *Schistosoma*.

Viruses Microorganisms smaller than bacteria which can only replicate within the cells of other living organisms. Viruses cause many common human infections; for example, HIV, hepatitis, influenza and dengue fever.

Vital statistics Demographic data on births, deaths, marriages and divorces.

Zoonosis An infectious disease that can be transmitted from a vertebrate animal to humans.

References and further reading

Abegunde, D., Mathers, C., Adam, T., Ortegon, M. and Strong, K. (2007). 'The burden and costs of chronic diseases in low-income and middle-income countries', *The Lancet*, 370: 1929–1938.

AbouZahr, C., Cleland, J., Coullare, F., Macfarlane, S.B., Notzon, F.C., Setel, P., Szreter, S., on behalf of the Monitoring of Vital Events (MoVE) (2007). 'The way forward', *The Lancet*, 370: 1791–1799.

Access Economics (2006). *Dementia in the Asia Pacific Region: The Epidemic is Here*. http://www.alz.co.uk/research/files/apreport.pdf

Access Economics (2009). *Keeping Dementia Front of Mind: Incidence and Prevalence 2009-2050*. Report for Alzheimer's Australia. http://www.accesseconomics.com.au/publicationsreports/showreport.php?id=214

Ali, S.H. and Keil. R. (eds) (2008). *Networked Disease: Emerging Infections in the Global City*, Malden, MA: Wiley-Blackwell.

Alley, D. and Crimmins, E. (2010). 'Epidemiology of ageing', in D. Dannefer and C. Phillipson (eds) *The SAGE Handbook of Social Gerontology*, London: Sage, pp. 75–95.

Allotey, P. and Zwi, A. (2007). 'Population movements', in I. Kawachi and S. Wamala (eds) *Globalization and Health*, Oxford: Oxford University Press, pp. 158–170.

Alwan, A. and Maclean, D.R. (2009). 'A review of non-communicable disease in low- and middle-income countries', *International Health*, 1(1): 3–9.

Alzheimer's Association (2011). *Generation Alzheimer's: The Defining Disease of the Baby Boomers*, New York: Alzheimer's Association.

Alzheimer's Association (2012). *2012 Alzheimer's Disease Facts and Figures*, New York: Alzheimer's Association.

Alzheimer's Disease International (2009). *World Alzheimer Report 2009*, London: ADI. http://www.alz.co.uk/research/files/WorldAlzheimerReport.pdf

Alzheimer's Disease International (2010). *World Alzheimer Report 2010: The Global Economic Impact of Dementia*, London: ADI. http://www.alz.co.uk/research/files/WorldAlzheimerReport2010.pdf

Alzheimer's Disease International (2011). *World Alzheimer Report 2011*, London: ADI. http://www.alz.co.uk/research/world-report-2011

Alzheimer's Society (2011). 'The later stages of dementia', Fact Sheet 417, London: Alzheimer's Society. http://alzheimers.org.uk/site/scripts/documents_info.php?documentID=101

Ambio (1982). Special issue on 'Nuclear War: The Aftermath', 11(2/3).

American Cancer Society (2010). *The Global Economic Cost of Cancer*, American Cancer Society. http://www.globalhealth.org/images/pdf/2010_cancer_report.pdf

American Veterinary Medical Association (2008). *One Health: A New Professional Imperative*, One Health Initiative Task Force: Final Report. http://www.avma.org/onehealth/onehealth_final.pdf

Arias, E. (2010). *United States Life Tables by Hispanic Origin*, Vital and Health Statistics Series 2, Number 152, Hyattsville, MD: US Department of Health and Human Services.

Ashdown, P. (2011). *Humanitarian Emergency Response Review*, London: HERR. http://www.dfid.gov.uk/emergency-response-review

Australian Bureau of Statistics (2007). 'Work-related injuries', in *Australian Social Trends 2007*, Canberra: Australian Bureau of Statistics, pp. 137–141.

Australian Bureau of Statistics (2009). *Experimental Life Tables for Aboriginal and Torres Strait Islander Australians, 2005–2007*, Canberra: Australian Bureau of Statistics.

Australian Bureau of Statistics (2011). *Causes of Death, Australia, 2009*, Canberra: Australian Bureau of Statistics.

Australian Institute of Health and Welfare (M. de Looper and P. Magnus) (2005). 'Australian health inequalities 2: trends in male mortality by broad occupational group', *Bulletin*, No. 25, Canberra: AIHW.

Axios (2010). 'On World Cancer Day, experts see growing global cancer gap as critical obstacle to progress against the disease'. http://www.axios-group.com/x/File/WCD2010ReleaseEN.pdf

Baltes, P.B. (1987). 'Theoretical propositions of life-span developmental psychology: on the dynamics between growth and decline', *Developmental Psychology*, 23: 611–696.

Baltes P.B., Staudinger, U.M. and Lindenberger, U. (1999). 'Lifespan psychology: theory and application to intellectual functioning', *Annual Review of Psychology*, 50: 471–507.

Banks, J., Marmot, M., Oldfield, Z. and Smith, J.P. (2006). 'Disease and disadvantage in the United States and England', *Journal of the American Medical Association*, 295: 2037–2047.

Banta, J. E. (2001). 'From international to global health,' *Journal of Community Health*, 26: 73–76.

Barrett, H.R. and Mulugeta, B. (2010). 'Human Immunodeficiency Virus (HIV) and migrant "risk environments": the case of the Ethiopian and Eritrean immigrant community in the West Midlands of the UK', *Psychology, Health and Medicine*, 15(3): 357–369.

Barriopedro, D., Fischer, E.M., Luterbacher, J., Trigo, R.M. and Garcia-Herrera, R. (2011). 'The hot summer of 2010: redrawing the temperature record map of Europe', *Science*, 332: 220–224.

Bartlett, J.D. (2011). 'Top 10 infectious diseases hot topics: 2010–2011', *Medscape News Today*. http://www.medscape.com/viewarticle/735126

Basch, P.F. (1999). *Textbook of International Health*, 2nd edition, New York: Oxford University Press.

Bassani, D.G. and Roth, D.E. (2011). 'China's progress in neonatal mortality', *The Lancet*, early online publication, 15 September. http://www.lancet.com/journals/lancet/article/PIIS0140-6736(11)61257-9/fulltext

BBC (2009). 'Seas threaten 20m in Bangladesh', BBC News, 7 September. http://news.bbc.co.uk/2/hi/8240406.stm

BBC (2010). 'Bhopal trial: Eight convicted over India gas disaster', BBC News, 7 June. http://news.bbc.co.uk/2/hi/south_asia/8725140.stm

BBC (2011a). 'Outrage as Pakistan's rape victim's attackers released', BBC News, 27 April. http://www.bbc.co.uk/news/world-south-asia-13205535

BBC (2011b). 'Rising food prices increase squeeze on poor: Oxfam', BBC News, 31 May. http://www.bbc.co.uk/news/world-13597657

Beaglehole, R. and Bonita, R. (2010). 'What is global health?', *Global Health Action*, 3: 5142.

Becares, L., Coope, C., Kelly, Y. and Karlsen, S. (2010). *Ethnicity and Health*, ICLS Briefing Note 2, London: International Centre for Lifecourse Studies.

Beggs, P.J. and Bennett, C.M. (2011). 'Climate change, aeroallergens, natural particulates, and human health in Australia: state of the science and policy', *Asia-Pacific Journal of Public Health*, Supplement to 23(2): 46S–53S.

Bell, F.C. and Miller, M.L. (2005). *Life Tables for the United States Social Security Area 1900–2100*, Washington, DC: Social Security Administration, Office of the Chief Actuary.

Beltz, L.A. (2011). *Emerging Infectious Diseases: A Guide to Diseases, Causative Agents, and Surveillance*, San Francisco: Jossey-Bass.

Benetar, S.R. and Singer, P.A. (2000) 'A new look at international research ethics', *British Medical Journal*, 321: 824–826.

Benetar, S.R. and Singer, P.A. (2010) 'Responsibilities in international research: a new look revisited', *Journal of Medical Ethics*, 36: 194–197.

Berger, K.S. (2007). *The Developing Person Through the Lifespan*, 7th edition, New York: Worth.

Berger, K.S. (2012). *The Developing Person Through the Lifespan*, 8th edition, New York: Worth.

Berman, P.A. and Bossert, T.J. (2000). 'A decade of health sector reform in developing countries: what have we learned?' Paper for Appraising a Decade of Health Sector Reform in Developing Countries, Washington, DC, 15 March. http://www.hsph.harvard.edu/ihsg/publications/pdf/closeout.pdf

Bilukha, O.O., Brennan, M. and Woodruff, B.A. (2003). 'Death and injury from landmines and unexploded ordnance in Afghanistan', *Journal of the American Medical Association*, 290(5): 650–653.

Birn, A.E., Pillay, Y. and Holtz, T.H. (2009). *Textbook of International Health: Global Health in a Dynamic World*, 3rd edition, Oxford: Oxford University Press.

Black, R.E., Allen, L.H., Bhutta, Z.Q.A., Caulfield, L.E., de Onis, M., Ezzati, M., Mathers, C. and Rivera, J. for the Maternal and Child Undernutrition Study Group (2008). 'Maternal and child undernutrition: global and regional exposures and health consequences', *The Lancet*, 371: 243–260.

Black, R.E., Cousens, S., Johnson, H.L., Lawn, J.E., Rudan, I., Bassani, D.G., Jha, P., Campbell, H., Walker, C.F., Cibulskis, R., Eisele, T., Liu, L. and Mathers, C. for the Child Health Epidemiology Reference Group of WHO and UNICEF (2010). 'Global, regional, and national causes of child mortality in 2008: a systematic analysis', *The Lancet*, 375(9730): 1969–1987.

Bloom, B.R., Michaud, C.M., La Montagne, J.R. and Simonsen, L. (2006). 'Priorities for global research and development of interventions', in D.T. Jamison *et al*. (eds) *Disease Control Priorities in Developing Countries*, 2nd edition, New York: Oxford University Press, pp. 103–118.

Board on International Health, Institute of Medicine (1997). *America's Vital Interest in Global Health*, Washington, DC: National Academy Press.

Boland, P.B. (2001). *Drug Resistance in Malaria*, Geneva: WHO.

Bond, J.B.A., Coleman, P.G. and Peace, S.M. (eds) (2007). *Ageing in Society: An Introduction to Social Gerontology*, 3rd edition, London: Sage.

Bongaarts, J. (2006). 'How long will we live?', *Population and Development Review*, 32(4): 605–628.

Bonita, R., Beaglehole, R. and Kjellstrom, T. (2006). *Basic Epidemiology*, 2nd edition, Geneva: WHO.

Boucher, H.W., Talbot, G.H., Bradley, J.S., Edwards, J.E., Gilbert, D., Rice, L.B., Scheld, M., Spellberg, B. and Bartlett, J. (2009). 'Bad bugs, no drugs: no ESKAPE! An update from the Infectious Diseases Society of America', *Clinical Infectious Diseases*, 48(1): 1–12.

Boyle, P. (2006). 'The globalisation of cancer', *The Lancet*, 368(9536): 629–630.

Boyle, P. and Howell, A. (2010) 'The globalisation of breast cancer', *Breast Cancer Research*, 12 (Suppl. 4): S7.

Boyle, P. and Levin, B. (eds) (2008). *World Cancer Report*, Geneva: WHO.

Braveman, P. and Tarimo, E. (2002). 'Social inequalities in health within countries: not only an issue for affluent nations', *Social Science and Medicine*, 54: 1621–1635.

Breman, J.G., Mills, A., Snow, R.W., Mulligan, J.-A., Lengeler, C., Mendis, K., Sharp, B., Morel, C., Marchesini, P., White, N.J., Steketee, R.W. and Doumbo, O.K. (2006). 'Conquering malaria', in D.T. Jamison *et al*. (eds) *Disease Control Priorities in Developing Countries*, 2nd edition, New York: Oxford University Press, pp. 413–431.

Brockerhoff, M. and Hewett, P. (2000). 'Inequality of child mortality among ethnic groups in sub-Saharan Africa', *Bulletin of the World Health Organization*, 78(1): 30–41.

Brown, T.M., Cueto, M. and Fee, E. (2006). 'The World Health Organization and the transition from "international" to "global" public health', *American Journal of Public Health*, 96(1): 62–72.

Brownstein, J.S., Freifeld, C.C. and Madoff, L.C. (2009). 'Digital disease detection – harnessing the web for public health surveillance', *New England Journal of Medicine*, 360(21): 2153–2157.

Bruce-Jones, E. and Itaborahy, L.P. (2011). *ILGA State-sponsored Homophobia Report: A World Survey of Laws Prohibiting Same Sex Activity between Consenting Adults*. http://old.ilga.org/Statehomophobia/ILGA_State_Sponsored_Homophobia_2011.pdf

Brundtland, G.H. (2003). 'The globalization of health', *Whitehead Journal of Diplomacy and International Relations*, 4(2): 7–12.

Brunkard, J., Namulanda, G. and Ratard, R. (2008) 'Hurrican Katrina deaths, Louisiana, 2005', *Disaster Medicine and Public Health Preparedness*, 2: 215–223.

Burd-Sharps, S., Lewis, K. and Martins, E.B. (eds) (2008). *The Measure of America: American Human Development Report 2008–09*. http://www.measureofamerica.org/wp-content/uploads/2008/10/american_hd_index_by_state.xls

Byass, P. (2007). 'Who needs cause-of-death data?', *PLoS Medicine*, 4(11): 1715–1716.

Caldwell, J.C. and Caldwell, B.K. (2003). 'Was there a Neolithic mortality crisis?', *Journal of Population Research*, 20(2): 153–168.

Caldwell, J., Findley, S., Caldwell, P., Santow, G., Crawford, W., Brand, J. and Broers-Freeman, D. (eds) (1990). *What We Know about Health Transition: The Cultural, Social and Behavioural Determinants of Health*, Canberra: Australian National University Printing Service.

Cameron, M., Gibson, J., Helmers, K., Lim, S., Tressler, J. and Vaddanak, K. (2010). 'The value of statistical life and cost–benefit evaluations of landmine clearance in Cambodia', *Environment and Development Economics*, 15(4): 395–416.

Campbell-Lendrum, D. and Corvalan, C. (2007). 'Climate change and developing-country cities: implications for environmental health and equity', *Journal of Urban Health: Bulletin of the New York Academy of Medicine*, 84(1): i109–i117.

Carnes, B.A., Olshansky, S.J. and Grahn, D. (2003). 'Biological evidence for limits to the duration of life', *Biogerontology*, 4(1): 31–45.

Carr, D. (2004). 'Improving the health of the world's poorest people', *Health Bulletin* 1, Washington, DC: Population Reference Bureau.

Cassels, A. (1995). 'Health sector reform: key issues in less developed countries', *Journal of International Development*, 7(3): 329–347.

Centers for Disease Control and Prevention (CDC) (2011a). 'Children and diabetes', Diabetes Public Health Resource, Atlanta: CDC. http://www.cdc.gov/diabetes/projects/cda2.htm

Centers for Disease Control and Prevention (CDC) (2011b). *Seasonal Influenza*. http://www.cdc.gov/flu/

Centers for Disease Control and Prevention (CDC) (2012). 'Progress in global measles control, 2000–2010', *Morbidity and Mortality Weekly Report*, 61(4): 73–78. http://www.cdc.gov/mmwr/preview/mmwrhtml/mm6104a3.htm?s_cid=mm6104a3_w

Central Bureau of Health Intelligence – India. (2010). *National Health Profile (NHP) of India – 2010*. http://www.cbhidghs.nic.in/index2.asp?slid=1125&sublinkid=929

Centre for Neglected Tropical Diseases, Liverpool School of Tropical Medicine (2012). *About NTDs*. http://www.cntd.org/index.htm

Chatterjee, P. (2009). 'Sex ratio imbalance worsens in Vietnam', *The Lancet*, 374(9699): 1410.

Chau, P.H., Woo, J., Chan, K.C., Weisz, D. and Gusmano, M.K. (2011). 'Avoidable mortality pattern in a Chinese population – Hong Kong, China', *European Journal of Public Health*, 21: 215–220.

Chau, P.H., Chen, J., Woo, J., Cheung, W.L., Chan, K.C., Cheung, S.H., Lee, C.H. and McGhee, S. (2011). *Trends of Disease Burden Consequent to Chronic Lung Disease in Older Persons in Hong Kong*, Hong Kong: Hong Kong Jockey Club.

Checchi, F. (2010) 'Estimating the number of civilian deaths from armed conflicts', *The Lancet*, 375(9711): 255–257.

Chivian, E. (ed.) (2002). *Biodiversity: Its Importance to Human Health: Interim Executive Summary*, Boston: Centre for Health and the Global Environment, Harvard Medical School.

Chopra, M. (2005). 'Inequalities in health in developing countries: challenges for public health research', *Critical Public Health*, 15(1): 19–26.

Christensen, K., Doblhammer, G., Rau, R. and Vaupel, J.W. (2009). 'Ageing populations: the challenges ahead', *The Lancet*, 374(9696): 1196–1208.

Chuma, J., Musimbi, J., Okungu, V., Goodman, C. and Molyneux, C. (2009). 'Reducing user fees for primary health care in Kenya: policy on paper or policy in practice?', *International Journal for Equity in Health*, 8. http://www.equityhealthj.com/content/8/1/15

Cliff, A.D., Haggett, P. and Smallman-Raynor, M.R. (2004). *World Atlas of Epidemic Diseases*, London: Arnold.

Cliff, A.D. and Smallman-Raynor, M.R., with Haggett, P., Stroup, D.F. and Thacker, S.B. (2009). *Emergence and Re-emergence: Infectious Diseases: A Geographical Analysis*, Oxford: Oxford University Press.

Coalition to Stop the Use of Child Soldiers (2008). *Child Soldiers Global Report 2008*. http://www.child-soldiers.org/coalition/the-coalition

Coalition to Stop the Use of Child Soldiers (2011). *Home site*. http://www.child-soldiers.org/coalition/the-coalition

Cockerham, G.B. and Cockerham, W.C. (2010). *Health and Globalization*, Cambridge: Polity Press.

Coleman, M.P., Quaresma, M., Berrino, F., Lutz, J.-M., De Angelis, R., Capocaccia, R., Baili, P., Rachet, B., Gatta, G., Hakulinen, T., Micheli, A., Sant, M., Weir, H.K., Elwood, J.M., Tsukuma, H., Koifman, S., Azevedo e Silva, G., Francisci, S., Santaquilani, M., Verdecchia, A., Storm, H.H., Young, J.L. and the CONCORD Working Group (2008). 'Cancer survival in five continents: a worldwide population-based study (CONCORD)', *The Lancet Oncology*, 9(8): 730–756.

Council for International Organizations of Medical Sciences (CIOMS) (2002). *International Ethical*

Guidelines for Biomedical Research Involving Human Subjects, prepared by CIOMIS in collaboration with the World Health Organization, Geneva: CIOMS.

Commission on Social Determinants of Health (CSDH) (2008). *Closing the Gap in a Generation: Health Equity through Action on the Social Determinants of Health: Final Report of the Commission on Social Determinants of Health*, Geneva: WHO.

Committee on Abrupt Climate Change, National Research Council (2002). *Abrupt Climate Change: Inevitable Surprises*, Washington, DC: National Academies Press.

Committee on the US Commitment to Global Health (2009). *The US Commitment to Global Health: Recommendations for the New Administration*, Washington, DC: National Academies Press.

Confalonieri, U., Menne, B., Akhtar, R., Ebi, K.L., Hauengue, M., Kovats, R.S., Revich, B. and Woodward, A. (2007). 'Human health', in M.L. Parry, O.F. Canziani, J.P. Palutikof, P.J. van der Linden and C.E. Hanson (eds) *Climate Change 2007: Impacts, Adaptation and Vulnerability. Contribution of Working Group II to the Fourth Assessment Report of the Intergovernmental Panel on Climate Change*, Cambridge: Cambridge University Press, pp. 391–431.

Costello, A., Abbas, M., Allen, A., Ball, S., Bell, S., Bellamy, R., Friel, S., Groce, N., Johnson, A., Kett, M., Lee, M., Levy, C., Maslin, M., McCoy, D., McGuire, B., Montgomery, H., Napier, D., Pagel, C., Patel, J., de Oliviera, J.A.P., Redclift, N., Rees, H., Rogger, D., Scott, J., Stephenson, J., Twigg, J., Wolff, J. and Patterson, C. (2009). 'Managing the health effects of climate change', *The Lancet*, 373: 1693–1733.

Crimmins, E.M., Hayward, M.D., Hagedorn, A., Saito, Y. and Brouard, N. (2009). 'Change in disability-free life expectancy for Americans 70 years old and older', *Demography*, 46(3): 627–646.

Crisp, N. (2010). *Turning the World Upside Down: The Search for Global Health in the 21st Century*, London: Royal Society of Medicine Press.

Curson, P. and McRandle, B. (2005). *Plague Anatomy: Health Security from Pandemics to Bioterrorism*, Barton: Australian Strategic Policy Institute.

Daily, G.C. and Ehrlich, P.R. (1996). 'Global change and human susceptibility to disease', *Annual Review of Energy and the Environment*, 21: 125–144.

Danaei, G., Finucane, M.M., Lu, Y., Singh, G.M., Cowan, M.J., Paciorek, C.J., Lin, J.K., Farzadfar, F., Khang, Y.-H, Stevens, G.A., Rao, M., Ali, M.K., Riley, L.M., Robinson, C.A. and Ezzati, M. for Global Burden of Metabolic Risk Factors of Chronic Diseases Collaborating Group (Blood Glucose) (2011). 'National, regional, and global trends in fasting plasma glucose and diabetes prevalence since 1980: systematic analysis of health examination surveys and epidemiological studies with 370 country-years and 2.7 million participants', *The Lancet*, 378(9785): 31–40.

Dannefer, D. and Daub, A. (2009). 'Extending the interrogation: life span, life course, and the constitution of human aging', *Advances in Life Course Research*, 14(1–2): 15–27.

Dannefer, D. and Phillipson, C. (eds) (2010). *The SAGE Handbook of Social Gerontology*, London: Sage.

Desselberger, U. (2000). 'Emerging and re-emerging infectious diseases', *Journal of Infection*, 40, 3–15.

Dhandapany, P.S., Sadayappan, S., Xue, Y., Powell, G.T., Rani, D.S., Nallari, P., Rai, T.S., Khullar, M., Soares, P., Bahl, A., Tharkan, J.M., Vaideeswar, P., Rathinavel, A., Narasimhan, C., Ayapati, D.R., Ayub, Q., Mehdi, S.Q., Oppenheimer, S., Richards, M.B., Price, A.L., Patterson, N., Reich, D., Singh, L., Tyler-Smith, C. and Thangaraj, K. (2009). 'A common MYBPC3 (cardiac myosin binding protein C) variant associated with cardiomyopathies in South Asia", *Nature Genetics*, 41(2): 187–191.

Diamond, J. (1998). *Guns, Germs and Steel*, New York: Norton Press.

Disease Control Priorities Project (2007). *Developing Countries Can Reduce Occupational Hazards*, fact sheet. http://www.dcp2.org/file/139/DCPP-OccupationalHealth.pdf

Disease Control Priorities Project (2008a). *Breathing Easier: Preventing Chronic Respiratory Diseases in Adults*, fact sheet. http://www.dcp2.org/file/221/dcpp-respiratorydisease-web.pdf

Disease Control Priorities Project (2008b). *Sex, Gender, and Women's Health: Why Women Usually Come Last*, fact sheet. http://www.dcp2.org/file/222/dcpp-gender-web.pdf

Dooley, K.E. and Chaisson, R.E. (2009). 'Tuberculosis and diabetes mellitus: convergence of two epidemics', *The Lancet Infectious Diseases*, 12: 737–746.

Dorfman, M. and Rosselot, K.S. (2011). *Testing the Waters: A Guide to Water Quality at Vacation Beaches*, New York: Natural Resources Defence Council.

Dumont, J.-C., Spielvogel, G. and Widmaier, S. (2010). *International Migrants in Developed, Emerging and Developing Countries: An Extended Profile*, OECD Social, Employment and Migration Working Papers No. 114, Paris: OECD.

Duncan, B.N., West, J.J., Yoshida, Y., Fiore, A.M. and Ziemke, J.R. (2008). 'The influence of European pollution on ozone in the Near East and northern Africa', *Atmospheric Chemistry and Physics*, 8: 2267–2283.

Dye, C., Bourdin, T.B., Lönnroth, K., Roglic, G. and Williams B.G. (2011). 'Nutrition, diabetes and tuberculosis in the epidemiological transition', *PLoS ONE*, 6(6). http://www.ncbi.nlm.nih.gov/pubmed/21712992

Ebil, K.L. and McGregor, G. (2008). 'Climate change, tropospheric ozone and particulate matter, and health impacts', *Environmental Health Perspectives*, 116(11): 1449–1455.

Elder, G.H. (1974). *Children of the Great Depression*, Chicago: University of Chicago Press.

Enserink, M. (2011). 'First specific drugs raise hopes for Hepatitis C,' *Science*, 332: 159–160.

Equality and Human Rights Commission (2010). *How Fair is Britain? 2010 Our First Triennial Review*. http://www.equalityhumanrights.com/key-projects/how-fair-is-britain/

Etches, V., Frank, J., Ruggiero, E.D. and Manuel, D. (2006). 'Measuring population health: a review of indicators', *Annual Review of Public Health*, 27: 29–55.

Evans, J.G. (1997). 'The rationing debate: rationing health care by age: the case against', *British Medical Journal*, 314: 822–825.

Evans, R.G. and Stoddart, G.L. (1994). 'Producing health, consuming health care', in R.G. Evans, M.L. Barer and T.R. Marmor (eds) *Why Are Some People Healthy and Others Not? The Determinants of Health of Populations*, New York: Aldine de Gruyter, pp. 27–64.

Expert Group on Climate Change and Health in the UK (2001). *Health Effects of Climate Change in the UK – 2001/2002 Report*, London: Department of Health.

Ezzati, M., Friedman, A.B., Kulkarni, S.C. and Murray, C.J.L. (2008). 'The reversal of fortunes: trends in county mortality and cross-county mortality disparities in the United States', *PLoS Medicine*, 5(4): 557–568.

Feachem, R., Yamey, G, and Schrade, C. (2010). 'Editorial: moment of truth for global health', *British Medical Journal*; 340: c2869.

Fendall, R. (1985). 'Myths and misconceptions in primary health care', *Third World Planning Review*, 3: 387–401.

Ferri, C.P. and Prince, M. (2010). '10/66 Dementia Research Group: recently published survey data for seven Latin America sites', *International Psychogeriatrics*, 22(1): 158–159.

Fine, A., Kotelchuck, M., Adess, N. and Pies, C. (2009). *Policy Brief: A New Agenda for MCH Policy and Programs: Integrating a Life Course Perspective*, Martinez, CA: Contra Costa Health Services. http://cchealth.org/groups/lifecourse/pdf/2009_10_policy_brief.pdf

Finucane, M.M., Stevens, G.A., Danaei, G., Lin, J.K., Paciorek, C.J., Singh, G.M, Gutierrez, H.R., Lu, Y., Bahalim, A.N., Farzadfar, F., Leanne M Riley, L.M., Ezzati, M. for Global Burden of Metabolic Risk Factors of Chronic Diseases Collaborating Group (Body Mass Index) (2011). 'National, regional, and global trends in body-mass index since 1980: systematic analysis of health examination surveys and epidemiological studies with 960 country-years and 9.1 million participants', *The Lancet*, 377(9765): 557–567.

Food and Agricultural Organization (FAO) (2010). *The State of Food Insecurity in the World 2010*, Rome: WFP and FAO.

Food and Agricultural Organization (FAO) (2011). *Global Forest Resources Assessment 2010: Main Report*, FAO Forestry Paper 163, Rome: FAO.

Food and Agricultural Organization, Fisheries and Aquaculture Department (2010). *The State of World Fisheries and Aquaculture 2010*, Rome: FAO.

Franca, E., de Abreu, D.A., Rao, C. and Lopez, A.D. (2008). 'Evaluation of cause-of-death statistics for Brazil, 2002–2004', *International Journal of Epidemiology*, 37: 891–901.

Frank, R. (2007). 'What to make of it? The (re)emergence of a biological conceptualization of race in health disparities research,' *Social Science and Medicine*, 64: 1977–1983.

Frederiksen, H. (1969). 'Feedbacks in economic and demographic transition', *Science*, 166(3907): 837–847.

Freedman, V.A., Martin L.G. and Schoeni, R.F. (2004). 'Disability in America', *Population Bulletin*, 59(3): 1–32.

Frenk, J. (2010). 'Globalization of health and health services', *The Journal* (AARP), Winter: 19–22.

Frenk, J., Bobadilla, J.L., Sepulveda, J. and Cervantes, M.L. (1989). 'Health transition in middle-income countries: new challenges for health care', *Health Policy and Planning*, 4(1): 29–39.

Fries, J.F. (1980). 'Aging, natural death, and the compression of morbidity', *New England Journal of Medicine*, 303(3): 130–135.

Fries J.F. (2003). 'Measuring and monitoring success in compressing morbidity', *Annals of Internal Medicine*, 139: 455–459.

Frost, L.J. and Reich, M.R. (2009). 'Creating access to health technologies in poor countries', *Health Affairs*, 28: 4962–4973.

Fujimura, J.H., Duster, T. and Rajagopalan, R. (2008). 'Introduction: race, genetics, and disease: questions of evidence, matters of consequence,' *Social Studies of Science*, 38(5): 643–656.

Garrett, L. (2000). *Betrayal of Trust: The Collapse of Global Public Health*, New York: Hyperion.

Garrett, L. (2007). 'The challenge of global health', *Foreign Affairs*, 86(1): 14–38.

Gates, S. and Reich, S. (eds) (2009). *Child Soldiers in the Age of Fractured States*, Pittsburg, PA: University of Pittsburgh Press.

Gettleman, J. (2011). 'Congo study sets estimates for rapes much higher', *New York Times*, 11 May. http://www.nytimes.com/2011/05/12/world/africa/12congo.html

Gill, A. and Mitra-Kahn, T. (2009). 'Explaining daughter devaluation and the issue of missing women in South Asia and the UK', *Current Sociology*, 57(5): 684–703.

Giuliani, G., De Bono, A., Kluser, S. and Peduzzi, P. (2004). 'Overfishing, a major threat to the global marine ecology', *Environment Alert Bulletin 4*, Rome: United Nations Environment Programme.

Gleick, P.H., Singh, A. and Shi, H. (2001). *Threats to the World's Freshwater Resources*, Oakland, CA: Pacific Institute for Studies in Development, Environment and Security.

Global Action on Aging (2010a). Newsletter, 17–21 May. http://www.globalaging.org/quickgo.htm

Global Action on Aging (2010b). *Older People in Emergencies and Disasters*. http://www.globalaging.org/armedconflict/countryreports/general/index.htm

Global Health Council (2010). *The Burden of Cancer in Developing Countries*, Washington, DC: Global Health Council.

Global Humanitarian Forum (2009). *Human Impact Report: Climate Change – The Anatomy of a Silent Crisis*, Geneva: Global Humanitarian Forum.

Goesling, B. and Firebaugh, G. (2004). 'The trend in international health inequality', *Population and Development Review*, 30(1): 131–146.

Gold, M.R., Stevenson, D. and Fryback, D.G. (2002). 'HALYs and QALYs and DALYs, oh my: similarities and differences in summary measures of population health', *Annual Review of Public Health*, 23: 115–134.

Gracey, M. and King, M. (2009). 'Indigenous health part 1: determinants and disease patterns', *The Lancet*, 374: 65–75.

Gragnolati, M, Shekar, M., Das Gupta, M., Bredenkamp, C. and Lee, Y.-K. (2005). *India's Undernourished Children: A Call for Reform and Action*, Health, Nutrition and Population (HNP) discussion paper, Washington, DC: World Bank.

Grand Challenges in Global Health (2011/2012). 'The grand challenges initiative'. http://www.grandchallenges.org/about/Pages/Overview.aspx

Gray, R., Headley, J., Oakley, L., Kurinczuk, J.J., Brocklehurst, P. and Hollowell, J. (2009). 'Towards an understanding of variations in infant mortality rates between different ethnic groups in England and Wales', *Inequalities in Infant Mortality Project Briefing Paper No. 3*, Oxford: National Perinatal Epidemiology Unit, pp. 1–10.

Griffith, L., Raina, P., Wu, H.-M., Zhu, B. and Stathokostas, L. (2010). 'Population attributable risk for functional disability associated with chronic conditions in Canadian older adults', *Age and Ageing*, 39(6): 738–745.

Grifo, F. and Rosenthal, J. (eds) (1997). *Biodiversity and Human Health*, Washington, DC: Island Press.

Groenewald, P., Bradshaw, D., Nojilana, B., Bourne, D., Nixon, J., Mahomed, H. and Daniels, J. (2003). *Cape Town Mortality, 2001. (Part I: Cause of Death and Premature Mortality; Part III: Cause of Death Profiles for Each Sub-district)*, Cape Town: City of Cape Town, South African Medical Research Council, University of Cape Town.

Gualvez, B.F. (2010). 'How do Philippine provinces fare in terms of human development?', *Philippine Institute for Development Studies Policy Notes No. 2010-01*, Makati: Philippine Institute for Development Studies.

Gusmano, M.K., Rodwin, V.G. and Weisz, D. (2010). *Health Care in World Cities*, Baltimore, MD: Johns Hopkins University Press.

Gustavsson, A., Jonsson, L., Rapp, T., Reynish, E., Ousset, P.J., Andrieu, S., Cantet, C., Winblad, B., Vellas B. and Wimo, A. (2010). 'Differences in resource use and costs of dementia care between European countries: baseline data from the ICTUS study', *Journal of Nutrition, Health & Aging*, 14(8): 648–654.

Haines, A., Kovats, R.S., Campbell-Lendrum, D. and Corvalan, C. (2006). 'Climate change and human health: impacts, vulnerability, and mitigation', *The Lancet*, 367: 2101–2109.

Halfon, N. and Hochstein, M. (2002). 'Life-course health development: an integrated framework for developing health, policy, and research', *Milbank Quarterly*, 80: 433–479.

Halpern, B.S., Walbridge, S., Selkoe, K.A., Kappel, C.V., Micheli, F., D'Agrosa, C., Bruno, J.F., Casey, K.S., Ebert, C., Fox, H.E., Fujita, R., Heinemann, D., Lenihan, H.S., Madin, E.M.P., Perry, M.T., Selig, E.R., Spalding, M., Steneck, R. and Watson, R. (2008). 'A global map of human impact on marine ecosystems', *Science*, 319: 948–952.

Hammond, C. (2011). 'How teenage health affects adult life', *Health Check*, BBC World Service, 4 May. http://www.open.ac.uk/openlearn/profiles/health-check-on-bbc-world-service

Hammond, C. (2011). 'How to raise survival rates for children with cancer in developing countries', *Health Check*, BBC World Service, 30 March. http://www.bbc.co.uk/programmes/p00fvj47

Harper, S. and Howse, K. (2008). 'An upper limit to human longevity?', *Population Ageing*, 1: 99–106.

Hawkins, J.S. and Emanuel, E.J. (eds) (2008). *Exploitation and Developing Countries: The Ethics of Clinical Research*, Princeton: Princeton University Press.

He, G.X., Wang, H.Y., Borgdorff, M.W., van Soolingen, D., van der Werf, M.J., Liu, Z.M., Li, X.Z., Guo, H., Zhao, Y.L., Varma, J.K., Tostado, C.P. and van den Hof, S. (2011). 'Multidrug-resistant tuberculosis, People's Republic of China, 2007–2009', *Emerging Infectious Diseases*, 17(10): 1831–1838.

Health Canada (2002). *The Economic Burden of Illness in Canada, 1998*. Ottawa: Health Canada.

Heilig, G.K. (2004). *RAPS-China: A Regional Analysis and Planning System*, CD-ROM, Laxenburg: International Institute for Applied Systems Analysis.

Herndon, C.N. and Butler, R.A. (2010). 'Significance of biodiversity to health', *Biotropica*, 42(5): 558–560.

Hill, K., Lopez, A.D., Shibuya, K. and Jha, P. on behalf of the Monitoring of Vital Events (MoVE) writing group (2007). 'Interim measures for meeting needs for health sector data: births, deaths, and causes of death', *The Lancet*, 370: 1726–1735.

HM Government (2008). *Health is Global: A UK Government Strategy 2008–2013*, London: Central Office of Information for the Department of Health.

HM Government (2011). *Health is Global: An Outcomes Framework for Global Health 2011–2015*, London: Global Health Team, Department of Health. http://www.dh.gov.uk/prod_consum_dh/groups/dh_digitalassets/documents/digitalasset/dh_125671.pdf

Hofkin, B. (2010). *Living in a Microbial World*, New York: Taylor and Francis.

Hogan, M.C., Foreman, K.J., Naghavi, M., Ahn, S.Y., Wang, M.R., Makela, S.M., Lopez, A.D., Lozano, R. and Murray, C.J.L. (2010). 'Maternal mortality for 181 countries, 1980–2008: a systematic analysis of progress towards Millennium Development Goal 5', *The Lancet*, 375(9726): 1609–1623.

Hooyman, N.R. and Kiyak H.A. (2010). *Social Gerontology: A Multidisciplinary Perspective*, 9th edition, Boston: Allyn and Bacon.

Howitt, R., McCracken, K. and Curson, P. (2005). 'Australian indigenous health: what issues contribute to a national crisis and scandal?', *GeoDate*, 18(1): 8–15.

Hutton, D. (2008). *Older People in Emergencies: Considerations for Action and Policy Development*, Geneva: WHO.

Institute of Medicine (IOM) (2010). *Antibiotic Resistance: Implications for Global Health and Novel Intervention Strategies – Workshop Summary*, Washington, DC: IOM and National Academies Press.

Institute of Medicine (IOM) (2011). *The Health of Lesbian, Gay, Bisexual and Transgender People:*

Building a Foundation for Better Understanding, Washington, DC: National Academies Press. http://www.ncbi.nlm.nih.gov/books/NBK53627/pdf/nap13128.pdf

Intergovernmental Panel on Climate Change (IPCC) (2007). 'Summary for policymakers', in S. Solomon, D. Qin, M. Manning, Z. Chen, M. Marquis, K.B. Averyt, M. Tignor and H.L. Miller (eds) *Climate Change 2007: The Physical Science Basis. Contribution of Working Group I to the Fourth Assessment Report of the Intergovernmental Panel on Climate Change*, Cambridge and New York: Cambridge University Press, pp. 1–18.

International Atomic Energy Agency (IAEA) (2003). *A Silent Crisis: Cancer Treatment in Developing Countries*, Vienna: IAEA.

International Atomic Energy Agency (IAEA) (2011). *Fukushima Nuclear Accident Update Log*, Vienna: IAEA. http://www.iaea.org/newscenter/news/tsunamiupdate01.html

International Committee of the Red Cross (ICRC) (2010). *Anti-personnel Landmines: Overview*, Geneva: International Committee of the Red Cross.

International Committee of the Red Cross (ICRC) (2011). *Somalia: War Wounded in Mogadishu Referral Hospitals Reach New Peak*, 27 January. http://www.icrc.org/eng/resources/documents/news-footage/somalia-tvnews-2011-01-27.htm

International Diabetes Federation (2003). *IDF Diabetes Atlas*, 3rd edition, Brussels: IDF.

International Diabetes Federation (2009). *IDF Diabetes Atlas*, 4th edition, Brussels: IDF.

International Diabetes Federation (2010). *National Diabetes Prevention Plans*, Brussels: IDF. http://www.idf.org/national-diabetes-prevention-plans

International Diabetes Federation (2011). *IDF Diabetes Atlas*, 5th edition, Brussels: IDF.

International Federation of Red Cross and Red Crescent Societies (IFRC) (2010). *World Disasters Report 2010: Focus on Urban Risk*, Geneva: IFRC.

International Federation of Red Cross and Red Crescent Societies (IFRC) (2011). *World Disasters Report 2011: Focus on Hunger and Malnutrition*, Geneva: IFRC.

International Labour Office. (2002). *A Future without Child Labour*, Geneva: International Labour Office.

International Network for Cancer Treatment and Research (2008). *Cancer – a Neglected Health Problem in Developing Countries*. http://www.inctr.org/about-inctr/cancer-in-developing-countries/

International Network for Cancer Treatment and Research (2010). *Cancer – an Increasingly Important Cause of Death in Developing Countries*. http://oerc-international.org/index.php?option=com_content&view=article&id=66:canceran-increasingly-important-cause-of-death-in-developing-countries&catid=95:cancer-control-&Itemid=100143

Ivanic, M., Martin, W. and Zama, H. (2011). *Estimating the Short-run Poverty Impacts of the 2010–11 Surge in Food Prices*, Policy Research Working Paper 5633, Washington, DC: Development Research Group, Agriculture and Rural Development Team, World Bank.

Jacobsen, K.H. (2008). *Introduction to Global Health*, Sudbury, MA: Jones and Bartlett.

Jamison, D.T., Breman, J.G., Measham, A.R., Alleyne, G., Claeson, M., Evans, D.B., Jha, P., Mills, A. and Musgrove, P. (eds) (2006). *Priorities in Health*, Washington, DC: World Bank.

Jamison, D.T., Breman, J.G., Measham, A.R., Alleyne, G., Claeson, M., Evans, D.B., Jha, P., Mills, A. and Musgrove, P. (eds) (2006). *Disease Control Priorities in Developing Countries*, 2nd edition, Washington, DC: World Bank.

Jemal, A., Center, M.M., DeSantis, C., and Ward, E.M. (2010). 'Global patterns of cancer incidence and mortality rates and trends', *Cancer Epidemiology, Biomarkers and Prevention*, 19(8): 1893–1907.

Jeffreys, M., Lawlor, D.A., Galobardes, B., McCarron, P., Kinra, S., Ebrahim, S. and Davey Smith, G. (2006). 'Lifecourse weight patterns and adult-onset diabetes: the Glasgow Alumni and British Women's Heart and Health studies', *International Journal of Obesity*, 30: 507–512.

Jenkins, C.D. (2003). *Building Better Health: A Handbook of Behavioural Change*, Scientific and Technical Publication No. 590, Washington, DC: Pan American Health Organization.

Jia, Z.-B., Tian, W.-H., Liu, W.-Z., Cao, Y., Yan, J. and Shun, Z.-S. (2010). 'Are the elderly more vulnerable to psychological impact of natural disaster? A population-based survey of adult survivors of the 2008 Sichuan earthquake', *BMC Public Health*, 10: 172.

Jones, G., Tay-Straughan, P. and Chan, A. (eds) (2008). *Ultra-low Fertility in Pacific Asia: Trends, Causes and Policy Issues*, New York: Routledge.

Jorm, A.F., Korten, A.E. and Henderson, A.S. (1987). 'The prevalence of dementia: a quantitative integration of the literature', *Acta Psychiatrica Scandinavica*, 76: 465–479.

Joseph, A.E. and Phillips, D.R. (1984). *Accessibility and Utilization: Geographical Perspectives on Health Care Delivery*, London: Harper and Row.

Judge, K., Mulligan, J. and Benzeval, M. (1998). 'Income inequality and population health', *Social Science and Medicine*, 46(4–5): 567–579.

Kahn, L.H. (2006). 'Confronting zoonoses, linking human and veterinary medicine', *Emerging Infectious Diseases*, 12(4): 556–561.

Kaiser Permanente (2010). 'Extreme obesity affecting more children at younger ages', Kaiser Permanente News Center, 18 March. http://xnet.kp.org/newscenter/pressreleases/nat/2010/031810extremeobesity.html

Kaplan, R.M. (1990). 'The General Health Policy model: an integrated approach', in B. Spilker (ed.) *Quality of Life Assessment in Clinical Trials*, New York: Raven Press, pp. 131–149.

Kaufman, F. (2007). 'Preventing type 2 diabetes in children – a role for the whole community', *Diabetes Voice*, 52: 35–38.

Kawachi, I. and Wamala, S.P. (eds) (2007). *Globalization and Health*, New York: Oxford University Press.

Kawachi, I., Subramanian, S.V. and Almeida-Filho, N. (2002). 'A glossary for health inequalities', *Journal of Epidemiology and Community Health*, 56: 647–652.

Kerber, K.K., Graft-Johnson, J.E., Bhutta, Z.A., Okong, P., Starrs, A. and Lawn, J.E. (2007). 'Continuum of care for maternal, newborn, and child health: from slogan to service delivery', *The Lancet*, 370(9595): 1358–1369.

Kikbusch, I. and Lister, G. (eds) (2006). *European Perspectives on Global Health: A Policy Glossary*, Brussels: European Foundation Centre.

King, D. (2011). 'The future challenge of obesity', *The Lancet*, 378(9793): 743–744.

King, M., Smith, A. and Gracey, M. (2009). 'Indigenous health part 2: the underlying causes of the health gap', *The Lancet*, 374(9793): 76–85.

Kinsella, K.G. (1992). 'Changes in life expectancy 1900–1990', *American Journal of Clinical Nutrition*, 55: 1196S–1202S.

Kinsella, K. and He, W. (2009). *An Aging World: 2008*, US Census Bureau International Population Reports P95/09-1, Washington, DC: US Government Printing Office.

Kinsella, K. and Phillips, D.R. (2005). 'Global aging: the challenge of success', *Population Bulletin*, 60(1): 1–40.

Knaul, F.M., Frenk, J. and Shulman, L. for the Global Task Force on Expanded Access to Cancer Care and Control in Developing Countries (2011). *Closing the Cancer Divide: A Blueprint to Expand Access in Low and Middle Income Countries*, Boston: Harvard Global Equity Initiative.

Koebnick, C., Smith, N., Coleman, K. J., Getahun, D., Reynolds, K., Quinn, V.P., Porter, A. H., Der-Sarkissian, J. K., Jacobsen, S. J. (2010). 'Prevalence of extreme obesity in a multiethnic cohort of children and adolescents', *Journal of Pediatrics*, 157(1): 26–31.

Koplan, J.P., Bond, T.C., Merson, M.H., Reddy, K.S., Rodriguez, M.H., Sewankambo, N.K. and Wasserheit, J.N. for the Consortium of Universities for Global Health Executive Board (2009). 'Towards a common definition of global health', *The Lancet*, 373(9679): 1993–1995.

Koplan, J.P., Wang, K.A and Lam, R.M.K. (2010). 'Hong Kong: a model of successful tobacco control in China', *The Lancet*, 375 (9723), 1330–1331.

Kovats, S. (ed.) (2008). *Health Effects of Climate Change in the UK 2008: An Update of the Department of Health Report 2001/2002*, London: Department of Health and the Health Protection Agency.

Krishnan, M. (2011). 'Violent crimes against women in India becoming a political issue', *DW-World*, 26 June. http://www.dw-world.de/dw/article/0,,6554770,00.html

Kumar, P. and Clark, M. (eds) (2009) *Kumar and Clark's Clinical Medicine*, 7th edition, Edinburgh: Elsevier.

Kumarasamy, K.K., Toleman, M.A., Walsh, T.R., Bagaria, J., Butt, F., Ravikumar Balakrishnan, R. *et al.* (2010). 'Emergence of a new antibiotic resistance mechanism in India, Pakistan, and the UK: a molecular, biological, and epidemiological study', *The Lancet Infectious Diseases*, 10(9): 597–602.

Labonté, R., Mohindra, K., Schrecker, T. and Stroebenau, K. (eds) (2011). *Global Health*, four-volume reference set, London: Sage.

Labonté, R. and Torgerson, R. (2005). 'Interrogating globalisation, health and development: towards a comprehensive framework for research, policy and political action', *Critical Public Health*, 15(2): 157–179.

Lafortune, G., Balestat, G. and the Disability Study Expert Group Members (2007). *Trends in Severe Disability among Elderly People: Assessing the Evidence in 12 OECD Countries and the Future Implications*, OECD Health Working Papers No. 26, Paris: OECD.

The Lancet (2009). 'Urgently needed: new antibiotics', *The Lancet*, 374(9705): 1868.

The Lancet (2011). 'Urgently needed: a framework convention for obesity control', *The Lancet*, 378(9793): 741.

Landsbergis, P.A. (2010). 'Assessing the contribution of working conditions to socioeconomic disparities in health: a commentary', *American Journal of Industrial Medicine*, 53: 95–103.

Levy, S. (2006). *Progress against Poverty: Sustaining Mexico's Progresa-Oportunidades Program*, Washington, DC: Brookings Institution Press.

Lewis, K. and Burd-Sharps, S. (2010). *A Century Apart: New Measures of Well-being for US Racial and Ethnic Groups*, New York: Social Science Research Council.

Li, J., Luo, C. and de Klerk, N. (2008). 'Trends in infant/child mortality and life expectancy in indigenous populations in Yunnan Province, China', *Australian and New Zealand Journal of Public Health*, 32(3): 216–223.

Liu, W.J., Lin, R., Liu, A.L., Du, L. and Chen, Q. (2010). 'Prevalence and association between obesity and metabolic syndrome among Chinese elementary school children: a school-based survey', *BMC Public Health*, 10: 780. http://www.biomedcentral.com/1471-2458/10/780

Lopez, A.D., Mathers, C.D., Ezzati, M., Jamison, D.T. and Murray, C.J.L. (2006). *Global Burden of Disease and Risk Factors*, Washington, DC: World Bank.

López-Ibor, J.J., Christodoulou, G., Maj, M., Sartorius, N. and Okasha, A. (2005). *Disasters and Mental Health*, Chichester: Wiley.

Lu, M.C. and Halfon, N. (2003). 'Racial and ethnic disparities in birth outcomes: a life-course perspective', *Maternal and Child Health Journal*, 7(1): 13–30.

Lucas, R., McMichael, T., Smith, W. and Armstrong, B. (2006). *Solar Ultraviolet Radiation: Global Burden of Disease from Solar Ultraviolet Radiation*, Environmental Burden of Disease Series No. 13, Geneva: WHO.

Lynch, J. and Smith, G.D. (2005). 'A life course approach to chronic disease epidemiology', *Annual Review of Public Health*, 26: 1–35.

MacArthur, C. (2009). 'Traditional birth attendant training for improving health behaviours and pregnancy outcomes: RHL commentary (last revised: 1 June)', in *WHO Reproductive Health Library*, Geneva: World Health Organization.

McCormick, D.P., Sarpong, K., Jordan, L., Ray, L.A. and Jain, S. (2010). 'Infant obesity: are we ready to make this diagnosis?', *Journal of Pediatrics*, 15(1): 15–19.

McCoy, M.A. and Salerno, J.A. (2010). *Assessing the Effects of the Gulf of Mexico Oil Spill on Human Health: A Summary of the June 2010 Workshop*, Washington, DC: Institute of Medicine and the National Academies Press.

McCracken, K. and Phillips, D.R. (2005). 'International demographic transitions', in G.J. Andrews and D.R. Phillips (eds) *Ageing and Place*, London: Routledge, pp. 36–60.

McCracken, K. and Phillips, D.R. (2009). 'Epidemiological transition', in R. Kitchin and N. Thrift (eds) *International Encyclopaedia of Human Geography*, Oxford: Elsevier, Vol. 3, pp. 571–579.

Macdonald, K. (2010). 'Part 1: Indigenous peoples and development goals: a global snapshot', in G. Hall and H. Patrinos (eds) *Indigenous Peoples, Poverty and Development*, discussion paper circulated by the World Bank, Washington, DC: World Bank.

Macdonald, V. (1998). 'Passive smoking doesn't cause cancer – official', *Electronic Telegraph*, 1017, 8 March. http://www.forces.org/articles/files/passive1.htm

McGinnis, J.M. and Foege, W.H. (1993). 'Actual causes of death in the United States', *Journal of the American Medical Association*, 270(18): 2207–2212.

MacIntyre, S., Ellaway, A. and Cummins, S. (2002). 'Place effects on health: how can we conceptualise, operationalise and measure them?', *Social Science and Medicine*, 55: 125–139.

Mackay, J., Jemal, A., Lee, N.C. and Parkin, D.M. (2006). *The Cancer Atlas*, Atlanta, GA: American Cancer Society.

Mackenbach, J.P. (2002). 'Income inequality and population health', *British Medical Journal*, 324: 1–2.

McKenzie, R.L., Aucamp, P.J., Bais, A.F., Bjorn, L.O., Ilyas, M. and Madronich, S. (2011). 'Ozone depletion and climate change: impacts on UV radiation', *Photochemical and Photobiological Sciences*, 10: 182–198.

McKeown, T. (1976). *The Modern Rise of Population*, London: Arnold.

McKinzie, J.P. (2007). 'Injury and global health', in W.H Markle, M.A. Fisher and R.A. Smego (eds) *Understanding Global Health*, New York: McGraw-Hill, pp. 200–207.

McMichael, A.J. (2001). *Human Frontiers, Environments and Disease: Past Patterns, Uncertain Futures*, Cambridge: Cambridge University Press.

McMichael, A., Githeko, A., Akhtar, R., Carcavallo, R., Gubler, D., Haines, A., Kovats, R.S., Martens, P., Patz, J. and Sasaki, A. (2001). 'Human health', in J.J. McCarthy, O.F. Canziani, N.A. Leary, D.J. Dokken and K.S. White (eds) *Climate Change 2001: Impacts, Adaptation and Vulnerability. Contribution of Working Group II to the Third Assessment Report of the Intergovernmental Panel on Climate Change*, Cambridge: Cambridge University Press, pp. 453–485.

McMichael, A.J., Woodruff, R.E. and Hales, S. (2006). 'Climate change and human health: present and future risks', *The Lancet*, 367: 859–869.

McNeil, D.G. (2011). 'New tick-borne disease is discovered', *New York Times*, 19 September. http://www.nytimes.com/2011/09/20/health/20tick.html

McNeill, W. (1976). *Plagues and People*, Middlesex: Penguin.

Mahapatra, P., Shibuya, K., Lopez, A.D., Coullare, F., Notzon, F.C., Rao, C. and Szreter, S. on behalf of the Monitoring of Vital Events (MoVE) writing group (2007). 'Civil registration systems and vital statistics: successes and missed opportunities', *The Lancet*, 370: 1653–1663.

Manton, K.G., Gu, X.-L. and Lamb, V.L. (2006). 'Change in chronic disability from 1982 to 2004–5 as measured by long-term changes in function and health in the US elderly population', *Proceedings of the National Academy of Science*, 103(48): 18374–18379.

Markle, W.H., Fisher, M.A. and Smego, R.A. (eds) (2007). *Understanding Global Health*, New York: McGraw-Hill.

Marmot, M. and Wilkinson, R.G. (eds) (2006). *Social Determinants of Health*, 2nd edition, Oxford: Oxford University Press.

Mason, J.K. and Laurie, G.T. (2011). *Mason and McCall Smith's Law and Medical Ethics*, Oxford: Oxford University Press.

Mathers, C.D., Fat, D.M., Inoue, M., Rao, C. and Lopez, A.D. (2005). 'Counting the dead and what they died from: an assessment of the global status of cause of death data', *Bulletin of the World Health Organization*, 83: 171–177.

Mathers, C.D. and Loncar, D. (2006). 'Projections of global mortality and burden of disease from 2002 to 2030', *PLoS Medicine*, 3(11): 2011–2030.

Mausner, J.S. and Kramer, S. (1985). *Mausner and Bahn: Epidemiology – an Introductory Text*, 2nd edition, Philadelphia, PA: W.B. Saunders Company.

Mayer, K. U. (2003). 'The sociology of the life course and life span psychology – diverging or converging pathways?', in U.M. Staudinger U. and Lindenberger (eds) *Understanding Human Development: Lifespan Psychology in Exchange with Other Disciplines*, Dordrecht: Kluwer Academic, pp. 463–482.

Merson, M.H., Black, R.E. and Mills, A.J. (eds) (2006). *International Public Health: Diseases, Programs, Systems and Policies*, 2nd edition, Sudbury, MA: Jones and Bartlett.

Micheli, A., Ciampichini, R., Oberaigner, W., Ciccolallo, L., de Vries, E., Izarzugaza, I., Zambon, P., Gatta, G. and De Angelis, R., the EUROCARE Working Group (2009). 'The advantage of women in cancer survival: an analysis of EUROCARE-4 data', *European Journal of Cancer*, 45: 1017–1027.

Midwifery Association of Pakistan (n.d.) *Midwifery in Pakistan*. http://www.midwifepak.org.pk/Midwifery_in_Pakistan.htm

Miller, R.A. (2002). 'Extending life: scientific prospects and political obstacles', *Milbank Quarterly*, 80: 155–174.

Mills, A., Bennett, S. and Russell, S. (2001). *The Challenge of Health Sector Reform*, London: Palgrave.

Ministry of Health, Government of Pakistan and World Health Organization (2010). *Weekly Epidemiological Bulletin: Flood Response in Pakistan*, 1(6), 27 September.

Ministry of Health, New Zealand (2011) *Antibiotic Resistance*. http://www.moh.govt.nz/moh.nsf/pagesmh/3345

Mission Readiness (2009). *Ready, Willing and Unable to Serve*, Washington, DC: Mission Readiness.

Montgomery, M.R. (2009). 'Urban poverty and health in developing countries', *Population Bulletin*, 64(2): 1–16.

Moody, H. (2010) *Aging: Concepts and Controversies*, Thousand Oaks, CA: Pine Forge Press/Sage.

Morens, D.M. and Taubenberger, J.K. (2011). 'Pandemic influenza: certain uncertainties', *Reviews in Medical Virology*, 21(5): 262–284.

Moser, K., Shkolnikov, V. and Leon, D.A. (2005). 'World mortality 1950–2000: divergence replaces convergence from the late 1980s', *Bulletin of the World Health Organization*, 83(3): 202–209.

Moyo, D. (2009). *Dead Aid: Why Aid Makes Things Worse and How There is Another Way for Africa*, London: Allen Lane.

Muntoni, S., Cocco, P., Aru, G., Cucca, F., and Muntoni, S. (2000). 'Nutritional factors and worldwide incidence of childhood type 1 diabetes', *American Journal of Clinical Nutrition*, 71(6): 1525–1529.

Murray, C.J.L., Ezzati, M., Lopez, A.D., Rodgers, A. and Vander Hoorn, S. (2003). 'Comparative quantification of health risks: conceptual framework and methodological issues', *Population Health Metrics*, 1(1). http://www.pophealthmetrics.com/content/1/1/1

Murray, C.J.L., King, G., Lopez, A.D., Tomijima, N. and Kru, E.G. (2002). 'Armed conflict as a public health problem', *British Medical Journal*, 324(7333): 346–349.

Murray, C.J.L., Rosenfeld, L.C., Lim, S.S., Andrews, K.G., Foreman, K.J., Haring, D., Fullman, N., Naghavi, M., Lozano, R. and Lopez, A.D. (2012). 'Global malaria mortality between 1980 and 2010: a systematic analysis', *The Lancet*, 379 (9814): 413–431.

Murthy, R.S. and Lakshminarayana, R. (2006). 'Mental health consequences of war: a brief review of research findings', *World Psychiatry*, 5(1): 25–30.

Myers, S.S. (2009). *Worldwatch Report 181: Global Environmental Change: The Threat to Human Health*, Washington, DC: Worldwatch Institute.

Naiman, A., Glazier, R.H. and Moineddin, R. (2010). 'Association of anti-smoking legislation with rates of hospital admission for cardiovascular and respiratory conditions', *Canadian Medical Association Journal*, 182(8): 761–767. http://www.cmaj.ca/cgi/reprint/182/8/761

National Center for Health Statistics (NCHS) (2011). *Health, United States, 2010*, Hyattsville, MD: US Department of Health and Human Services.

National Institute on Aging (NIA) (2007). *Why Population Aging Matters: A Global Perspective*, Washington, DC: National Institutes of Health.

National Intelligence Council (NIC) (2000). *The Global Infectious Disease Threat and Its Implications for the United States*, Washington, DC: NIC.

National Research Council (NRC) (1999). *From Monsoons to Microbes: Understanding the Ocean's Role in Human Health*, Washington, DC: National Academies Press.

National Research Council (2003). *Malaria Control During Mass Population Movements and Natural Disasters*, Washington, DC: National Academies Press.

National Statistical Coordination Board (2005) *Philippine Statistical Yearbook*, CD-ROM, Manila: National Statistical Coordination Board.

Neria, Y., Galea, S. and Norris, F.H. (eds) (2009). *Mental Health and Disasters*, Cambridge: Cambridge University Press.

Neumann, A.K. and Lauro, P. (1982). 'Ethnomedicine and biomedicine linking', *Social Science and Medicine*, 16: 1817–1824.

New Internationalist (1999). 'Landmines: the facts', fact sheet, Oxford: New Internationalist Cooperative. http://www.newint.org/easier-english/landmine/lmfacts.html

Ngozo, C. (2011). 'Malawi: uncertainty over role for traditional birth attendants', Global Issues Inter-Press Service, 15 March. http://www.globalissues.org/news/2011/03/15/8880

Niño-Zarazú, M. (2010). *Mexico's Progresa-Oportunidades and the Emergence of Social Assistance in Latin America*, BWPI Working Paper 142, Manchester: Brooks World Poverty Institute, University of Manchester.

Nolte, E. and McKee, M. (2004). *Does Health Care Save Lives? Avoidable Mortality Revisited*, London: Nuffield Trust.

Norval, M., Lucas, R.M., Cullen, A.P., de Gruijl, F.R., Longstreth, J., Takizawa, Y. and van der Leun, J.C. (2011). 'The human health effects of ozone depletion and interactions with climate change', *Photochemical & Photobiological Sciences*, 10: 199–225.

Notestein, F.W. (1945). 'Population – the long view', in T.W. Schultz (ed.) *Food for the World*, Chicago: University of Chicago Press, pp. 36–69.

Nzegwu, M.A., Banjo, A.A.F., Akhiwu, W., Aligbe, J.U. and Nzegwu, C.O. (2008). 'Morbidity and mortality among road users in Benin-city, Nigeria', *Annals of African Medicine*, 7(3): 102–106.

Öberg, M., Jaakkola, M.S., Woodward, A., Peruga, A. and Prüss-Ustün, A. (2011). 'Worldwide burden of disease from exposure to second-hand smoke: a retrospective analysis of data from 192 countries', *The Lancet*, 377(9760): 139–146.

Oceanography (2006). Special issue on 'The Oceans and Human Health', 19(2).

Oeppen, J. and Vaupel, J.W. (2002). 'Broken limits to life expectancy', *Science*, 296: 1029–1031.

Office of the High Commissioner for Human Rights (OHCHR). (2011). *Ending 'Son Preference' to Promote Gender Equality*, joint declaration, 15 July. http://www.ohchr.org/EN/NewsEvents/Pages/GenderEquality.aspx

Office of the Inspector General (2000). *The Globalization of Clinical Trials: A Growing Challenge in Protecting Human Subjects*. Boston: US Department of Health and Human Service, OIG, Office of Evaluation and Inspections, Boston Regional Office. http://oig.hhs.gov/oei/reports/oei-01-00-00190.pdf

Ofili, A.N. and Okojie, O.H. (2005). 'Assessment of the role of traditional birth attendants in maternal health care in Oredo Local Government Area, Edo State, Nigeria', *Journal of Community Medicine and Primary Health Care*, 17(1): 55–60.

Olshanky, S.J. and Ault, A.B. (1986). 'The fourth stage of the epidemiologic transition: the age of delayed degenerative diseases', *Milbank Quarterly*, 64(3): 355–391.

Olshansky, S.J. (2004). 'The future of human life expectancy', in United Nations, Department of Economic and Social Affairs, *World Population to 2300*, New York: United Nations, pp 159–164.

Omran, A.R. (1971). 'The epidemiologic transition: a theory of the epidemiology of population change', *Milbank Memorial Fund Quarterly*, 49(4): 509–538.

Ong, C.K., Bodeker, G., Grundy, C., Burford, G. and Shein, K. (2005). *WHO Global Atlas of Traditional, Complementary and Alternative Medicine*, Kobe: WHO Centre for Health Development.

Organization for Economic Cooperation and Development (OECD). (2007). 'Immigrant health workers in OECD countries in the broader context of highly skilled migration', in *International Migration Outlook 2007*, Paris: OECD, pp. 161–228.

Organization for Economic Cooperation and Development (OECD). (2009). *Measuring Aid to Health*, Paris: OECD. http://www.oecd.org/dataoecd/44/35/44070071.pdf

Organization for Economic Cooperation and Development (OECD). (2010a). *Health at a Glance: Europe 2010*, Paris: OECD. http://www.oecd-ilibrary.org/social-issues-migration-health/health-at-a-glance-europe-2010_health_glance-2010-en;jsessionid=97mmen2q2f5hr.delta

Organization for Economic Cooperation and Development (OECD). (2010b). *Health at a Glance: Asia/Pacific 2010*, Paris: OECD.

Organization for Economic Cooperation and Development (OECD). (2010c). *Obesity and the Economics of Prevention: Fit Not Fat*, Paris: OECD. http://www.oecd.org/document/31/0,3343,en_2649_33929_45999775_1_1_1_1,00.html#Executive_Summary

Organization for Economic Cooperation and Development (OECD). (2011a). *Focus on Aid to Health*, Paris: OECD. http://www.oecd.org/document/44/0,3746,en_2649_34631_24670956_1_1_1_1,00.html

Organization for Economic Cooperation and Development (OECD). (2011b). *OECD at 50 – International Migration Outlook 2011*, Paris: OECD.

Osler, M. (2006). 'The life course perspective: a challenge for public health research and prevention', *European Journal of Public Health*, 16(3): 230.

Osterholm, M.T. (2007). 'Unprepared for a pandemic', *Foreign Affairs*, 86(2): 47–57.

Oxfam. (2011a). *East Africa Food Crisis*, Oxford: Oxfam International. http://www.oxfam.org/eastafrica

Oxfam (2011b). *Growing a Better Future: Food Justice in a Resource-constrained World*, Oxford: Oxfam International. http://www.oxfam.org/sites/www.oxfam.org/files/growing-a-better-future-010611-en.pdf

Pan, C.X., Chai, E. and Faber, J. (2007). *Myths of the High Medical Cost of Old Age and Dying*, New York: International Longevity Center.

Pan American Health Organization (PAHO) (2000). *Natural Disasters: Protecting the Public's Health*, Scientific Publication 575, Washington, DC: PAHO.

Pathak, A., Desania, N.L. and Verma, R. (2008). 'Profile of road traffic accidents and head injury in Jaipur (Rajasthan)', *Journal of Indian Academy of Forensic Medicine*, 30(1): 6–9.

Patz, J.A. and Olson, S.H. (2006). 'Malaria risk and temperature: influences from global climate change and local land use practices', *Proceedings of the National Academy of Sciences*, 103(15): 5635–5636.

Patz, J.A., Engelberg, D. and Last, J. (2000). 'The effects of changing weather on public health', *Annual Review of Public Health*, 21: 271–307.

Patz, J.A., Olson, S.H. and Gray, A.L. (2006). 'Climate change, oceans, and human health', *Oceanography*, 19(2): 52–59.

Patz, J.A., Olson, S.H., Uejio, C.K. and Gibbs, H.K. (2008). 'Disease emergence from global climate and land use change', *Medical Clinics of North America*, 92: 1473–1491.

Pedersen, D. (2002). 'Political violence, ethnic conflict, and contemporary wars: broad implications for health and social well-being', *Social Science and Medicine*, 55(2): 175–190.

Percival, V. and Sondorp, E. (2010). 'A case study of health sector reform in Kosovo', *Conflict and Health*, 4: 7. http://www.conflictandhealth.com/content/4/1/7

Peterman, A., Palermo, T. and Bredenkamp, C. (2011). 'Estimates and determinants of sexual violence in the Democratic Republic of the Congo', *American Journal of Public Health*, 101(6): 1060–1067.

Peters, D.H., El-Saharty, S., Siadat, B., Janovsky, K. and Vujicic, M. (eds) (2009). *Improving Health Service Delivery in Developing Countries: From Evidence to Action*, Washington, DC: World Bank.

Peterson, S. (2002–03). 'Epidemic disease and national security', *Security Studies*, 12(2): 43–81.

Phillips, D.R. (1990). *Health and Health Care in the Third World*. London: Longman.

Phillips, D.R., Rosenberg, M.W. and Wilson, K. (2007). 'Medical geography', in M. Sala (ed.) *Geography* (e-book), *Encyclopedia of Life Support Systems*, Oxford: EOLSS Publishers/UNESCO, Vol. 2, pp. 141–158.

Phillips, D.R. and Siu, O.-L. (2012). 'Global aging and aging workers', in J.W. Hedge and W.C. Borman (eds) *Oxford Handbook of Work and Aging*, New York: Oxford University Press.

Phillipson, C. and Baars, J. (2007). 'Social theory and social ageing', in J. Bond, S. Peace, F. Dittmann-Kohli and G. Westerhof (eds) *Ageing in Society*, 3rd edition, London: Sage, pp. 68–84.

Plomer, A. (2005). *The Law and Ethics of Medical Research: International Bioethics and Human Rights*, Oxford: Cavendish.

Popkin, B.M. (2002). 'An overview on the nutrition transition and its health implications: the Bellagio meeting', *Public Health Nutrition*, 5(1A): 93–103.

Popkin, B.M. (2006). 'Global nutrition dynamics: the world is shifting rapidly toward a diet linked with noncommunicable diseases', *American Journal of Clinical Nutrition*, 84: 289–298.

Population Foundation of India and Population Reference Bureau (2007). *The Future Population of India*. http://www.prb.org/pdf07/futurepopulationofindia.pdf

Population Reference Bureau (2010). 'Population Reference Bureau receives funding for raising the visibility of malnutrition', press release, Washington, DC: PRB. http://www.prb.org/Journalists/PressReleases/2010/renew.aspx

Rapp, T. (2010). 'Health economics and health policy issues in Alzheimer's Disease', *Journal of Nutrition, Health & Aging*, 14(8): 630–632. http://www.springerlink.com/content/4106u635024h2807/fulltext.pdf

Ratzan, S.C., Filerman, G.L. and LeSar, J.W. (2000). 'Attaining global health: challenges and opportunities', *Population Bulletin*, 55(1): 1–48.

Redfoot, D.L. and Houser, A. (2010). *More Older People with Disabilities Living in the Community: Trends from the National Long-term Care Survey, 1984–2004*, AARP Public Policy Institute Research Report No. 2010-08, Washington, DC: AARP Public Policy Institute.

Relman, D.A., Choffnes, E.R. and Mack, A. (2010). *Infectious Disease Movement in a Borderless World: Workshop Summary*, Washington, DC: National Academies Press.

Remennick, L. (2006). 'The challenge of early breast cancer detection among immigrant and minority women in multicultural societies', *Breast Journal*, 12 (Supplement 1): S103–S110.

Requejo, J. (2010). *Countdown to 2015 – Decade Report (2000–2010): Taking Stock of Maternal, Newborn and Child Survival*, Geneva: Countdown Group. http://www.countdown2015mnch.org/reports-publications/2010-report/2010-report-downloads

Richel, T. (2003). 'Will human life expectancy quadruple in the next hundred years? Sixty geron-tologists say public debate on life extension is necessary', *Journal of Anti-Aging Medicine*, 6(4): 309–314.

Riley, J.C. (2005a). 'Estimates of regional and global life expectancy, 1800–2001', *Population and Development Review*, 31(3): 537–543.

Riley, J.C. (2005b). 'The timing and pace of health transitions around the world', *Population and Development Review*, 31(4): 741–764.

Riley, J.C. (2005c). 'Bibliography of works providing estimates of life expectancy at birth and estimates of the beginning period of health transitions in countries with a population in 2000 of at least 400,000'. http://www.lifetable.de/RileyBib.htm

Robert Woods Johnson Foundation (2008). 'A look at obesity trends nationwide', Princeton: RWJF. http://www.rwjf.org/files/research/obesitytrends95to06.pdf

Rockett, I.R.H. (1999). 'Population and health: an introduction to epidemiology (2nd edition)', *Population Bulletin*, 54(4): 1–44.

Rodwin, V.G. and Gusmano, M.K. (eds) (2006). *Growing Older in World Cities: New York, London, Paris, and Tokyo*, Nashville, TN: Vanderbilt University Press.

Royal College of Physicians (2010). *Passive Smoking and Children: A Report of the Tobacco Advisory Group of the Royal College of Physicians*, London: RCP. http://www.rcplondon.ac.uk/professional-Issues/Public-Health/Documents/Preface-to-passive-smoking-and-children-March-2010.pdf

Ruit, S., Tabin, G.C. and Wykoff, C.C. (2006). *Fighting Global Blindness: Improving World Vision through Cataract Elimination*, Washington DC: American Public Health Association.

Sankaranarayanan, R., Swaminathan, R., Brenner, H., Chen, K., Chia, K.S, Chen, J.G., Law, S.C.K, Ahn, Y.-O., Xiang, Y.B., Yeole, B.B., Shin, H.R., Shanta, V., Woo, Z.H., Martin, N., Sumitsawan, Y., Sriplung, H., Barboza, A.O., Eser, S., Nene, B.M., Suwanrungruang, K., Jayalekshmi, P., Dikshit, R., Wabinga, H., Esteban, D.B., Laudico, A., Bhurgri, Y., Bah, E. and Al-Hamdan, N. (2010). 'Cancer survival in Africa, Asia, and Central America: a population-based study', *The Lancet Oncology*, 11(2): 165–173.

Sankaranarayanan, R. and Swaminathan, R. (2011). *Cancer Survival in Africa, Asia, the Caribbean and Central America*, IARC Scientific Publication No. 162, Lyon: IARC and WHO.

Sargent, R.P., Shepard, R.M. and Glantz, S.A. (2004). 'Reduced incidence of admissions for myocardial infarction associated with public smoking ban: before and after study', *British Medical Journal*, 328: 977–980.

Save the Children (2011). 'Report on global birth attendance', BBC World Service, 1 April. http://www.savethechildren.org.uk/

Schlein, L. (2012). 'WHO stands by its numbers on malaria deaths', *Voice of America*, 3 February. http://www.voanews.com/english/news/health/WHO-Stands-By-Its-Numbers-On-Malaria-Deaths-138651424.html

Schneider, M.J. (2011). *Introduction to Public Health*, 3rd edition, Sudbury, MA: Jones and Bartlett.

Seeman, T.E., Merkin, S.S., Crimmins, E.M. and Karlamangla, A.S. (2010). Disability trends among older Americans: National Health and Nutrition Examination surveys, 1988–1994 and 1999–2004, *American Journal of Public Health*, 100(1): 100–107.

Sen, G., George, A. and Östlin, P. (eds) (2002). *Engendering International Health: The Challenge of Equity*, Cambridge, MA: MIT Press.

Setel, P.W., Macfarlane, S.B., Szreter, S., Mikkelsen, L., Jha, P., Stout, S. and AbouZahr, C. on behalf of the Monitoring of Vital Events (MoVE) writing group (2007). 'A scandal of invisibility: making everyone count by counting everyone', *The Lancet*, 370: 1569–1577.

Shabila, N.P., Taha, H.I. and Al-Hadithi, T.S. (2010). 'Landmine injuries at the Emergency Management Center in Erbil, Iraq', *Conflict and Health*, 4: 15. http://www.conflictandhealth.com/content/4/1/15

Shanghai Daily (2011) 'Hospital births spur huge drop in deaths', *Shanghai Daily*, 17 September, p. A3.

Sims, M., Maxwell, R., Bauld, L. and Gilmore, A. (2010). 'Short term impact of smoke-free legislation in England: retrospective analysis of hospital admissions for myocardial infarction', *British Medical Journal*, 340(c2161). http://www.bmj.com/content/340/bmj.c2161.abstract

Skolnik, R.L. (2008). *Essentials of Global Health*, Sudbury, MA: Jones and Bartlett.

Skolnik, R.L. (2012). *Global Health 101* (2nd edition of Skolnik, 2008), Burlington, MA: Jones and Bartlett.

Slate (2001) 'How does Alzheimer's kill?' http://www.slate.com/articles/news_and_politics/explainer/2001/04/how_does_alzheimers_kill.html

Smallman-Raynor, M. and Phillips, D. (1999). 'Late stages of epidemiological transition: health status in the developed world', *Health and Place*, 5(3): 209–222.

Smet, J. de, Charlton, J.E. and Meynadier, J. (1998). 'Pain and rehabilitation from landmine injury', *Pain Clinical Updates*, 6(2). http://www.iasp-pain.org/AM/AMTemplate.cfm?Section=Home, Home,Home,Home&CONTENTID=7590&TEMPLATE=/CM/ContentDisplay.cfm&SECTIO N=Home,Home,Home,Home

Smylie, J. and Adomako, P. (eds) (2009). *Indigenous Children's Health Report: Health Assessment in Action*, Toronto: Centre for Research on Inner City Health, Li Ka Shing Knowledge Institute.

Soleman, N., Chandramohan, D. and Shibuya, K. (2006). 'Verbal autopsy: current practices and challenges', *Bulletin of the World Health Organization*, 84: 239–245.

Soltesz, G., Patterson, C. and Dahlquist, G. (2009). 'Diabetes in the young: a global perspective – global trends in childhood type 1 diabetes', in International Diabetes Federation, *IDF Diabetes Atlas*, 4th edition, Brussels: IDF, pp. 1–36. http://www.idf.org/diabetesatlas/downloads/backgroundpapers

Sonnega, A. (2006). 'The future of human life expectancy: have we reached the ceiling or is the sky the limit?', *Research Highlights in the Demography and Economics of Aging*, 8: 1–4.

Sparks, B.T. (2004). 'A descriptive study of the changing roles and practices of traditional birth attendants in Zimbabwe', in E. van Teijlingen, G. Lowis, P. McCaffery and M. Porter (eds) *Midwifery and the Medicalization of Childbirth*, New York: Nova Science, pp. 245–257.

Sproston, K. and Mindell, J. (eds) (2006). *Health Survey for England 2004. Volume 1: The Health of Minority Ethnic Groups*, Leeds: The Information Centre.

Statistics Canada (2006). *Life Tables, Canada, Provinces and Territories: 2000 to 2002*. http://www.statcan.gc.ca

Statistics New Zealand (2009). *New Zealand Life Tables: 2005–07*. http://www.stats.govt.nz

Stephens, C., Porter, J., Nettleton, C. and Willis, R. (2006). 'Disappearing, displaced, and under-valued: a call to action for Indigenous health worldwide', *The Lancet*, 367: 2019–2028.

Stevens, G., Dias, R.H., Thomas, K.J.A., Rivera, J.A., Carvalho, N., Barquera, S., Hill, K. and Ezzati, M. (2008). 'Characterising the epidemiological transition in Mexico: national and subnational burden of diseases, injuries, and risk factors', *PLoS Medicine*, 5(6): 900–910.

Stevens, P. (2009). 'Bias in WHO report on the social determinants of health', *The Lancet*, 373: 298.

Sturm R. (2002). 'The effects of obesity, smoking, and problem drinking on chronic medical problems and health care costs', *Health Affairs*, 21(2): 245–253.

Surrency, A.B., Graitcer, P.L. and Henderson A.K. (2007). 'Key factors for civilian injuries and deaths from exploding landmines and ordnance', *Injury Prevention*, 13(3): 197–201.

Swinburn, B.A., Sacks, G., Hall, K.D., McPherson, K., Finegood, D., Moodie, M.L. and Gortmaker, S.L. (2011). 'The global obesity pandemic: shaped by global drivers and local environments', *The Lancet*, 378(9793): 804–814.

Taubenberger, J.K. and Morens, D.M. (2010). 'Influenza: the once and future pandemic', *Public Health*, 125(Supplement 3): 16–26.

Thames Water (2011). 'London Tideway Improvements: Frequently Asked Questions: Are the Thames and Lee Tunnels Really Needed?' http://www.thameswater.co.uk/cps/rde/xchg/corp/hs.xsl/8877.htm

Thun, M.J., DeLancey, J.O., Center, M.M., Jemal, A. and Ward, E.M. (2009). 'The global burden of cancer: priorities for prevention', *Carcinogenesis*, 31(1): 100–110.

Toon, O.B., Robock, A., Turco, R.P., Bardeen, C., Oman, L. and Stenchikov, G.L. (2007). 'Consequences of regional-scale nuclear conflicts', *Science*, 315: 1224–1225.

Tracey, E., Barraclough, H., Chen, W., Baker, D., Roder, D., Jelfs, P. and Bishop, J. (2007). *Survival from Cancer in NSW: 1980 to 2003*. Sydney: Cancer Institute NSW.

Turrell, G., Oldenburg, B., McGuffog, I. and Dent, R. (1999). *Socioeconomic Determinants of Health: Towards a National Research Program and a Policy and Intervention Agenda*, Canberra: Queensland University of Technology, School of Public Health, Ausinfo.

Ungoed-Thomas, J. and Krause, S. (2010). 'How our beaches are polluted by thousands of sewage spills', *Sunday Times*, 23 May. http://www.timesonline.co.uk/tol/news/environment/article7134009.ece

United Kingdom Parliamentary Office of Science and Technology (2003). 'Childhood obesity', *Postnote* No. 205: 1–4.

United Kingdom Office for National Statistics (2010). *Period and Cohort Expectation of Life Tables (2008-based)*. http://www.statistics.gov.uk/downloads/theme_population/Interim_Life/period_cohort_tables_index08.pdf

United Kingdom Office for National Statistics (2011). *Trends in Life Expectancy by National Statistics Socio-economic Classification (NS-SEC), 1982-2006*. http://www.ons.gov.uk/ons/publications/re-reference-tables.html?edition=tcm%3A77-247704

United Nations (1962) *The Situation and Recent Trends of Mortality in the World*, Population Bulletin of the United Nations No.6, New York: United Nations.

United Nations (2001). *Stockholm Convention on Persistent Organic Pollutants*. http://www.pops.int/documents/convtext/convtext_en.pdf

United Nations (2011). *"Ending 'Son Preference' to Promote Gender Equality"*, Joint declaration, UN Human Rights Office (OHCHR), 15 July. http://www.ohchr.org/EN/NewsEvents/Pages/GenderEquality.aspx

United Nations Children's Fund (UNICEF) (2008). *The State of the World's Children 2009: Maternal and Newborn Health*, New York: United Nations. http://www.unicef.org/sowc09/

United Nations Children's Fund (UNICEF) (2009). 'Global child mortality continues to fall', 10 September. http://www.unicefusa.org/news/releases/global-child-mortality.html

United Nations Convention to Combat Desertification (UNCCD) (2011). *Background Document: High-level Meeting on Addressing Desertification, Land Degradation and Drought in the Context of Sustainable Development and Poverty Eradication* (advanced unedited text), New York: UNCCD.

United Nations Department of Economic and Social Affairs (UNDESA) (2008). *Regional Dimensions of the Ageing Situation*, New York: United Nations.

United Nations Department of Economic and Social Affairs (UNDESA) (2010). *The World's Women 2010: Trends and Statistics*, New York: United Nations. http://unstats.un.org/unsd/demographic/products/Worldswomen/WW_full%20report_color.pdf

United Nations Department of Economic and Social Affairs (UNDESA) (2011). *The Millennium Development Goals Report 2011*, New York: United Nations.

United Nations Department of Economic and Social Affairs, Population Division (UNDESA-PD) (2009). *World Population Prospects: The 2008 Revision*, New York: United Nations.

United Nations Department of Economic and Social Affairs, Population Division (UNDESA-PD) (2010). *World Urbanisation Prospects: The 2009 Revision*, New York: United Nations. http://esa.un.org/unpd/wup/index.htm

United Nations Department of Economic and Social Affairs, Population Division (UNDESA-PD) (2011). *World Population Prospects: The 2010 Revision*, New York: United Nations. http://esa.un.org/unpd/wpp/index.htm

United Nations Department of Public Information (1996). *Women and Violence: Human Rights*, New York: United Nations. http://www.un.org/rights/dpi1772e.htm

United Nations Development Programme (1994). *Human Development Report 1994*, New York: Oxford University Press.

United Nations Development Programme (2009). *Human Development Report 2009: Overcoming Barriers: Human Mobility and Development*, New York: United Nations.

United Nations Development Programme (2010). *What Are the Millennium Development Goals?* http://www.undp.org/mdg/basics.shtml

United Nations Foundation (2009). 'Global measles deaths drop by 78%, but resurgence likely', press release. http://www.unfoundation.org/press-center/press-releases/2009/global-measles-deaths-drop-by-78-percent.html

United Nations General Assembly (1997). *Report of the Economic and Social Council for 1997*, New York: United Nations.

United Nations General Assembly (2011). *Political Declaration of the High-level Meeting of the General Assembly on the Prevention and Control of Non-communicable Diseases*, New York: United Nations.

United Nations High Commissioner for Refugees (2011). *Statistics and Operational Data*. Geneva: UNHCR. http://www.unhcr.org/pages/4a324fcc6.html

United Nations Inter-agency Group for Child Mortality Estimation (2007). *Levels and Trends of Child Mortality in 2006: Estimates Developed by the Inter-agency Group for Child Mortality Estimation*, New York: UNICEF.

United Nations Inter-agency Group for Child Mortality Estimation (2010). *Levels and Trends in Child Mortality: Report 2010. Estimates Developed by the Inter-agency Group for Child Mortality Estimation*, New York: UNICEF.

United Nations Inter-agency Group for Child Mortality Estimation (2011). *Levels and Trends in Child Mortality: Report 2011. Estimates Developed by the Inter-agency Group for Child Mortality Estimation*, New York: UNICEF.

United Nations in Vietnam (2011). 'Speech at the meeting with officials of the National Assembly on Sex Ratio at Birth Imbalance', press statement, 8 November. http://www.un.org.vn/en/news-centre/speeches/153-unfpa-speeches/2001-speech-of-ms-mandeep-obrien-unfpa-officer-in-charge-at-the-meeting-with-officials-of-the-national-assembly-on-sex-ratio-at-birth-imbalance.html

United Nations Joint Programme on HIV/AIDS (UNAIDS) (2005). *In the Front Line: A Review of Policies and Programmes to Address AIDS among Peacekeepers and Uniformed Services*, New York: UNAIDS.

United Nations Population Fund (UNFPA) (2009). *UNFPA Strategy and Framework for Action to Addressing Gender-based Violence 2008–2011*, New York: UNFPA.

United Nations Population Fund (UNFPA) (2011a). *The State of the World's Midwifery 2011*. New York: United Nations. http://www.stateoftheworldsmidwifery.com

United Nations Population Fund (UNFPA) (2011b). *Stop Sex Selection: A Threat to Lives of Women and Girls*, fact sheet, 10 June, Hanoi: UN in Vietnam.

United Nations Population Fund (UNFPA) and Population Reference Bureau (PRB) (2009). *Healthy Expectations: Celebrating Achievements of the Cairo Consensus and Highlighting the Urgency for Action: International Conference on Population and Development in Cairo 15 Years Later*, New York: UNFPA and Washington, DC: PRB.

United States Department of State (2010). *Country Reports on Terrorism 2010*, Washington, DC: Department of State.

United States Social Security Administration (2011). *2011 Trustees Report*. http://www.ssa.gov/oact/tr/2011/lr5a3.html

Van de Poel, E., Hosseinpoor, A.R., Speybroeck, N., Van Ourti, T. and Vega, J. (2008). 'Socioeconomic inequality in malnutrition in developing countries', *Bulletin of the World Health Organization*, 86(4): 282–291.

Varmus, H., Klausner, R., Zerhouni, E., Acharya, T., Daar, A.S. and Singer, P.A. (2003). 'Grand challenges in global health', *Science*, 302, 17: 398–399.

Vellas, B. and Aisen, P.S. (2010). 'Early Alzheimer's trials: new developments', *Journal of Nutrition, Health & Aging*, 14(4): 293.

Verbrugge, L. (1984). 'Longer life but worsening health? Trends in health and mortality of middle-aged and older persons', *Milbank Memorial Fund Quarterly*, 62(3): 475–519.

Victor, C. (2010). 'The demography of ageing', in D. Dannefer and C. Phillipson (eds) *The SAGE Handbook of Social Gerontology*, London: Sage, pp. 61–74.

Waage, J., Banerji, R., Campbell, O., Chirwa, E., Collender, G., Dieltiens, V., Dorward, A., Godfrey-Faussett, P., Hanvoravongchai, P., Kingdon, G., Little, A., Mills, A., Mulholland, K., Mwinga, A., North, A., Patcharanarumol, W., Poulton, C., Tangcharoensathien, V. and Unterhalter, E., (2010) 'The Millennium Development Goals: a cross-sectoral analysis and principles for goal setting after 2015', *The Lancet*, 376(9745): 991–1023.

Waidmann, T.A. and Manton, K.G. (1998). *International Evidence on Disability Trends among the Elderly*, Report for the Office of the Assistant Secretary for Planning and Evaluation, US Department of Health and Human Services, Office of Disability, Aging and Long-Term Care, Washington, DC.

Walsh, J.A. and Warren, K.S. (1979). 'Selective primary health care: an interim strategy for disease control in developing countries', *New England Journal of Medicine*, 301(18): 967–974.

Wang, S.J., Salihu, M., Rushiti, F., Bala, L. and Modvig, J. (2010). 'Survivors of the war in the

Northern Kosovo: violence exposure, risk factors and public health effects of an ethnic conflict', *Conflict and Health*, 4: 11. http://www.biomedcentral.com/content/pdf/1752-1505-4-11.pdf

War Victims Monitor (2011). 'Six die in roadside bomb blast in Mogadishu'. http://warvictims. wordpress.com/tag/somalia/

Watson, J.T., Gayer, M. and Connolly, M.A. (2007) 'Epidemics after natural disasters', *Emerging Infectious Diseases*, 13(1): 1–5.

Wellcome Trust (2009) 'Flu: your guide to H1N1 and other pandemics', *Big Picture*, Special issue, October.

Wen, C.P., Tsai, S.P., Shih, Y.-T. and Chung, W.-S.I. (2004). 'Bridging the gap in life expectancy of the aborigines in Taiwan', *International Journal of Epidemiology*, 33: 320–327.

Wethington, E. and Johnson-Askew, W.L. (2009). 'Contributions of the life course perspective to research on food decision-making', *Annals of Behavioral Medicine*, 38 (Supplement 1): S74–S80.

Whitehead, M. (1990). *The Concepts and Principles of Equity and Health*, Copenhagen: World Health Organization Regional Office for Europe.

Wilcox, B.A. and Gubler, D.J. (2011). 'Environmental change and new infectious diseases', *Environment Times: Poverty Times*, 4. http://www.grida.no/publications/et/ep4/page.aspx

Wilkinson, R. and Marmot, M. (eds) (2003). *Social Determinants of Health: The Solid Facts*, 2nd edition, Copenhagen: World Health Organization Regional Office for Europe.

Wilkinson, R.G. and Pickett, K. (2009). *The Spirit Level: Why More Equal Societies Almost Always Do Better*, London: Allen Lane.

Williams, A. (1997). 'The rationing debate: rationing health care by age: the case for', *British Medical Journal*, 314: 820–822.

Wilmoth, J.R. (1998). 'The future of human longevity: a demographer's perspective', *Science*, 280: 395–397.

Wojcicki, J.M. and Heyman, M.B. (2010). 'Let's move – childhood obesity prevention from pregnancy and infancy onward', *New England Journal of Medicine*, 362(16): 1457–1459.

Wolf, D.A., Hunt, K. and Knickman, J. (2005). 'Perspectives on the recent decline in disability at older ages', *Milbank Quarterly*, 83(3): 365–395.

Woodward, D., Drager, N., Beaglehole, R. and Lipson, D. (2001). 'Globalization and health: a framework for analysis and action', *Bulletin of the World Health Organization*, 79: 875–881.

World Bank (2007). *The Study of Traffic Accident Costs in Thailand*, Washington, DC: World Bank. http://web.worldbank.org/WBSITE/EXTERNAL/COUNTRIES/EASTASIAPACIFICEXT/EXTEAPREGTOPTRANSPORT/0,,contentMDK:21700813~menuPK:3969695~pagePK:2865114~piPK:2865167~theSitePK:574066,00.html

World Bank (2010). *The MDGS After the Crisis: Global Monitoring Report 2010*, Washington, DC: World Bank. http://publications. worldbank.org/index.php?main_page=product_info&cPath=0&products_id=23794

World Health Organization (WHO) (2000). *World Health Report 2000 – Health Systems: Improving Performance*, Geneva: WHO.

World Health Organization (WHO) (2001). *World Health Report 2001 – Mental Health: New Understanding, New Hope*, Geneva: WHO.

World Health Organization (WHO) (2002). *World Report on Violence and Health*, Geneva: WHO.

World Health Organization (WHO) (2003). *Climate Change and Human Health: Risks and Responses. Summary*, Geneva: WHO, WMO, UNEP.

World Health Organization (WHO) (2004). *World Report on Road Traffic Injury Prevention*, Geneva: WHO. http://whqlibdoc.who.int/publications/2004/9241562609.pdf (accessed 20 March, 2012).

World Health Organization (WHO) (2005). *WHO Multi-country Study on Women's Health and Domestic Violence Against Women*, Geneva: WHO.

World Health Organization (WHO) (2007a). *A Conceptual Framework for Action on the Social Determinants of Health*, discussion paper, Commission on Social Determinants of Health. http://www.who.int/social_determinants/resources/csdh_framework_action_05_07.pdf (accessed 31 March, 2010).

World Health Organization (WHO) (2007b). 'The health of indigenous peoples', Fact Sheet No. 326, Geneva: WHO.

World Health Organization (WHO) (2007c). *Verbal Autopsy Standards: Ascertaining and Attributing Cause of Death.* http://www.whqlibdoc.who.int/publications/2007/9789241547215_eng.pdf (accessed 8 June, 2009).

World Health Organization (WHO) (2008a). *2008–2013: Action Plan for the Global Strategy for the Prevention and Control of Noncommunicable Diseases*, Geneva: WHO. http://whqlibdoc.who.int/publications/2009/9789241597418_eng.pdf (accessed 28 October, 2011).

World Health Organization (WHO) (2008b). *The Global Burden of Disease: 2004 Update*, Geneva: WHO. http://www.who.int/healthinfo/global_burden_disease/GBD_report_2004update_full.pdf (accessed 6 September, 2009).

World Health Organization (WHO) (2008c). *Closing the Gap in a Generation: Health Equity through Action on the Social Determinants of Health*, Geneva: WHO.

World Health Organization (WHO) (2008d). *Older People in Emergencies: An Active Ageing Perspective*, Geneva: WHO.

World Health Organization (WHO) (2008e). *Traditional Medicine*, Fact Sheet No. 134, Geneva: WHO. http://www.who.int/mediacentre/factsheets/fs134/en/ (accessed 25 May, 2011).

World Health Organization (WHO) (2009a). *Global Health Risks: Mortality and Burden of Disease Attributable to Selected Major Risks*, Geneva: WHO. http://whqlibdoc.who.int/publications/2009/9789241563871_eng.pdf (accessed 22 October, 2010).

World Health Organization (WHO) (2009b). *Women's Health.* Fact Sheet No. 334, Geneva: WHO. http://www.who.int/mediacentre/factsheets/fs334/en/index.html (accessed 28 October, 2011).

World Health Organization (WHO) (2009c). *Global Status Report on Road Safety: Time for Action*, Geneva: WHO. http://whqlibdoc.who.int/publications/2009/9789241563840_eng.pdf (accessed 29 February, 2012).

World Health Organization (WHO) (2009d). *Protecting Health from Climate Change: Global Research Priorities*, Geneva: WHO.

World Health Organization (WHO) (2009e). *Mortality and Burden of Disease Estimates for WHO Member States in 2004*, Geneva: WHO. http://www.who.int/healthinfo/global_burden_disease/gbddeathdalycountryestimates2004.xls (accessed 11 February, 2011).

World Health Organization (WHO) (2010a). *World Health Report 2010 – Health Systems Financing: The Path to Universal Coverage*, Geneva: WHO. http://www.who.int/whr/2010/en/index.html (accessed 15 September, 2011).

World Health Organization (WHO) (2010b). *Preventing Noncommunicable Diseases – Advocacy Pack*, Manila: WHO, Western Pacific Region.

World Health Organization (WHO) (2010c). *Medicines: Spurious/Falsely-Labelled/ Falsified/Counterfeit (SFFC) Medicines*, Fact Sheet No. 275, Geneva: WHO.

World Health Organization (WHO) (2011a). *World Health Statistics, 2011*, Geneva: WHO.

World Health Organization (WHO) (2011b). *Decade of Action for Road Safety 2011–2020: Saving Millions of Lives.* http://www.who.int/violence_injury_prevention/publications/road_traffic/saving_millions_lives_en.pdf (accessed 8 June, 2011).

World Health Organization (WHO) (2011c). *World Report on Disability*, Geneva: WHO. http://www.who.int/disabilities/world_report/2011/report.pdf (accessed 29 October, 2011).

World Health Organization (WHO) (2011d) *Global Plan for Artemisinin Resistance Containment (GPARC)*, Geneva: WHO. http://www.who.int/malaria/publications/atoz/artemisinin_resistance_containment_2011.pdf (accessed 7 September, 2011).

World Health Organization (WHO) (2011e). *Malaria*, Fact Sheet No. 94, Geneva: WHO. http://www.who.int/mediacentre/factsheets/fs094/en/index.html (accessed 26 October, 2011).

World Health Organization (WHO) (2011f). *Pandemic Influenza Preparedness: Sharing of Influenza Viruses and Access to Vaccines and Other Benefits*, Geneva: WHO. http://apps.who.int/gb/ebwha/pdf_files/WHA64/A64_8-en.pdf (accessed 26 October, 2011).

World Health Organization (WHO) (2011g) *WHO The Abuja Declaration Ten Years On*, Geneva: WHO. http:// www.who.int/healthsystems/publications/abuja_report_aug_2011.pdf (accessed 20 March, 2012).

World Health Organization (WHO) (2011h) *Cancer*, Fact Sheet No. 297, Geneva: WHO. http://www.who.int/mediacentre/factsheets/fs297/en/index.html (accessed 28 October, 2011).

World Health Organization (WHO) (2011i) *Neglected Tropical Diseases*, Geneva: WHO. http://www.who.int/neglected_diseases/faq/en/index.html (accessed 26 October, 2011).

World Health Organization (WHO) (2011j). *Global Partnerships: A Network of Networks*, Geneva: WHO. http://www.who.int/csr/about/partnerships/en/ (accessed 26 September, 2011).

World Health Organization (WHO) (2011k). 'Antibiotics may lose their power to cure disease, WHO warns', press release, 7 April. http://www.wpro.who.int/media_centre/press_releases/pr20110711.htm (accessed 12 March, 2012).

World Health Organization (WHO) (2011l). *Preventing Gender-biased Sex Selection.* An interagency statement OHCHR, UNFPA, UNICEF, UN Women and WHO. Geneva: WHO.

World Health Organization (WHO) (2012a). *Measles Mortality Reduction: A Successful Initiative*, Geneva: WHO. http://www.who.int/immunization/newsroom/measles/en/ (accessed 15 February, 2012).

World Health Organization (WHO) (2012b). *Accelerating Work to Overcome the Global Impact of Neglected Tropical Diseases: A Roadmap for Implementation*, Geneva: WHO. http://www.whqlibdoc.who.int/hq/2012/WHO_HTM_NTD_2012.1_eng.pdf (accessed 28 February, 2012).

World Health Organization/UNICEF (WHO/UNICEF) (2010). *Progress on Sanitation and Drinking Water: 2010 Update*, Geneva: WHO/UNICEF.

World Health Organization (WHO) and China State Council DRC (2005). *China: Health, Poverty and Economic Development*, Beijing: WHO and China State Council.

World Health Organization/UN-HABITAT (WHO/UN-HABITAT) (2010). *Hidden Cities: Unmasking and Overcoming Health Inequities in Urban Settings*, Geneva: WHO/UN-HABITAT.

Yach, D. and Bettcher, D. (1998a). 'The globalization of public health, I: threats and opportunities', *American Journal of Public Health*, 88: 735–738.

Yach, D. and Bettcher, D. (1998b). 'The globalization of public health, II: the convergence of self-interest and altruism', *American Journal of Public Health*, 88: 738–741.

Yang, W.Y., Lu, J.M., Weng, J.P., Jia, W.P., Ji, L., Xiao, J.Z., Shan, Z.Y., Liu, J., Tian, H.M., Ji, Q.H., Zhu, D.L., Ge, J.P., Lin, L.X., Chen, L., Guo, X.H., Zhao, Z.G., Li, Q., Zhou, Z.G., Shan, G.L. and He, J. for the China National Diabetes and Metabolic Disorders Study Group (2010). 'Prevalence of diabetes among men and women in China', *New England Journal of Medicine*, 362(12): 1090–1101.

You, D.Z., Jones, G., Hill, K., Wardlaw, T. and Chopra, M. (2010). 'Levels and trends in child mortality, 1990–2009', *The Lancet*, 376(9745): 931–933.

Yu, R., Chau, P.H., McGee, S., Cheung, W.L., Chan, K.C., Cheung, S.H. and Woo, J. (2010). *Dementia Trends: Impact of the Ageing Population and Societal Implications for Hong Kong*, Hong Kong: Hong Kong Jockey Club.

Zhang, Y.W. (2008). *Encyclopedia of Global Health*, New York: Sage.

Zinsser, H. (1935). *Rats, Lice and History*, Boston: Little, Brown & Co.

Websites

Coalition to Stop the Use of Child Soldiers. http://www.child-soldiers.org/coalition/the-coalition

Dementia Research Group. http://www.alz.co.uk/1066/

Demographic and Health Surveys. http://www.measuredhs.com/countries/

Eurostat Database. http://epp.eurostat.ec.europa.eu/portal/health/public_health/database

Gapminder. http://www.gapminder.org/

Gates Foundation. http://www.gatesfoundation.org/Pages/home.aspx

GAVI Alliance. http://www.gavialliance.org/

Global Action on Aging. http://www.globalaging.org/index.htm

Global Health Council. http://www.globalhealth.org/

Global Viral Forecasting (GVF). http://www.gvfi.org/

International Agency for Research on Cancer (IARC). *CANCERMondial*. http://www-dep.iarc.fr/

International Agency for Research on Cancer (IARC). *CI5: Cancer Incidence in Five Continents*. http://ci5.iarc.fr/

International Diabetes Federation. http://www.idf.org/

International Federation of Red Cross and Red Crescent Societies (IFRC). http://www.ifrc.org/

National Institute of Allergy and Infectious Diseases (NIAID). http://www.niaid.nih.gov/topics/emerging/Pages/list.aspx

OECD. *OECD Health Data 2011*. http://www.oecd.org/health/healthdata

Population Reference Bureau. http://www.prb.org

Statistics Japan. *Prefecture Comparisons*. http://stats-japan.com

Training Programs in Epidemiology and Public Health Interventions Network (TEPHINET). http://www.tephinet.org/

UNAIDS (Joint United Nations Programme on HIV/AIDS). http://www.unaids.org/

United Kingdom Department of Health. *Health Survey for England*. http://www.dh.gov.uk/en/Publicationsandstatisticsics/PublishedSurvey/HealthSurveyForEngland/index.htm

United Nations. *Human Development Reports Annual*. http://hdr.undp.org/en/

United Nations. *Millennium Development Goals Indicators*. http://mdgs.un.org/unsd/mdg/ Default.aspx

United Nations Children's Fund (UNICEF). *The State of the World's Children Annual*. http://www.unicef.org/ sowc/

United Nations Department of Economic and Social Affairs, Population Division (UNDESA-PD). *World Population Prospects*. http://esa.un.org/unpd/wpp/index.htm

United Nations Department of Economic and Social Affairs, Population Division (UNDESA-PD). *World Urbanization Prospects*. http://esa.un.org/unpd/wup/index.htm

United Nations Development Programme (UNDP). http://www.beta.undp.org/undp/en/home.html

United Nations Population Fund (UNFPA). http://www.unfpa.org/public/

United States Census Bureau. *International Database*. http://www.census.gov/population/international/data/idb/informationGateway.php

United States Centers for Disease Control and Prevention. http://www.cdc.gov/

United States Department of State. *Country Reports on Terrorism*. http://www.state.gov/s/ct/rls/crt/

United States National Center for Health Statistics. http://www.cdc.gov/nchs/

University of California, Berkeley, and Max Planck Institute for Demographic Research. *The Human Mortality Database*. http://www.mortality.org/

World Bank. *Food Crisis*. http://www.worldbank.org/foodcrisis/

World Bank. *World Development Indicators*. http://data.worldbank.org/data-catalog/world-development-indicators

World Health Organization (WHO). http://www.who.int/

World Health Organization (WHO). *Cancer*. http://www.who.int/cancer/en/

World Health Organization (WHO). *Burden of Disease Associated with Urban Outdoor Air Pollution for 2008*. http://www.who.int/phe/health_topics/outdoor/databases/burden_disease/en/

World Health Organization (WHO). *Global Alert and Response*. http://www.who.int/csr/disease/en/

World Health Organization (WHO). *Global Burden of Disease (GBD)*. http://www.who.int/healthinfo/global_burden_disease/en/

World Health Organization (WHO). *Life Tables for WHO Member States*. http://www.who.int/healthinfo/statistics/mortality_life_tables/en/

World Health Organization (WHO). *Outdoor Air Pollution*. http://www.who.int/gho/phe/outdoor_air_pollution/en/index.html

World Health Organization (WHO). *The World Health Report*. http://www.who.int/whr/en/

World Health Organization (WHO). *World Health Statistics*. http://www.who.int/whosis/whostat/en/index.html

World Health Organization (WHO). *World Health Survey*. http://www.who.int/healthinfo/survey/en/

World Health Organization (WHO). *World Malaria Report 2010*. http://www.who.int/malaria/world_malaria_report_2010/en/ (accessed 28 February, 2012).

World Health Organization (WHO). *World Malaria Report 2011*. http://www.who.int/malaria/world_malaria_report_2011/en/ (accessed 28 February, 2012).

Index